Handling the Young Child
with Cerebral Palsy at Home

This book is dedicated to the late Berta Bobath.

Handling the Young Child with Cerebral Palsy at Home

Nancie R. Finnie   FCSP

with contributions by

J. Bavin MB, BS, BSc, FRC Psych, DPM
M. Bax DM, FRCP
Marian Browne BMedSci (SP), Reg MRCSLT
Mary Gardner Bsc(Econ), DipEd, DipPsych
Helen A. Mueller, Speech and Language Therapist
Diana Thornton, RMTh, MA (Oxon)

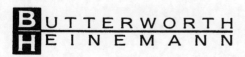

Butterworth-Heinemann
Linacre House, Jordan Hill, Oxford OX2 8DP
225 Wildwood Avenue, Woburn, MA 01801-2041
A divison of Reed Educational and Professional Publishing Ltd

℞ A member of the Reed Elsevier plc group

OXFORD   AUCKLAND   BOSTON
JOHANNESBURG   MELBOURNE   NEW DELHI

First published 1968
Reprinted 1969, 1971
Second edition 1974
Reprinted 1976, 1978, 1981, 1984, 1986, 1987, 1989, 1990, 1991, 1994
Third edition 1997
Reprinted 1998, 1999 (twice), 2000

British Library Cataloguing in Publication Data
A Catalogue record for this book is available from the British Library

Library of Congress Cataloguing in Publication Data
A catalogue record for this book is available from the Library of Congress

ISBN 0 7506 0579 0

Printed and bound in Great Britain by Martins of Berwick, Berwick upon Tweed

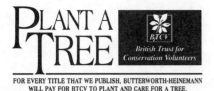

Contents

Preface   vii

Contributors   ix

Foreword   xi

Acknowledgements   xii

Introduction   xiii

Part I   Communication with parents
1   The importance of communication – parents and professionals   3
2   Medical aspects of cerebral palsy   8
    Martin Bax
3   Parents' problems   18
    Jack Bavin
4   Psychological guidance   34
    Mary Gardner

Part II   Basic information
5   Understanding movement and development   47
6   Basic principles of handling   65
7   Early stages of hand function   80
8   Equipment as an adjunct to rehabilitation   96

Part III   Integration of treatment and handling
9   The parents' contribution to early learning   107
10   Speech   112
    Helen A. Mueller
11   Communication and technology   118
    Marian Browne
12   Music and music therapy   125
    Diana Thornton
13   Play   127

Part IV   Handling during routine activities
14   Sleeping   163
15   Toilet training   173
16   Bathing   180
17   Dressing   190
18   Feeding   209
    Helen A. Mueller
19   Carrying   222
20   Chairs, pushchairs and car seats   231
21   Aids to mobility   247

Part V   Additional information
22   The management of contractures and deformities   257
23   Going into hospital   263
24   Recreational activities   265

Appendices
I   Illustrations of some of the terms used   269
II   An overview of the early stages of sensorimotor development   278
III   Glossary for parents – the terms we use   284
IV   Suppliers of equipment   288
V   Useful addresses: general; communication and technology; toys; social services   290

Further reading for parents   292

Index   293

Preface

The third edition of this book is intended, as with previous editions, to be a practical manual for parents whose child has cerebral palsy. The age group covered is from infancy up to 5 years – a time when a child is handled and taught mainly by his parents.

The purpose of the book is to:

- explore the parents' **central** role in the management of their child, with professionals and parents working in close partnership with one another
- help parents understand some of the medical aspects of cerebral palsy, including associated problems that may be present, and the reasons why their child could be delayed or arrested in certain areas of his development
- answer some of the questions parents often raise following the initial shock of hearing that their child has cerebral palsy
- provide practical suggestions for parents regarding the handling of their child during routine activities.

In preparing this edition I have revised the text, rewritten a number of chapters and added new chapters. The sections on equipment have been updated. As equipment is expensive and unobtainable in some countries, I have included from the second edition some simple equipment that parents can make themselves. I have also included the majority of the sketches drawn by Margaret Inkpen from the second edition, as I feel that these and the new sketches drawn by Carolyn Panter do so much to illuminate the text.

Cerebral palsy is a complex subject and one is always aware that inevitably many aspects of concern and importance to parents will not be covered. I have, however, been very fortunate that a number of experts working in the field of cerebral palsy agreed, despite their busy schedules, to contribute chapters for this edition which has enabled me to extend and strengthen the scope of the book.

The children mentioned in this book are almost always referred to as 'he', to avoid clumsy sentences involving 'he or she' or even 's/he'. However, to counterbalance this unintended sexism, workers in the field, such as therapists, are designated 'she'. Those caring for the child at home are called 'parents' or 'mother and father', terms intended to include any 'partners'.

Contributors

Martin Bax DM, FRCP
Consultant Paediatrician
Chelsea and Westminster Hospital
London

Jack Bavin MB, BS, BSc, FRC Psych, DPM
Former Consultant Psychiatrist to Leavesden Hospital,
Charing Cross Hospital, Hammersmith Hospital and
Gloucestershire Area Health Authority

Mary Gardner BSc (Econ), DipEd, DipPsych
Honorary Child Psychologist, Charing Cross Hospital
London

Helen A. Mueller
Speech and Language Therapist
Zurich
Switzerland

Marian Browne BMedSci (SP), Reg MRCSLT
Speech and Language Therapist
The Bobath Centre for Children with Cerebral Palsy
London

Diana Thornton RMTh, MA (Oxon)
Registered Music Therapist
London

Artwork used from second edition by **Margaret Inkpen**, OTR, Edmonton, Canada
Additional artwork for third edition by **Carolyn Panter**, MCSP, Superintendent Community
Paediatric Physiotherapist, North Middlesex Hospital Trust, London

Foreword

Of every thousand children that are born about 2 have cerebral palsy. A large district general hospital might deliver 4000 babies in a year, which means that about 8 children in that district will be diagnosed each year. There may be about 200 children and young adults with cerebral palsy in their parents' homes and in the schools in the area.

Most parents have children that do not have cerebral palsy, so there is an immediate sense of isolation for parents who become aware that their child is different. Unfortunately not all health professionals are able to give good advice. Even doctors and therapists who know a lot about child development have difficulty in being certain about the diagnosis in the first few months of life. At this time of uncertainty about the future, parents are subjected to all sorts of information and opinion from relatives, friends, newspapers, magazines and television programmes. Does anybody really know how to treat the child?

The main author of this book, Nancie Finnie, is an expert. The first edition distilled the knowledge and experience accumulated during years of working with the parents of children who have cerebral palsy. The book also drew on the experience of other experts – in particular Dr. and Mrs. Karel Bobath, the originators of Neuro-Developmental Treatment for cerebral palsy.

The third edition has been up-dated and further improved by the contributions of other specialists and has been reorganized so that the chapters on communication with parents are rightly concentrated at the beginning. The detailed practical advice comes later – this is where parents can learn what they can do with their own hands. The aim is to support parents and strengthen their ability to help their child and enjoy life together. The hope is that support for the family will maintain the happiness of a normal home as much as is humanly possible.

Although this book is written for parents, it is used by therapists, doctors, nurses and teachers. It has become an essential manual for those who are working with parents as part of a team to give the best possible treatment for children with cerebral palsy. These children have varied and complex needs, so the task of learning may seem daunting. However the chapters are well written and clearly organized, with illustrations that amplify and support the excellent text. Finally there is advice about further sources of information and support, so that parents who read the book should not feel isolated or ignored.

Chris Verity, MA, FRCP, DCH
Consultant Paediatric Neurologist
Addenbrooke's Hospital
Cambridge, UK

Acknowledgements

I would like to extend my sincere thanks to all the contributors for sharing their knowledge and giving so generously of their time: Martin Bax, on medical aspects of cerebral palsy (Chapter 2), Marian Browne, on communication and technology (Chapter 11), Diana Thornton, on music and music therapy (Chapter 12) and Carolyn Panter for the many hours she spent doing the new drawings throughout the various chapters.

My thanks also to my colleagues, Jack Bavin, Mary Gardner and Helen A. Mueller for revising and updating their chapters from the second edition. I am also most grateful to Jane Park who so patiently typed and retyped the manuscript, and to Dr C.M. Verity for kindly agreeing to write the foreword to this edition.

Finally, my gratitude is extended to all my colleagues for their support and encouragement during the writing of this book, and to the many parents and their children I have been privileged to meet over the years, from whom I have learned so much.

Introduction

This book is written to help parents of a child with cerebral palsy assist their child towards achieving his potential for independence in movement and functional activities. It is intended to show how by using the normal parenting skills, which inevitably means guiding and exposing their child to learning through challenging experiences, the child with cerebral palsy will also learn. It is also intended to help parents handle their child, during routine daily tasks, in such a way that both they and their child can enjoy as many of the daily experiences together as possible, without encountering the barriers often presented by the aberrant motor behaviour of their child.

The book is not prescriptive, nor is it intended to supplant or substitute the intervention of the several professional therapists that will almost certainly be responsible for your child's treatment. Therefore, throughout the text there is little emphasis on diagnostic categories such as hemiplegia, diplegia or total involvement, although these terms are explained. Rather the emphasis is on how the child presents to his parents, and on the difficulties most commonly met in respect of the presence or absence of abnormal postural tone and motor behaviour, resulting in poor head control, asymmetry and postural instability, affecting the child's ability to coordinate his movements and function effectively. As there will also be a wide variation in the pressures within a family and between families, we have tried to address the needs of the child **while at the same time** taking into account the needs of the family.

The best analogy during the early years (0–5 years of age), I think, is that of a kaleidoscope, an ever-changing picture of motor performance, emotional, intellectual, communication and social development of the child. A time when lots of good things are happening but often clouded by the child's difficulties, a time for parents when the hours at home without the benefit of the therapist's guiding hand can appear to make even simple tasks a burden.

For most parents the knowledge that their child has suffered some degree of brain damage and is therefore diagnosed as having cerebral palsy is not only a grievous shock but also gives them a sense of panic. They ask themselves inner questions like 'What is cerebral palsy?', 'How can I help my child?', 'I don't know anything about it, what can we expect?' Visits to the clinics to see the various professional staff responsible for the treatment and management of their child can be both reassuring and at the same time a little terrifying. There always seems so much to learn. By introducing a new chapter by Martin Bax on medical aspects and Jack Bavin's revised chapter on parents' problems from the second edition, I hope that the reader will be reassured, first, that they are not alone in these feelings and, secondly, that all the members of the multidisciplinary team responsible for the management of their child's care expect to respond to your many questions.

The treatment and management of a child with cerebral palsy involves tackling a wide range of problems, due to the variability in the degrees of impairment that can range from minimal to severe involvement, variations in abnormal postural tone, plus any associated problems that may be present.

All children with cerebral palsy have a difficulty in moving purposefully and efficiently, but **no two**

children experience exactly the same difficulties; for example:

- a child with increased postural tone (hypertonia/spasticity) will have a paucity of movements which are stereotyped, consisting mainly of patterns of flexion and extension
- a child with fluctuations in postural tone, involuntary movements and intermittent spasms (athetosis), although he can move, does so in a disorganized manner lacking both postural control and stability
- a child with low postural tone (hypotonia/ataxia) will have excessive incoordination of voluntary movements and difficulty in timing and grading movements.

There may also be associated handicaps of vision, hearing, speech, and possibly learning and behavioural problems, with a wide spectrum of intelligence ranging from normal to subnormal. Furthermore, in a number of children chronological age may not correspond with their developmental age, sometimes being generally lower in all aspects of their development, at other times a 'scatter' in their achievements.

A child of 4 years, for example, may not progress in all areas of his development beyond that of a 2 year old, whereas another child may be within normal limits as regards gross motor skills but have difficulty using his hands for fine motor skills and have a problem with his speech.

Of course, not all the difficulties described will necessarily apply to any one child.

All babies need the same daily care to be washed, fed, bathed and carried – tasks that are often demanding at a time when a mother is developing her own mothering skills. However, she is rewarded by the warm bond that gradually develops between herself and her baby, both parents taking pleasure in each new skill their child achieves. The same joy is there for the mother of a baby with cerebral palsy, but the presence of abnormal postural tone and exaggerated or absent responses may make the daily, repetitious tasks mentioned more difficult for her to do and creates barriers to learning together. The major part of this book is therefore dedicated to showing how these tasks may be accomplished in a way that makes handling easier and at the same time facilitates the child's potential for learning.

Repetition and overlap between the content of the various chapters are at times unavoidable: first because different aspects of the same problem will be seen from a different perspective by the several contributors, depending on their professional background; secondly, because there is a naturally occurring overlap in activity as development proceeds. For example, when discussing the early interaction between a mother and her baby, the important role she plays in helping him develop early basic skills and pre-linguistic communication is also discussed in the chapter on speech. We have deliberately not edited out any repetition, as many readers will not necessarily tackle reading the chapters in the order in which they have been presented, and in addition it often serves to remind the reader that there is a carryover of learning from one situation to another.

Over the many years since I wrote the first edition of this book, ideas on appropriate therapy(ies) have changed and developed, and new concepts underpinning therapeutic intervention have evolved. Similarly, opinion on early intervention with therapeutic programmes has changed and the method of delivery of service has moved away from centralization to home-based or community provision. The emphasis remains, however, on a holistic approach to the child's needs, seeing his difficulties in relation to his overall development as the unique person he is from childhood to adulthood. Although this text is only intended to cover the early years, i.e. from birth to approximately 5 years of age, the tasks and activities described are those which are fundamental to his eventually reaching independence in adulthood. Like all professionals, my own development and practice has grown over time, being modified by learning and experience; however, the concepts of handling on which this book is based remain those that I adopted during the 13 years that I worked as deputy to the late Mrs Berta Bobath. She and her husband, Dr Karel Bobath, as the worldwide respected clinicians and innovators that they were, modified, changed and developed their concept of the approach to treatment over the years, and I was privileged to enjoy their friendship and the possibility to discuss new ideas with them until their death in 1991.

The choice of the word 'Handling' in the title of the book is intended to signify clearly that the methods and ideas proposed in this text are not directly treatment strategies, but ways in which parents can handle their child to enable him to practise newly acquired motor skills throughout the day, to integrate part of one skill with another, so building his repertoire of competence and achievements. Approaching the child's day in this way means that the beneficial effects of structured therapy sessions will be enhanced and reinforced as the mother handles her child during routine daily activities.

It is for this reason that I have not included specific reference to the child born prematurely with cerebral palsy, although sadly it is the increased numbers in this group that probably account for the failure to see a reduction in the incidence of cerebral palsy in Western nations. The tremendous advances in neonatal care have meant that the gestational age at which babies survive has fallen and many babies born prematurely who would not previously have survived the early weeks of postnatal life now do so. Although I was fortunate to spend the past five years working with preterm infants who had cerebral damage, the specific differences in treatment were more appropriate to the therapeutic intervention by the therapist.

Suggestion on how to use this book

The reader who has taken this book from the shelf has his or her own motivation for doing so, most probably because he or she has suddenly been confronted with the difficulties of a child with cerebral palsy.

Part I provides important and often essential information for the parent about the wider aspects of cerebral palsy and the implications for the parents and family. The section on basic information (Part II), as its name suggests, is included to give the reader a framework in which to place the more

specific and detailed suggestions on handling made in the remainder of the text. Depending on the individual's previous knowledge, whether their child with cerebral palsy is the first child in the family and individual style of learning will all influence whether this section is read in its entirety at the beginning or dipped into and returned to at different times. The chapters on understanding movement and early stages of hand function included in this section are not intended to be complete and definitive in detail, but rather an introduction to the subject. For the parent who wishes to seek more precise information, there are many such books available. The illustrations in this section have been included to highlight the important areas of head control, symmetry, stability and sensory input that we emphasize throughout the various chapters.

Parts III and IV are self-descriptive and there to be used as problems are encountered. They are not prescriptive, so there will be times when the difficulties described will not be those necessarily experienced by any one child. It is therefore important to read carefully the reasons given why a certain technique of handling is recommended, so that you are able to adapt your handling to meet the specific needs of your child. As you learn to understand more about the problems of your child you will soon find different ways of your own of handling and encouraging your child to achieve more on his own. We are always learning from parents, so do share any new ideas with your therapist, to give her the opportunity of passing them on to other parents.

Part V describes some contractures and deformities seen as secondary problems to cerebral palsy, and the methods used for their correction. A chapter giving practical advice on allaying the anxiety of a child going into hospital precedes the final chapter on some stimulating recreational activities for the child with cerebral palsy.

In the appendices you will find a brief outline of the early stages of normal motor development, which is included to give the reader an idea of how each stage of development prepares for and overlaps with the next, including that of vision, hearing and speech. The terminology used by professionals is gradually introduced, so that for the lay reader these should not present a problem. A glossary of terminology and illustrations of the terms mentioned will also be found at the end of the book.

In conclusion, always remember that if your child is to achieve some degree of independence, however limited that may be, he must be given **every opportunity and encouragement** whenever there is a possibility of him succeeding – to move, communicate and use his hands, practising new skills as he acquires them, throughout the day.

Part I
Communication with parents

Chapter 1

The importance of communication – parents and professionals

- At the time of diagnosis
- At the time of assessment
- At the formulation of a management programme
- Integrating therapy into daily activities
- Using videotape recording

I feel strongly that any programme of intervention for the child with cerebral palsy can only be successful when, from the beginning, it is based on a sound foundation of communication between parents and professionals. Only in this way will we be able to address the needs and changing priorities of both the child and the family.

What do we mean by communication? At the very least, communication has two parts – speaking and listening. But of course this does not bring understanding, unless the several participants use the same code to decipher the idea or message being transmitted. This is of the utmost importance in the relationship between parents and professionals, where assumptions about understanding are often made that are untrue. The reality is that both parents and professionals have much to contribute to the treatment/management programme of the child with cerebral palsy. When there is a communication gap it is to the detriment of the child's total management programme; that is why it is so important to work towards establishing a partnership of mutual understanding and respect for what each can bring to the child's care.

To illustrate this point, a few years ago I attended a seminar where the mother of a child with cerebral palsy was speaking to an audience of medical students about her experience of attend-

ing doctors' clinics and hospital departments with her child for routine tests and appointments. At the end of the mother's presentation, the chairman asked if she would give her audience of future doctors a final message. She replied: '**Please listen to us**, the parents.' How right she was! It was a message I have always tried to remember.

Exchange of information

Parents' reactions when they receive their child's initial diagnosis of cerebral palsy varies greatly, and these reactions go through many phases during the ensuing days, weeks and months. In my experience most, if not all, parents will reach a stage where they want more information, clarification and will have countless questions. The questions often relate to the diagnosis, the meaning of some clinical tests and, possibly most important, a desire to know their child's prognosis.

I do urge you to ask your paediatrician, therapist or other professional and go on asking until you understand, rather than keeping any anxieties and worries within the family or trying to find answers by asking family and friends. To make sure that you do not forget the questions in the hurly-burly of the clinic, I suggest you write them down and take the list with you. It is clear that the answers to some of these questions will have an impact on the whole family; for example, you may want a clearer picture of your child's prognosis and what demands a treatment/management programme may make on your time, in order that you can plan to integrate this with other commitments that you may have, such as work or activities with other members of the family. The answers may also affect later decisions in relation to employment opportunities or choice of house, its type and location.

I would also caution you about the well-meaning advice which will doubtless be offered to you by friends and other family members who suddenly seem to have heard of a new therapy programme that claims to offer great benefit, if not a miracle cure. It is wise simply to note these and discuss them with your paediatrician at the next follow-up appointment **before** embarking on a new programme. Professionals will always be willing to discuss the advantages and disadvantages of a new approach. This will be far more satisfactory than 'shopping around' on your own.

As therapists, we have skills and expertise which enables us to analyse your child's problems with movement and identify his potential for development. We do this through successive assessments, in order to monitor the child's changing needs, with the parents of course being active and full participants in the programme. One of the therapist's roles is to guide the parents in **how to modify** their normal care-giving activities, so that each daily task, whether it is bathing, feeding or dressing, etc., is used to **reinforce the improved motor patterns their baby/child has learned during his therapy sessions**. For the older child this will mean identifying specific motor skills and self-help tasks that he finds difficult and then breaking them down into small steps, thus making it easier for him to learn. Our role as professionals is to give you guidance and support, **not to make you expert therapists or to supplant your role as parents**.

It is essential therefore that you should be involved from the very beginning in any decision-making regarding your child's management, which underlines once more the importance of the two-way flow of communication between you the parents and us the professionals.

During the early sessions with your therapist it is important that you share with her the wealth of knowledge that you have about your child. The type of information she will need will come in response to some of the following questions.

- What is it about your baby/child's development that makes you think he is behind or different in his development?
- What do you feel are his main problems?
- Has he ever done something that you had previously thought was beyond his ability?
- Has it ever occurred to you or other members of the family that if you did less for your baby/child he might achieve more on his own?

Assessing the motor ability of a baby with cerebral palsy

For techniques of handling to be effective, the criteria for using them must first be clearly understood. During the assessment process you will be aware that the therapist is documenting different aspects of your baby's behaviour: this will include presence or absence of physiological reactions, changes in muscle tone, the baby's behaviour and his response to being handled. However, another very important part of the assessment process is learning about the baby's motor behaviour by the simple, unsophisticated method of observation, as the way he moves spontaneously as he interacts with you while you talk and play with him speaks volumes about his level of competence. Through the eyes of your therapist you will soon learn to recognize and understand that although your child may have little difficulty in moving he cannot do so skilfully, i.e. purposefully and efficiently. You may observe that his movements are poorly coordinated and therefore abnormally executed, his abnormal patterns of posture and movement affecting all aspects of his development and preventing him from functioning effectively.

A typical day in the life of the baby

Any programme of management will inevitably make extra demands of time and effort on the parents, particularly on the mother. For this reason, I think it is important before putting any plan into action that therapists and professionals involved in the care of the child should know how **you** previously organized **your** time as a family, and how **you** would now like to plan your day. They can then structure the treatment/management programme around your day, so that handling your child does not become intrusive. I have found that the best way of doing this is to ask parents to take me though '**a typical day in the life of the family**', then together we can structure a programme that puts minimal strain on the mother while at the same time addresses the needs of her baby and the family.

This is invaluable information that tells me something about the family's routine, the baby's routine, the way he expresses himself, his likes and dislikes, and **the time when he is most susceptible to being handled**.

The following are a few examples to illustrate this approach.

How the day starts

For many families, especially when there are other children, the start to the day is usually described as a 'mad rush' – a time when mother, having fed the baby and got herself dressed is then busy seeing to the needs of the family. Perhaps preparing breakfast, getting the other children ready for school and seeing her husband off to work. This is a time when **their** needs come first, certainly not one when she, or other members of the family, can be expected to give their undivided attention to the baby.

During the early months, the majority of babies sleep after a feed, and it is only when this pattern starts to change that some babies with cerebral palsy, unable to play and amuse themselves because of their immature motor behaviour, become bored and frustrated and demand attention.

We therefore need to ask ourselves why he is so distressed, and then find ways of organizing **this part of his day** so that we make sure that he has every opportunity to look, react and explore, and can practise and use those abilities which we know he is capable of using **without** our participation or supervision.

We need to be sure that the activities we expect of him, and the toys that we select, are at the baby's functional level and **not** necessarily his chronological age, so that every effort made on the baby's part is rewarded **by success**, in this way stimulating and sustaining his interest.

For example, the baby who with your help enjoys the experience of getting his hands together, feeling, looking and taking them to his mouth, may be able to practise doing this on his own if supported on his side or in a cut-out wedge (see Chapter 8). Alternatively he may enjoy the visual stimulus of focusing and following a moving object so that, by giving him a favourite mobile whose colour, movement and changing shape attracts his attention, he will not only become more visually alert, but happy and contented while on his own.

The baby who can reach out and grasp on the other hand, will need toys to play with that stimulate his interest while at the same time offering him the opportunity to practise these skills (see Chapters 7 and 13).

It is also worth remembering that even when a baby becomes skilful at using his hands, he will continue for quite a time to take toys to his mouth to explore them further. It is therefore worthwhile having a couple of toys near him or attached to his cot so that he can pull them towards himself, to suck, bite and explore further.

The baby's routine

Parents' description of a typical day also provides us with invaluable information about their baby's daily routine, the way he expresses himself, his likes and dislikes. When he is at his most alert and responsive. Whether he is a baby who is contented during the day but becomes unsettled during the evening or vice versa. Whether he has a prolonged period of responsiveness following a bath or a feed, or perhaps is a baby who immediately he is fed likes to doze? We can then channel our input into those activities he enjoys and avoid those he actively dislikes. This is particularly important in the beginning, as most babies do not welcome the extra handling and demands made on them.

Fortunately most routine activities, such as diaper (nappy) changing, are repeated throughout the day, which means that we can choose the time when he is most responsive to intervene. For example, if a mother describes her child as being niggly and unsettled towards the evening and that he is at his most active during times when she is changing his diaper, we would know that

● diaper-changing times offered an opportunity for learning
● the morning period was when he was most receptive.

Similarly, if a baby had reached the stage of starting to feed himself with a spoon, and if lunch time was the only meal when he really enjoyed his food, rather than having a battle on her hands, it would be sensible for the mother to concentrate on the one meal where she would be sure that he would be responsive, only introducing other mealtimes gradually.

It is important to remember that the same fundamental motor skills used in a particular activity are also used in other tasks but in a different position, and these also need to be practised in order that there is a carryover – an extension of learning.

Setting priorities and communicating goals

There is always the danger when discussing short- and long-term goals and the immediate priorities in treatment for your child, that by concentrating on one aspect of a baby's development we forget to explain that at the same time he should be given an opportunity of accomplishing motor activities and skills in a variety of positions. It is also of paramount importance to emphasize that all aspects of his development, and not only his motor achievements, must be considered in his total management.

I continue discussing with parents, from time to time, how their child spends his day, as I find it an excellent way of finding out whether **I** have been successful in communicating with parents. I might find, for example, that because our aim had been to help the child use his hands in sitting, he was now sitting most of the day, as I had not explained the importance of him **also** being on the floor and encouraged to move as he played. Activities with a baby while he was being dressed might not have been done because the handling techniques I had shown the mother were not clear. It also helps me to know how often and in which situations a piece of therapeutic equipment is being used.

Although we need to encourage and train a baby to develop hand skills in sitting before sitting balance has been achieved, if at the same time we limit his range of experience and opportunities to move and use his hands in other positions both his ability to balance in sitting and the quality and performance of his hand function will be slow to improve. There is also the danger that by the baby spending so much time in sitting, the muscles at the hips and behind the knees will become tight and contractures will develop.

The infant/child who is already limited in his ability to move around is then likely to become what I call a 'container baby', spending his day either sitting in his high chair, corner seat or specially adapted chair, and in some households in a baby swing. Or when taken out, sitting in his pushchair or car seat. I have on occasions found that **the only time** the baby is not sitting is when he is having his diaper changed or when in his cot.

The use of videotape recording as a means of communication

Observation and analysis of problems

Observing how a child moves is never easy and this is where videotape recording is a useful tool for recording the initial and sequential evaluations, enabling the child's progress to be monitored. Videotape recording, therefore, offers another way of facilitating communication between parents and professionals and between professionals.

Furthermore, the tape recording allows the parent to distance themselves from the child, often allowing them to see that their child was much more independent than they had given him credit for or to appreciate where he has difficulties.

Learning new techniques

When it is impossible for both parents to attend a therapy session, I think a videotape recording is invaluable in providing parents with an opportunity to review at home the child's performance and any modifications that have been made to his treatment programme. Through discussion together they can decide on any points they do not understand, disagree with or want clarified.

A short sequence of film can also act as a back-up for parents, for example, as a reminder of any special techniques they have been taught or to help them identify the different stages necessary for the acquisition of a particular skill.

The use of videotape recording also extends to helping parents learn particular handling skills. For example, I have often filmed a parent handling her child when she has just been taught a new technique. Then, together, we have been able to look at the sequence and make any changes that might be necessary.

Similarly a short sequence filmed at home by the parents of their child moving spontaneously in his own environment, or using a new piece of equipment, may offer a new insight to the doctor or therapist who only sees the child in the foreign environment of the clinic.

Two-way communication in the total management programme

Various professionals will evaluate your child's physical and social development, language, communication skills and response to learning. Based on these assessments, the total management programme embracing all these aspects is planned. The programme will inevitably have to be changed over time to reflect the changing needs and priorities of the child and family. However, I cannot overemphasize that these programmes are developed in partnership with you the parents. The professionals contribute their base knowledge of development, understanding of the child's problems and treatment skills, while you the parents bring to the partnership your expert knowledge of your child, knowledge of the needs and abilities of other members of the family and knowledge of your own needs and priorities. Partnership does not mean that there will always be total agreement, but **effective** communication should mean that there is an open door to resolving differences and reaching an understanding, whether this be on setting priorities, use of a particular technique or even accepting that long-term estimates of your child's potential for development are not possible at an early stage.

In summary, effective communication between parents and professionals, and between professionals of different disciplines, is essential in the assessment of the child's needs and in planning and implementing total management programmes.

I hope that the foregoing has made clear the need for a two-way flow of communication and emphasized the importance of the parents' contribution in this process.

Chapter 2

Medical aspects of cerebral palsy

Martin Bax

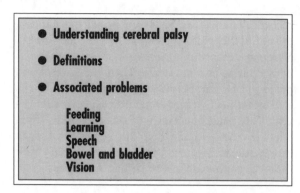

- Understanding cerebral palsy
- Definitions
- Associated problems

    Feeding
    Learning
    Speech
    Bowel and bladder
    Vision

What is cerebral palsy?

Cerebral palsy is a disorder of movement and posture. People with cerebral palsy often cannot carry out the big movements we make when walking, running, jumping, either at all or nearly as well as ourselves. Also, often the fine, manipulative movements that we make with our hands and fingers may be disturbed. Posture – the way we stand, sit or move – is also often abnormal. Instead of standing in a relaxed and symmetrical position, a person with hemiplegic (i.e. one-sided) cerebral palsy will have an inturned foot, and a bent elbow and wrist, so that the hand is held across the tummy instead of relaxed at the side. Others, with athetoid cerebral palsy (see later), find it very difficult to stand still at all and have constant unwanted movements.

Cerebral palsy is caused by damage to the immature brain and always starts in childhood. If adults have damage to the brain, particularly in older age, they have a stroke or haemorrhage and in some ways the consequences would not be all that dissimilar to that of the child with cerebral palsy. However, there is a very big difference in that the adult brain is mature and no longer growing, whereas in the child with cerebral palsy the brain is not yet fully functional and still growing and developing, so the **effect** of the damage is rather different from that seen in the adult. Once the damage (or lesion) to the brain has occurred in cerebral palsy it does not usually extend or become worse, whereas in some other disorders of movement in childhood, unfortunately, the child will get slowly worse as, for example, in muscular dystrophy. Thus, the cerebral palsied child has a **static lesion** which in itself will not become worse. However, because the child is very often born with it, the way the damage is apparent changes as he grows and develops. So cerebral palsy is a non-progressive but **not unchanging disorder of movement and posture** starting in the early years of life. A baby or young child who has had a head injury in a car accident may develop cerebral palsy. If the injury occurs when the child is older, it will be more like the injury that would appear in an adult.

What are the types of cerebral palsy?

Broadly, there are two types of cerebral palsy: those that primarily leave a child with weak, stiff limbs – the spastic type – and those in which there are unwanted movements, called athetoid or sometimes dyskinetic cerebral palsy. Another group of unwanted movements is found in the ataxic (i.e. having difficulty in coordinating movement) cerebral palsied child. The athetoid child has **constant unwanted movements**, even when trying to sit still, and these unwanted movements interfere with all the movements the child tries to make, such as walking or doing things with his hands. An ataxic child does not have unwanted movements when sitting still, but makes **clumsy and awkward voluntary movements**. On the other hand, the spastic child has **poor, weak movements** and indeed often has difficulty in moving at all.

In the athetoid and ataxic cerebral palsies, usually, though not invariably, all parts of the body are involved. But in spastic cerebral palsy, different parts of the body may be involved. In **hemiplegic cerebral palsy**, one half of the body is involved, i.e. the right arm and right leg, or the left arm and left leg. Spasticity usually affects the arm more than the leg, so virtually all hemiplegic children can walk, but the hand sometimes is not very useful and is simply used as a prop or helper to the unaffected hand.

In **diplegic cerebral palsy**, the lower limbs are more severely affected than the upper. Diplegic cerebral palsy is commoner in babies who are born early. In **quadriplegic cerebral palsy**, all four limbs are severely affected. Sometimes the word tetraplegia is used to describe this condition. Other, less commonly used terms are double hemiplegia, where all four limbs are involved, but the arms seem much more affected than the legs; triplegia, where three limbs are involved; and monoplegia, where only one limb is involved. These three terms describe the less common types of cerebral palsy.

As explained, what labels a child as having cerebral palsy is the fact that there is a disorder of movement and posture, and it is caused by brain damage. Virtually all the other functions of the brain may be involved in the condition, and all the other problems associated with it are discussed below. Nevertheless, the particular parts of the brain that are known to be involved with movement are those areas where one looks for the damage in cerebral palsy. They are in the cerebral cortex, which is the large area in the brain under the skull, in the spastic type of cerebral palsy; the deeper parts – the basal ganglia – in the athetoid type of cerebral palsy, and the area of the brain at the back of the head – the cerebellum – in ataxic

cerebral palsy. These are the classic descriptions written in textbooks, but very often the pattern in any one child is very individual and idiosyncratic, i.e. peculiar to that child.

What are the causes of cerebral palsy?

In Victorian times there were two main theories about the cause of cerebral palsy. One was partly put forward by the great psychoanalyst, Sigmund Freud, before he took up psychiatry. He thought that there was disorganization to the brain while it was developing before the child was born. Another great Victorian, an orthopaedic surgeon, William Little, thought the damage occurred at the time of birth, during the birth process. This latter idea, that a shortage of oxygen during the birth process was the principal cause of cerebral palsy, has probably been the most popular one in the past 20 or 30 years and has led to many sad parents (particularly in the USA) suing their obstetrician for mismanaging the labour.

It is now believed that babies are much more resistant to a shortage of oxygen during birth than once believed, and while undoubtedly there are instances where a baby is actually damaged during the birth process, this is probably much less common than was thought previously.

Something like 40–50% of babies with cerebral palsy are those born very early and very small. Such tiny babies are certainly at risk of becoming damaged after they are born. The blood vessels around the ventricles, or the cavities in the brain, have rather fragile walls at this early stage and it is relatively common for there to be some bleeding into the ventricles – an intraventricular haemorrhage. A minor bleed which is not very extensive is not serious, but a more extensive one, perhaps pushing back the wall of the ventricle and damaging the surrounding tissues, can cause serious disturbance of function. It is interesting that the area where this happens is also an area that we know sends messages about movement. In the most serious types of intraventricular haemorrhage, up to 90% of babies may develop cerebral palsy, so the monitoring of the newborn small baby is very important and with the use of ultra-sound scans (see below) we are able to watch what goes on in the ventricles and detect small, unimportant bleeds as well as those in the large, important ones. We can also see the damage extending into the tissues.

While haemorrhage into the ventricles is certainly an important cause of cerebral palsy, there are other causes that can affect the development of the brain before this. One of the striking things of the embryonic life of the baby is how much development happens so very quickly, so that by 12 or 13 weeks of pregnancy the fetus, though very small, has all the characteristics of a human and looks like a little person. Arms, legs, heart and so on are all present, but the brain at this point is still a fairly simple globe – an enormous amount of development goes on in the second two-thirds of pregnancy, and indeed a lot of development goes on after the child is born. The cells are not only dividing within the brain, but they are moving about, and fibre tracts are forming. Not surprisingly, these delicate operations in this very small organ can be interfered with. We know some of the things that can interfere with them. For example, alcohol and cocaine, and some infections, such as German measles (rubella) can also damage the brain. There are doubtless quite a lot of other things that might damage the brain that we do not know about yet.

Sometimes the damage can occur after birth. In hemiplegia we often know the mechanism of the damage if not what caused it, because what happens here is similar to an adult stroke. Damage occurs in the area supplied by one particular artery, and there may be either a haemorrhage – that is to say, all of the artery breaking down – or a thrombosis, which is a blockage in the artery. Some of the hemiplegias that are caused after birth are probably due to weakness in the walls of the blood vessels in the brain that for some reason have not formed perfectly during development.

We can now look at what areas of the brain have been damaged, by using new investigative techniques (see below), and the appearance may give us a good idea as to when that damage occurred, but it does not always help us to know what caused it.

In individual cases, one is often left explaining that 'this bit of the brain had been damaged, but we don't know why'.

How many people have cerebral palsy?

The number of children born with cerebral palsy in developed countries has not varied very much over the past 30 or 40 years. It went down a little in the 1970s and 1980s, but more recently it appears to have been going up. Rather more than 2 babies out of every 1000 born will have cerebral palsy.

Discovery and diagnosis

For some parents there will be anxiety about the baby from very early on. The staff in the special care baby unit will alert the parents that their baby may develop some difficulty. Other babies may become acutely ill with meningitis, or fits, and these could presage cerebral palsy. On the other hand, some parents may simply notice, when the child is 4, 5 or 6 months, that his movement development is delayed. In both instances this is a time when the doctors have to decide whether a child has cerebral palsy or not. To some extent the diagnosis is one of exclusion of other causes, which indeed might be more serious, such as tumours or degenerative diseases. Blood tests, which look for abnormal constituents of blood and also look at the chromosomes which carry the inherited information, should be carried out. Incidentally, cerebral palsy is very rarely inherited. There is a form of spastic paraplegia that does run in families, but this affects less than 1 in 20 cerebral palsied people and some doctors will exclude this from the diagnosis of cerebral palsy. In general, it may be sensible to ask for genetic advice before embarking on a further pregnancy, but the chances of having a second child with cerebral palsy are slight, although there may be a higher risk of having a small baby, for example. These issues can be discussed with the geneticist.

There are also 'imaging' studies that can be carried out. An X-ray of the skull will not tell very much about the brain, but other types of investigations such as the computerized tomography scan (CAT or CT scan), or magnetic resonance imaging (MRI), are both very commonly used to look at the brain of children to see whether a damaged part can be located. Ultrasound can be used in the young baby, but not after the skull is sealed, i.e. once the bones of the skull finally fuse.

More complicated methods of investigation, which involve looking at specific chemicals in the brain, are sometimes used, e.g. the positon emission tomography scan (PET scan), and undoubtedly more and more sophisticated ways of looking at the brain will be developed. Sometimes another investigation – the electroencephalogram (EEG) – may be useful, particularly if there is concern about the child having fits, although in cerebral palsy the EEG is often disorganized and sometimes not very helpful when deciding whether a particular event that has happened to the child is a fit or not.

Once all these investigations have been done, and other disorders eliminated, the diagnosis of cerebral palsy can firmly be established – this should usually be apparent within the first year or two of life. While the diagnostic tests are being made, this is obviously a very anxious time for the family. Equally when a diagnosis is conveyed, it is a very stressful time. Very often, families feel that doctors tell them about the diagnosis rather badly, and probably they do, but the shock of learning that there is something seriously wrong with one's child makes it difficult to absorb information, and it takes time to come to terms with the problem. It is helpful for both the family and the doctor if both parties write down what they say to each other. I always try to write down what I say at my interviews and let the family have this information. I then suggest the family write down the questions they want answered, as well as correcting me about errors I may have made in my notes about their child. At the same time as wanting to know what it all means, the family also very urgently want to do as much as possible to help their child improve. One important but sad thing to grasp at once is that there is no actual treatment for the brain damage, and there is no way at present that we can replace the damaged area of the brain with new brain cells. This may be something we may be able to do in the twenty-first century. On the other hand, there are lots of ways in which a child with cerebral palsy can be helped.

Other problems

Inevitably, as already stated, one part of the brain is damaged that deals with movement, but there may be other parts of the brain damaged that deal with other functions. The next section will deal with the other functions where children with cerebral palsy may have problems.

Of course, many children with cerebral palsy do not have associated problems, but it is important to outline them. An appropriate question is: how clever will the child be? Many children without cerebral palsy have learning disorders. People nowadays prefer not to use the label 'mental retardation', but rather they talk about mild, moderate or severe learning disorders. About half the population of cerebral palsied children will have moderate to severe learning disorders, which means that they will have difficulty for example in learning to read in school. Their intelligence quotient (IQ) will be below 70 or 80: the average IQ is 100, and someone who goes on to university usually has an IQ of above 120. Someone who has difficulty reading usually has an IQ of below 75. But cerebral palsied children may have unexpected learning difficulties. For example, a child who may seem to be good at several things may have problems with reading, which is sometimes called dyslexia, or may have difficulty with mathematics. Others may be very good at reading and maths, but be poor at shape perception, and have great difficulty drawing. Thus the process of learning for the cerebral palsied child needs to be monitored all the time. In all aspects of cerebral palsy there may be abnormal development or there may be slow development. The child with severe learning difficulties is often slow to learn to walk, and slow to learn to talk and then slow at activities when entering school.

Visual impairment

A small proportion of cerebral palsied children have damage to the nerves that run from the eyes to the part of the brain that initially interprets signals from the eyes: they are therefore blind. This is not very common, but on the other hand the disordered control of movement often affects the eye muscles, so cerebral palsied children are very likely to have squints, and this may occur in up to half this population. The squints need attention early on and can either be corrected by very minor surgery or sometimes by patching. In addition, small babies tend to have short-sightedness and so quite a lot of cerebral palsied children will need spectacles to correct this. Where there is disability it is very important that other disabilities are treated as effectively as possible. It is essential, therefore, for cerebral palsied children to have a good assessment of their vision by an ophthalmologist.

Hearing impairment

Children with cerebral palsy may have damage to the nerves from the ear and the parts of the brain that interprets the sound signals. Years ago, when athetoid cerebral palsy was associated with rhesus haemolytic disease (jaundice of the newborn), hearing problems were even more common. Hearing problems that involve the nerves from the ear and the parts of the brain concerned with hearing are called 'sensorineural' hearing loss to distinguish them from hearing loss that is very common in all children, caused by infections in the ear – the well-known so-called glue ear. This type of hearing loss, which is an association of the conduction of the sound waves to the inner ear to make nervous impulses, are called 'conductive' losses, and in general are treatable and sometimes preventable. Cerebral palsied children, who may get an ear infection and throat infection, may have higher rates of these conductive problems and again they need to be very carefully looked after.

Sensorineural hearing loss is more serious, as there is no way we can repair the damaged nerves.

Speech and language problems

Language is the way we think and is the inner symbolization of thought, and speech is one way or 'medium' of conveying what we wish to communicate. There are other ways or media for expressing our inner language, such as writing or morse code or sign language. What is important is to have the inner language and a good medium of conveying this. Some children with cerebral palsy have a lot of difficulty moving the muscles that control the sound-making operation; this is particularly common in children with athetoid cerebral palsy who sometimes have very good inner language and know exactly what they want to say but cannot say it. In quite a number of cerebral palsied children, speech and language is delayed. There is also a smaller group who have problems with speech development, and these are discussed in Chapter 10.

Epilepsy or fits

Cerebral palsied children are more likely than other children to have a fit or convulsion some time during their life. This may happen in about half the population with cerebral palsy. Some babies are liable to have neonatal convulsions. On the other hand, there are a number of cerebral palsied children who may have one or two fits in early childhood without any serious consequences. There are various types of fits and nowadays the old terms 'grand mal' and 'petit mal' have been superseded by rather more technical descriptions. In general, convulsions can be divided into the gross or generalized fits, when the whole body is liable to shake and the child loses consciousness, and more minor fits where there is a brief moment of loss of awareness, associated perhaps with rolling of the eyes, and where people may not be aware the fit is occurring. The interruption will, however, profoundly interfere with the child's learning because suddenly the child is unaware of what is going on for about 30 seconds, and such loss of awareness does not help in a learning situation.

There is now a wide range of drugs to treat the various types of convulsions that can occur. Some are more effective for one type of fit and some for another. In general, it is good to try to avoid the child being on anticonvulsants for long periods. Some of the older drugs, such as phenobarbitone, are known to interfere with the workings of the brain and particularly so in the brain-damaged child. Another general rule is that a combination of two or three drugs should be avoided as far as possible; instead, drugs should be tried singly and alternately before moving on to using two or more drugs in combination. If a fit does occur it is now possible to have suppositories of a drug available that can be given to the child at home by the parents. This usually stops the fit and is therefore a reassuring treatment to have available. Because of the unwanted movements seen in cerebral palsy, and the fact that the EEG is often disorganized in any event, it is sometimes difficult to decide if certain phenomena in a less able cerebral palsied child are epileptic fits or not. Careful observation, sometimes including video recording the child, may be necessary to be certain of the diagnosis.

Feeding

Many cerebral palsied children are difficult to feed. The problem may start in infancy when the child has difficulty in sucking, and continue when the child becomes older, where chewing is not possible. There may also be problems with swallowing. There are two types of swallowing in the normal child. The first is seen when the baby is being fed milk. Here, there is a spontaneous pressure on the teat, forcing the milk out along the tongue so that it reaches the back of the tongue and the top of the pharynx and then is rapidly and automatically swallowed. Sometimes two 'boluses' – or spurts of milk – will move back before the swallow is initiated, but the whole process seems very much an automatic one. The tongue stays in the mid-line and does not move around. Once the child moves on to mixed feeding, he begins to chew and explore the food with

the tongue. This second type of swallowing is more complicated: food is collected into a bolus by the tongue and then moved to the back of the mouth where again swallowing is initiated. Very often, this preparation by the tongue and the almost voluntary act of getting food from between the teeth and ready for swallowing is something that children with cerebral palsy find difficult to achieve. Instead they may continue with the primitive suck-and-swallow pattern of the infant.

Once food has progressed beyond the mouth, the cerebral palsied child may have other problems with the swallow. In the normal child the larynx that lets air into the lungs automatically closes as the swallow has started and the liquid or solid food goes down the oesophagus to the stomach. In the child with cerebral palsy, sometimes the rhythmic organization of closure of larynx and procedure of swallow does not take place and the food or liquid can get into the lungs – called aspiration. When this occurs there is a risk that, along with the food, germs will be carried into the lungs and the child can get repeated chest infection.

Finally, when the food has passed to the stomach there is the problem that also occurs in young normal infants, that the food is regurgitated. That is to say, when the stomach contracts, instead of pushing the food down the intestines, it may shoot it up the oesophagus again and it may appear as a small vomit. While this difficulty is common in the very young child, it is something that usually disappears early on, but is liable to persist in the child with cerebral palsy and can lead to problems. The stomach contents are acid, whereas the wall of the oesophagus, or pipe that leads down to the stomach, is not used to acid material. If there is frequent regurgitation, the oesophagus may become sore and be painful during swallowing, and may put the child off eating.

There are all sorts of ways one can help with these problems. A proper positioning of the child before feeding begins is very important. The child's head should be in a flexed forward position, which is the way most of us approach a spoon as we take food off it, and he should be sitting up. The texture of the food, if the child cannot chew, is very important and there are all sorts of textured foods available. If the child has difficulty with liquids, a material called Thick-and-Easy will make liquid into a kind of soup and may be easier for the child to swallow than actual liquid. It is essential to ensure that the child receives enough calories so that he has plenty of energy and also is growing normally. There are now available lots of high-caloric supplements – powders that can be added to food to increase the amount of nutrients that the child receives. It is also important to see that feeding starts off well and continues well, because if the child loses weight he may eat less and a vicious circle is set up.

Sometimes, despite all efforts, it may be impossible to get enough food down the child by ordinary feeding and in that case there are two ways in which we can help. For the short term, it is possible to pass a tube down the oesophagus, usually through the nose (a nasogastric tube) and food can thus be introduced to the stomach. This has been very popular in the past, but many people now feel that it is a mistake to have a nasogastric tube inserted for too long. It interferes with the child's ordinary swallowing and vomiting reflexes and may make ordinary feeding even more difficult to establish. A better way of providing extra food is through a gastrostomy, in which a small 'buttonhole' is made in the abdominal wall and a little tube inserted. This is less invasive than a nasogastric tube and also allows oral feeding to go on uninterrupted and to be developed while maintaining the nutrient state of the child. The gastrostomy tube can readily be closed off once ordinary feeding has been achieved.

There are other strategies that may be necessary to help with feeding. For example, the valve at the top of the stomach can be tightened, which reduces the reflux of the contents described above (gastro-oesophageal reflux). This operation is call **fundoplication**. Speech therapists in particular are keen to help with feeding, and the earlier the feeding pattern is established the better.

Drooling

Another problem in the area of the mouth is that children with cerebral palsy may have difficulty in controlling their saliva. All babies have a period of about six months when they dribble a lot and need to wear a bib, but shortly after this they learn to keep their mouths shut and swallow the saliva. The child with cerebral palsy may have difficulty in achieving lip closure and difficulty in achieving the regular swallowing of their saliva. It can be demeaning and distressing for an older child to have a constantly wet front from drooling. Again, there are various ways of helping with this problem now, both medical – with skin patches which reduce the amount of saliva produced – and minor surgery, where the ducts that introduce the saliva into the mouth are turned so that they face backwards for the saliva to drain down the throat rather than drip forward.

Teeth

Because the child with cerebral palsy may have difficulty with tongue movements, and particularly in those children who never get beyond the primitive suck-and-swallow pattern and cannot chew, food can very easily be stuck and stay caught around the teeth. These children are particularly likely to have decayed teeth. Obviously, prevention is better than letting this situation develop, and regular toothbrushing after every meal may be necessary to stop this occurring.

Bowel and bladder

Sometimes there are feeding difficulties in addition to a general lack of mobility, and cerebral palsied children may become constipated. Again, this is a problem that is very much more easily dealt with early on than at a later age when the child presents with a bowel habit that is very disturbed. Plenty of fluid keeps the faeces soft, and various fibrous-like materials will help to bulk it up. Suppositories may help with regular emptying of the bowel. One problem with the more severely affected child is that people may not be aware that he has a very full bowel, and regular examination early on is important, to see that the bowel is emptying/opening. Equally, children with cerebral palsy are more likely to have difficulty in learning bladder control, and a proportion go on to be incontinent. In children where continence has not been established, the bladder can be investigated using a range of techniques that are relatively non-intrusive. The danger with an incompletely empty bladder is that the child will get infections, and again prevention of this is very much better than cure.

Treating the motor disorder

Cerebral palsy is a disorder of movement, and most parents naturally find themselves focusing on this aspect of the child's development, particularly at the outset, hoping that he will be able to move in a more-or-less normal manner. One confusion for these families is to discover that there are many people who have different ideas about how a child is best helped with his movements. This book does not discuss these different treatments, but emphasizes practical ways of managing the child.

The doctor, in collaboration with therapeutic colleagues and you the child's parents, have to ensure that realistic goals are set for the child and that therapy does not interfere with all the normal activities that go on in a young child's life.

The first important thing to think about is the encouragement of normal movement. As we are well aware, in the animal kingdom the young are born with the ability to move. The piglet pops out of the sow and runs round to latch onto a nipple. The foal stands up and trots at his mother's side. The newborn baby apparently cannot walk, and most people therefore talk about the child learning to walk during the first year and a half of life. In fact, this is not the case. The child, as with the animal, walks when the brain has matured so that he can walk, and walking is not a learnt phenomenon but an aspect of the development of the brain. Actually, the newborn baby makes splendid stepping movements and the only reason he or she does not walk is because he cannot balance and falls over if unsupported. The balancing reactions do not emerge until between 6 and 10 months, and not until balance is achieved can independent

walking start. Before that, the child has usually found some other method of movement, such as crawling or sometimes sitting on his bottom and moving along in that manner. Sometimes the areas of the brain that need to develop for the integration of balance and the development of the walking reaction just do not develop and this can be seen because the child retains some of the primitive reflexes such as the asymmetric neck reflex – a curious position of the arms (see Chapter 5) – and it is not too difficult to make a prediction, when the child is about the age of 2 years, whether he will walk or not. Almost all hemiplegic children will be able to walk, but many of those with spastic diplegia and most with quadriplegia will never walk.

So too with the hand movements. This again is something that is not learnt, but follows the development of the central nervous system. Initially, the child grabs with the whole hand and only around the ninth or tenth month can we see the development of what is called the pincer grip, with the thumb opposite the first finger, enabling small objects such as beads or raisins to be picked up. This development occurs when certain long fibres coming from the cerebral cortex form junctions with other nerves in the spinal cord. The moment of joining occurs around about 8 months and then the child develops the pincer grip. If the pincer grip does not develop naturally, there is really no way that we can train the child to develop it, but the pincer grip is the basis on which all our fine skill motor movements are developed. Of course, after that stage we develop sophisticated 'skills' such as playing the piano or writing, but these are things we learn to achieve. Children with cerebral palsy may find learning to do these difficult.

The above might suggest that there is little that can be done to help the child with cerebral palsy to achieve movement, but this is not the case.

Preventing deformity

Firstly we can see that the effects of the brain damage do not affect the way the limbs and muscle grow. Because of the abnormalities within the motor system, if appropriate action is not taken further deformities may develop which may prevent movement. For example, the tendon attached to the big muscle at the back of the ankle (tendo Achilles) may not grow properly and will become shortened, and eventually the child stands on tiptoes and cannot walk because he trips over his own toes. If this stage is reached, it can be helped by a surgical operation to lengthen the tendo Achilles. But much better is to prevent the shortening of that muscle occurring, and this can be done by seeing that the foot is held in a normal position and not with pointing toes. This has to be done for several hours per day. Lightweight splints, called ankle–foot orthosis, achieve this. Similarly, all the handling of the child will affect the development of normal postural patterns and help the prevention and persistence of abnormal pattern, but this is really the focus of this whole book and I shall not elaborate upon it here.

Secondly there are various ways we can try to modify the effects of the brain damage and finally one can devise ways of handling the child so that the effects of the brain damage are mitigated as far as possible. (This last practice is, of course, the theme of this whole book.)

There are various surgical techniques that come to the fore from time to time that may help with spasticity. Some years ago the implantation of an electrode into the brain (cerebellar stimulation) was very popular, but more recently an operation called dorsal rhizotomy has become widely available and particularly favoured in the USA. In this operation the spinal nerves are identified and some of them cut, because these are the ones that make the muscles spastic. This procedure only works in a small number of cerebral palsied children, but it certainly can be helpful on occasion. However, most people would prefer to try less invasive procedures first. Another recent development has been the use of electrical stimulation to strengthen the muscles, because, although spastic, cerebral palsied muscles are also weak. This again is helpful in a number of children, but to select those children from whom it would be beneficial remains quite difficult and is something for discussion between you, the family, the doctors and the therapists.

Orthopaedic operations and drugs

If contractures do occur, and in various other circumstances, orthopaedic operations may help the child. As has already been mentioned, if the muscles are short the tendon can be artificially lengthened. Sometimes it may be helpful to transfer the attachment of a muscle from one place to another. Sometimes the surgeon may do bony operations; for example, he may fuse together some of the bones in the ankle to make the joint more stable. One particular area of concern for the orthopaedic surgeon is the development of the child's hips. The hip joint in children with cerebral palsy may not develop well, and the thigh bone may eventually not stay in the joint. In these circumstances the surgeon may decide to operate to make the joint stable. A lack of standing practice and staying in fixed postures can slowly lead to an increase in the hip problems as the child gets older.

Another possible way to help a child with cerebral palsy is to give him some medications. Drugs may help relax the spastic muscles. They may be taken orally or sometimes they are injected at particular points into the muscle. All these treatments try to modify the effects of the brain damage on movement (motor system). They cannot cure it.

Behaviour

There are some cerebral palsied children whose behaviour is more difficult than children without disabilities. For example, many have difficulties sleeping at night and there may be quite a lot of night-crying, and some seem particularly irritable in the early years of life. In general, the sorts of behaviour children with cerebral palsy show are similar to those shown by children without disability, but they are more likely to have behavioural problems. Thus they may have more temper tantrums, often set off by the same things that instigate tantrums in normal children. They may be highly active; and sometimes those who are immobile find it difficult to sustain attention for very long. In all young toddlers, attention span is rather short, but one of the things they learn during the first years of life is to lengthen this and they spend quite a long time exploring and playing with a toy. If this does not happen, the child cannot find out about the toy's quality. Overactivity and attention problems are all more common in the cerebral palsied child and there is a need to be aware of the child's diminished activity and develop the child's attention.

Normal development

It is often difficult to remember, when so much seems to be happening to help with the cerebral palsy of the child, that the affected child needs to do all the things that the normal child does as far as he is able. Sometimes the cerebral palsied child is not able to do things that the normal child can do, and will need help. For example, all normal children around the age of 5–6 months tend to pick up all sorts of objects and put them in their mouths, or crawl over to a chair and be seen sucking the cushion. Parents naturally discourage putting the less desirable objects into their mouths, but are not able to prevent them having a good chew at many things. Actually, this is probably very important to the child because he or she gets an idea of taste, texture and shape from exploring objects with the tongue and fingers. Most of us can imagine what the carpet or floor would taste like if we licked it with our tongue, although it is many years since we did this. If the cerebral palsied child is immobile, he is unable to crawl around and pick up objects to put in his mouth and therefore he may have to be given objects to taste and should be encouraged to do this.

As the normal child becomes older he may be encouraged to explore shapes with something like posting games, in which differently shaped items are put into holes of similar shapes to the items. But for the cerebral palsied child this may be difficult because of the movement problems.

However, the child may very much enjoy being helped to explore shapes and should be assisted to make a selection of which hole to put them in. If the child does not have the opportunity to do this exploration, there may not be development of ideas about space. Children begin to show affection toward dolls and teddy bears at a certain age, recognizing them as 'mock' or substitute humans. We see doll play from the age of 15 months or so by both boys and girls, but again if they cannot pick up the doll it is difficult to do things like putting the doll to bed or changing its nappy.

These are all just examples of things that go in the life of the normal child, but the child with cerebral palsy needs to experience them as well. There are hundreds of examples, such as water play and the pleasure the child takes in the bath, with splashing and pushing toys up and down, where a child with cerebral palsy may need help to experience something that occurs readily in children without a disability. The tendency is to concentrate so much on the exercises for the legs that all these normal activities that should be included tend to be forgotten. The child's disability should not overwhelm the fact that he is an ordinary child growing up with a disability, but who has need of as much normal experience as possible.

Cerebral palsy is a complex condition. It is difficult to understand all the aspects of the condition and much time and money have been and are being spent on trying to understand the nature of the condition. Much new research is being published every year, and our understanding of cerebral palsy changes all the time. Meanwhile, many of the needs of the child with cerebral palsy are the same as those of the normal child. They need the love and affection of their families, and the opportunity that a home gives to explore their full potential.

Chapter 3

Parents' problems

Jack Bavin

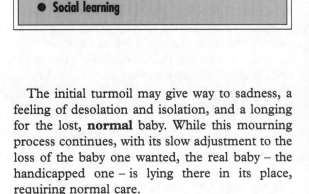

- Coping with the diagnosis
- Changing relationships
- Social development
- Bonding
- Mutual pleasure and play
- The rights of siblings
- Social learning

The problem of acceptance

No one wants a handicapped child. We all want fit, handsome, intelligent children who will do well in the competitive society we live in, and be 'a credit to us'. We even have baby competitions to find the most beautiful baby. It is small wonder, therefore, that parents worry during pregnancy about what sort of baby they are going to have, and become acutely distressed if they give birth to a damaged or imperfect child.

The parents' distress can be, and usually is, severe. At first, the feelings of anger, guilt, shame, despair and self-pity may be overwhelming, and give way to the agony of longing for a way out. In some, these feelings may even be accompanied by a resolve to end the baby's and their own life. If the distress of meeting the situation is intolerable, there may be total rejection of the child, or denial that there is anything wrong with him, or a belief that he belongs to someone else.

Torturing questions flood the mind: 'What did I do wrong? Why did it happen to me? What is wrong with me?' The answers are no less distressing: 'Perhaps I can't produce **normal** children. I damaged its brain because my pelvis is small – "they" said it is. I wish I had never got married. How I hate the other mothers who have **normal** babies.' And then, maybe, more questions such as: 'Oh, why am I thinking these terrible thoughts – what sort of person am I? He needs a mother to love him and yet we were going to abandon him.'

The initial turmoil may give way to sadness, a feeling of desolation and isolation, and a longing for the lost, **normal** baby. While this mourning process continues, with its slow adjustment to the loss of the baby one wanted, the real baby – the handicapped one – is lying there in its place, requiring normal care.

The way in which parents adjust to this apparently disastrous situation is crucial for the future welfare of not only the handicapped child, but the whole family. It is not surprising that many parents are ambivalent about the child; that is, they sometimes feel they love him as if he were normal, and at other times feel distressed, anxious and even rejecting. This is because they love and want the child, but do not want, and are distressed by, the handicaps. They may try to solve this problem by 'shopping around' for a doctor or hospital which will offer a miraculous cure. Parents who suffer severe guilt may attempt to relieve their distress, and to right the wrongs done to the innocent child, by one of two ways: they may either punish themselves by dedicating their whole life to unremitting slavery in caring for the child, or they may project the guilt onto their doctors, social workers and teachers, and angrily accuse them of neglect or mistakes. Sometimes they do both.

The reason that satisfactory adjustment must rapidly be achieved is because otherwise the handicapped child will become further handicapped, and a family's happiness and social life partly or totally destroyed.

Without skilled help, most distressed parents will tend to make an adjustment which reduces their distress, but at the cost of distorting their relationships with the handicapped child and the rest of the family. Ideally these relationships should remain emotionally and socially normal, but extra skills are needed to help the child overcome, as far as is possible, his handicaps.

This means that the child needs to be loved and accepted as a normal child would be – accepted as he is, with all his difficulties and problems, whatever they may be. Acceptance in the normal way, so that mutually enjoyable relationships are established between the child and his family, will allow the child's personality to grow in the most favourable environment. In the long run, it is the ability to face the world with self-confidence, to be friendly, helpful and useful, so that one is socially acceptable, that matters, not being physically perfect or very intelligent. Whether a child is normal or handicapped at birth, he will most easily achieve happiness and a satisfying adult social role if he is brought up in a happy, contented, united family. Even learning, in the strict educational sense, is greatly facilitated if the child is happy and secure in its first relationships within the family.

Adjustment

The first shock of being told of the child's handicaps is greatly lessened if the telling is done skilfully, and with compassion, by a doctor who offers to help the family through the early problem period. Many families do not receive this help even today, but things are slowly improving. If parents find they need more help than they are receiving they should contact SCOPE (formerly known as the Spastics Society), or MENCAP (in the UK), whose local branches may be able to arrange contact with the appropriate professional services.

As the initial distress lessens, the family must take stock of itself in relation to the task of doing the best for the new handicapped child. Perhaps the most important asset a family can have is a firmly united partnership between the parents. It is of the highest importance that **both** parents should accept their full share of the responsibility for the care of their child. Any tendency for one to blame the other, or to feel less involved, or on the other hand for one to accept the total responsibility, can be disastrous. Mothers are more likely to accept the full responsibility and fathers to allow this to happen. Mothers nurture the child for 9 months within their body, and are told of all the things they must do to keep their unborn child healthy, and all the things they must not do in order to prevent damage. Not unnaturally, therefore, they easily fall prey to feelings of guilt, or inadequacy as a wife and mother, and believe they have to suffer alone in caring for the child. Unfortunately, doctors sometimes reinforce this tendency by revealing the news to the father seen alone, and leave him to tell his wife as best he can, giving the impression that the child is really **her** problem, and the wife's distress is **his** problem.

Ideally both parents should draw closer together, and support each other by resolving to share fully the problems and the joys. Fathers should realize what an enormous comfort it is to their wives if they can speak openly about their attitudes to the child and each other, and if their feelings can be shared. Parents should also try to realize from the beginning that **they** also have needs as well as the child, and they should not stop enjoying themselves as a couple. They still need each other's companionship, leisure time spent together and separately, friends and social activities, sexual enjoyment, and a loving relationship with their other children. Nothing less than a normal family life is satisfactory for the handicapped child, its brothers and sisters, and for the parents themselves. The idea of sacrificing everybody in order to care better for the child should be thrown away. The handicapped child who has overburdened and over-caring parents suffers unnecessarily, and so does the rest of the family. At worst, the family may eventually disintegrate under the strain. Fathers who lose their place in their family may resent the handicapped child who has replaced them, and may even leave the family to find solace elsewhere. Brothers and sisters may take their pleasures outside the home dominated by the imagined needs of a handicapped sibling.

No: the handicapped child has the **same** emotional and social needs as other children. He needs love but not smothering; care but not over-indulgence; and above all opportunities for achievement, self-control and social growth towards an independent adult place in society.

Shame, embarrassment and social isolation

One problem facing parents, as soon as they have been told about their child's handicaps, is what to tell relatives, friends and neighbours. The answer is undoubtedly – the truth. You expect your doctor to tell you the truth, and you should do the same. Doctors sometimes misguidedly cover up the truth for fear of distressing parents, and parents often cover up in order to save themselves and their friends from embarrassment. Friends and neighbours are bound to enquire when you take the baby home from hospital, and failure to tell them at once of the child's disability is only to make it more difficult next time. Tell all enquirers, including your other children, as naturally as you can that the doctors think that the baby has weak arms and legs, or is severely mentally and physically handicapped, or that he has fits, and that treatment has begun. You have nothing to be ashamed of, and few people will fail to be helpful and sympathetic. On the other hand, once you have told someone that 'baby is fine', you have begun to lie, and to build a wall between you and your friends. As time goes by, it will be more and more difficult to meet people, who can see for themselves that something is wrong. They will wonder whether you know, and are too embarrassed to tell them, or whether you don't know, in which case they won't want to be the first to suggest it. Gradually you will become socially isolated, your embarrassment causing them and you to avoid each other.

Of course, some people's attempts to help may be a little misguided. Some may try to persuade you that the diagnosis must be wrong: 'How can they tell at such an early age?'; or 'He'll grow out of it'. You must let your friends be sympathetic, as

they are trying to be, and then help them to see that wishful thinking is not going to mend anything.

If you tell people in this straightforward way, you will quickly have a circle of helpful friends, relatives, neighbours and shopkeepers whose interest, enquiries and offers of help will be of the greatest support to you and your family. The alternative course, leading to gradually increasing social embarrassment, distress at having to face the outside world, and eventual social isolation and withdrawal of the family into itself, is harmful. If you maintain and even extend or strengthen your social contacts, you will be secure enough to be able to withstand the occasional rebuff or hurtful remark from the few people who lack understanding, knowledge or sympathy. Let **them** be the odd ones out – not **you**. Don't hate them for hurting you – try to help them to understand. The natural and normal behaviour of parents of handicapped children in the community is probably the greatest force we have for informing the public of their needs and dispelling the prejudice and ignorance which still exists.

Accepting help

Parents of older children often complain that no one wants to help. Many people will help, however, if given the chance. Right from the start – encourage them. Don't be too proud to ask for help, or to accept it if it is offered. Don't keep putting off the time when you return to going out in the evening together. Ask a friend to baby-sit, and then go out and enjoy yourselves. If you believe no one would want to help in this way; that no one but you can manage to look after your baby or child; that no one else could cope with a fit; or that you must always be with the baby in case something happens: in most cases you are already making unnecessary excuses.

You are overburdening yourself without benefit to the child, and jeopardizing the future happiness of the whole family. No family can be happy with a worn-out, overburdened, irritable mother (it is usually mothers who martyr themselves). Find some baby-sitters. If you do not know of any, your health visitor, GP or social worker may well be able to recommend one. Perhaps the local parents' group organizes arrangements for looking after one another's children. Explain to the baby-sitter what the child's needs are, what may happen, and how to cope. Even teenagers are capable of taking on this task (and often do so willingly) given the chance. The community will never really understand the problems of handicapped people or be sympathetic and helpful, if they are not given the chance to help.

Social acceptance – the ultimate objective

When parents have reached the stage when their distress is diminishing and they have resolved to do everything in their power to help the child, it is time to think carefully about what one is trying to do. The handicapped child is going to become an adult. As an adult, his happiness will depend on his social acceptance. If he has friends, can live and work in the community, and can actively participate in leisure and community activities – he will be happy. If, on the other hand, he has no friends and he is shunned by acquaintances and strangers alike because his behaviour is odd, infantile, aggressive or unpleasant – he will be unhappy. Nothing is more important for the parents than to realize at the beginning, and to remember all along, that the ultimate objective in rearing your child is to produce an adult who **behaves** like other adults, as far as this is possible with disabilities – and it is certainly far more possible than most people believe. Any form of bizarre behaviour, especially behaviour which is inappropriate to his age, will make real social acceptance difficult or impossible.

But, you may ask, what if the child is not intelligent enough to understand how he should behave? The answer is – do not believe it, because it is never true. Socially appropriate behaviour requires very little intelligence for its learning. It requires only consistent training which provides the child with clear-cut learning situations in which he is left in no doubt as to what is expected.

Establishing the first relationships

Social acceptance begins in the family group, where the child will establish his first, and most important, relationships. These experiences will colour his relationships with other people, and personality growth will be facilitated if the early social experiences are satisfactory. The handicapped child needs, from an emotional and social point of view, exactly the same as other children. He needs love and care, but not **more** love and care. He certainly does not need pitying, oversentimental, clinging, smothering, tearful, overprotective stroking and cuddling treatment for the rest of his life. At first, of course, he needs lots of physical contact, lots of gentle vocal stimulation, and total physical care. But even this is not likely to be satisfactory unless the baby is loved in a relaxed, joyful, accepting way, because babies are very sensitive to the mood of the mother, transmitted through her voice and physical handling.

Very quickly, however, the baby begins to establish himself as a person in his own right. He is not just helpless and passive, and if he is handicapped it is very important to observe and notice the little signs that he is beginning to listen and look, and to expect familiar experiences to be repeated. He is beginning to learn about you and the world already!

The changing relationship

It is very fashionable to talk of **child** development, and to emphasize its importance, but few people talk of **parent** development, which is equally important. It should be obvious that the normal parent–child relationship is constantly changing as time passes. What is appropriate parental behaviour towards a two-week baby is not appropriate for an infant of 6 months, or even more obviously for a child of 5 years. Beware the tendency to say: 'He's only a baby', or 'It's time enough for that later', or 'He can't understand'. It may well be that these remarks stem from a wish to deny the handicaps, with a consequent tendency to 'infantilize' the child, so that he is thought of as a baby (and treated as one) in order to explain his helplessness. Unfortunately such treatment **promotes** helplessness, so that the baby's development is retarded, even in areas where he could be making progress.

The more the child progresses in areas of development where he can, the more his remaining handicaps will be obvious by comparison, and it takes courage to be able to face up to the gradual unveiling of the true picture. On the other hand, to keep the child totally and uniformly helpless in order to hide his disabilities for a long time, is to deny the child his right to develop maximal independence. For optimal development of the child, you must gradually be changing your relationship with him, always gently encouraging every effort he makes to observe, to vocalize and to explore and manipulate the environment. Month by month and year by year he should therefore be learning to do things he could not previously do, and learning under your skilled and caring guidance. This, not keeping him dependent on you, is true parental love.

One day he is going to have to live without you, and even if he is grievously handicapped he will be better prepared for the parting if he has at least reached that stage in social development when he needs and enjoys the company of others, and is not still emotionally attached to his parents.

The ultimate objective of adult independence is reached, therefore, by starting from a basis of security resulting from your warm, tender, stimulating care, and moving gradually and steadily, with your encouragement of his efforts, towards self-confident achievement.

The mother as teacher

All infants need frequent, close and intimate contact with the mother in order to form the social bond which enables the mother, and later others, to influence the child's behaviour. The association between the feeding, warming and comforting tasks which the mother frequently and regularly performs in the early months of the child's life, with her actual presence, results in the infant starting to regard the mother as his primary source of pleasure. The mother's face, voice, smell and skin contact become highly rewarding and pleasurable in their own right, and therefore motivating. The infant therefore looks forward to this stimulation, seeks it, desires it, and becomes distressed if it is not frequently forthcoming. The fact that the baby's waking moments are often filled with the pleasure of contact with his mother makes him feel secure, so that a little later he can begin to investigate the rest of his environment for short periods, secure in the knowledge that she is close at hand to help, comfort or protect him if he gets into difficulties.

The importance of this process for the child's social development is obvious, but it is equally important for his **intellectual** development. Learning does not start at 5 years of age in school – it starts at birth (some say before birth). The most important teaching is done by the mother, often spontaneously and unknowingly. The frequent and close imposition of the 'talking face' in front of the baby teaches him the vital skill of concentrating on one set of meaningful and associated stimuli, rather than vaguely scanning the world in general. He learns to filter out confusing and irrelevant sensations, and to pay attention to one problem at a time. He also learns to be alert, to think, to anticipate, and later to explore, manipulate and experiment. He does this initially by becoming socially responsive, as he derives much pleasure from paying attention to his mother's face, which in turn responds to him and thus rewards him for his effort.

This process is essential for laying the foundation of all future learning. It is impossible to learn without paying attention to stimuli in a structured way. This means being able to concentrate on the relevant or linked stimuli, in order to discover the connection between them, without being distracted. The mother's face blots out the rest of the environment by its approach to a very close distance; it does this frequently in a way which nothing else does; it repeats the same pattern day after day, and yet it is moving and interesting; it consists of shapes, colour and the fascination of staring eyes; and it is accompanied by familiar sounds, smell and comforting skin contact. Imagine the contrast which exists for an unwanted baby, or one which the mother finds distressing or repulsive! He is left to lie alone for most of the time, not handled tenderly, not spoken to lovingly, and not frequently comforted. It is not surprising if such an understimulated baby becomes apathetic, incurious, miserable and socially unresponsive. Little useful learning will then be possible, and eventually no motivation will activate the baby to seek stimulation and experience.

Play

The importance of play for any child's development is well known, but even today few parents receive sufficient help in learning how to play with their children. Play can be defined as a pleasurable exploration of the environment. If a task is interesting and enjoyable, it will be actively pursued without apparent effort. If, on the other hand, it becomes boring, repetitive or too difficult, it will soon seem to be hard work, and require self-discipline, external pressure or reward to continue with it.

The essence of play for the child must be **pleasure** – mutual pleasure for parent and child. If the infant is smiling and excited by the adult, he is playing and learning. At first the games most likely to give pleasure are simple physical contact games (cuddling, tickling, stroking, rubbing noses, kissing); visual games (approach and retreat of your face, movements of your mouth, tongue and head, hiding and reappearing); and vocal games (singing, gentle talking, lip and tongue noises, blowing and puffing air). These lead on to simple nursery games of a more structured type, such as 'clap hands' and 'round and round the garden'. We must not forget that fathers also need to play with babies. They play differently and more roughly from the beginning – they talk in a deeper voice, look slightly different, and engage in antigravity play (see Chapter 6, Figures 6.26a–c). This provides the baby with excitement and variety of play, as well as getting him used to males and their different behaviour.

Noisy toys are useful – rattles, paper being crumpled, spoons banged on trays or cups –

because it is vital that the baby becomes interested in sounds. Always talk when you are with your baby – never handle him silently. Don't try to get him to imitate single words – let him hear the sing-song rhythm of normal speech, and the flow of normal language. He will later on try to imitate this, and you will be excited when he 'scribble-talks' in his own 'language'. Even if his cerebral palsy affects the muscles of his throat and mouth, he will understand more by hearing sentences spoken spontaneously than by listening to words repeated artificially.

When your baby makes a noise, imitate it – even a burp or a chuckle. Then wait a little while and repeat the noise again. Later on, the baby will listen for your response, and smile when he hears it. He is now playing with sounds! Still later he will make his noise in order to get you to copy, and in this way you are both 'throwing' sounds back and forwards like a ball, with enjoyment. You can then vary the sound and he will try to follow you, and you are teaching him to enjoy learning to control his speech organs in order to make the sounds he wants. He is well on the way to acquiring speech.

The point about **waiting for a response** from the baby is an important one during any form of play or learning. It is all too easy to be too impatient, and to keep showing a child what you want him to do, without giving him a chance to try himself. By waiting, after you have shown the child what to do, you increase the desire on his part to act in an effort to try for himself. You make it clear to him that you want him to participate. If and when he tries to imitate your play or voice, repeat the procedure and wait again, so that he knows that it is his turn. The more handicapped the child, mentally or physically (or both), the more one needs to wait in order to encourage him to participate. Too much hurry or repetition too quickly may deter him from trying to make an effort. He may then fall into a pattern of being a passive recipient of your efforts, and merely a spectator.

Self-help skills

The same principles apply here as for play. Every effort should be made to encourage the child to attempt tasks for himself. This requires not only patience but **time**. He must not be left to struggle too long unaided, so that he is discouraged by failure, nor must everything be done hurriedly for him, so that he becomes a passive doll. He must be shown the task, and then helped to go through the movements with his own hands or body. After a number of trials like this, he may be moving with you, or at least offering minimal resistance. At this point you should gradually withdraw your effort, **particularly at the end of a sequence of movements**, so that he tends to complete the task for himself. For example, when feeding with a spoon, put your hand over his hand when holding the spoon. Then take it to the food, fill it, take it to his mouth, and after a few trials withdraw your hand at the last point before the spoon goes into his mouth. The task is therefore easily understood, and **the tendency to complete the sequence is maximal**. In fact, it would almost require a positive desire to resist in order to avoid completion of the task.

This process of active encouragement of self-help and participation must start at birth. Encourage your baby to look at the bottle or breast and to open his mouth when it is touched by the teat or nipple. Don't just force it in! It is so easy to believe that the new baby is helpless and not able to understand, especially if you know he is handicapped. But failure to interest, stimulate and to motivate for exploration is in fact **discouragement**. The baby is learning, whether you like it or not. If he is not being taught to help himself, he is being taught to lie helplessly. It may give a parent satisfaction to feel that a child is totally dependent, and will always be so, but this is really a poor substitute for the joy of helping one's child to learn, to struggle and to overcome his handicaps.

Some guiding principles

During any teaching periods, attention to the following principles may be helpful in making your efforts more effective:

- The baby, infant or child should be keen to cooperate, and therefore be alert, happy,

responsive to you, and interested in the task. Teach, therefore, when he is most highly motivated; for example, feeding is best taught at the beginning of a meal when he is hungry, not at the end when he is satisfied and likely to play about or resist.

- The teaching period should be kept short, and ended at once if boredom or protest of any sort begins.

- No battling should occur – if it does you will always lose. The session must be fun for both of you.

- Demonstrate – wait – encourage – wait – demonstrate, and so on. Give him time to respond, and as soon as he makes any effort, encourage him by praise and smiling.

- Try to be **positive** – encourage every effort, rather than criticizing for clumsiness, messiness or failure to complete the whole task. Encouragement and praise for every little effort will help him to enjoy learning.

- Gradually work backwards from the **end** of a sequence. That is, get him to do the **last** bit, after you have done the rest; then, when this is well learnt, get him to learn the next-to-last step, and so on, so that he is working into areas which he can already do, and so that he gets the feeling of achievement as if he had done the whole job himself.

- **If you meet rebellion**, or negativism, do not respond with pressure, but instead terminate the session. Remember: the more important a thing is to you, the more likely he is to resist. Why? Because he doesn't like the pressure to conform to your wishes, and because he enjoys the power of being able to upset you by resisting. **Don't let him enjoy upsetting you.** If he won't eat his meal – calmly take it away (and don't relent later – he should get nothing till the next meal, so that it is clear that he upsets himself rather than you). Cruel? Not really – in the long run it is kinder to be firm. If the rules are crystal clear, then they will quickly be learnt.

- You must have both patience and **time**. Unless the slow, handicapped child has plenty of your calm, unhurried time, he may be unable to respond quickly enough, and may therefore look as if he is not understanding anything. This is particularly true if he is physically handicapped, because his physical responses may be slow, difficult or even impossible.

- If his limbs are paralysed completely, try to develop another way of knowing whether he understands, such as head-nodding for 'yes', and head-shaking for 'no'.
- Keep on trying if progress is very slow, and look for very small signs of progress. If you give up teaching him, he then has no possibility of learning. If you decide he can't do something, then he never will. Remember trying to learn to swim? For months one feels it is impossible, and one can't understand how people do it, then suddenly it comes, and one can't understand what the problem was.

Helping now

It is natural that parents should worry about the child's future. They often worry constantly about this, and are preoccupied with questions such as: 'Will he speak?'; 'Will he walk?'; 'Will he ever be able to work?'; 'What will happen to him when we die?' These questions should obviously be answered truthfully by the family's medical adviser, as far as it is possible to do so. But often they can only be answered in a very guarded fashion, as accurate prediction may be impossible, especially when the child is very young.

It is, however, most important that parents should concentrate on helping the child **now**, rather than worrying about the future. Worry is often **destructive** – it may prevent you the parents from making the best of present opportunities, and it may also be transmitted to the handicapped child, who may become unhappy as a result. What is needed is not even a blind acceptance of the somewhat vague prediction you may have been given of final performance, but a realistic look at the child's present state of development and a determination to help him develop to the maximum of his capabilities. Nothing is so healing of your distress as the certain knowledge that you are working steadily and expertly, day by day, to help your child overcome his handicaps. Progress, even very slow progress, keeps hope alive – realistic hope for another small step in his achievement. Read, listen, and learn from others about ways of helping your child. You are his principal teacher. The professionals help, but they cannot do your job. Learn from them, so that your child gets expert help all the time, not just for a few hours a week. And don't forget that **you** did the most expert and important job of all at the beginning, when he was a baby – you taught him to love people, to concentrate, to be curious, to explore the environment, and to want to learn.

Concentrate therefore on the present state of development and what needs to be done to reach the next stage – not on whether he will ever be completely normal. Regrets, recriminations, worry, sentimental sympathy, or painful longing for miracles, are not helpful. Effort is needed: informed, skilled, patient, determined, but relaxed effort, and not an excessive preoccupation with the child to the exclusion of your happiness and that of your family.

The task facing parents is like that of a mountaineer determined to scale Everest: he wants to reach the summit but he knows well that many have failed, and that he may fail. But he also knows that it is dangerous not to concentrate on his present position, and how to overcome the immediate obstacles in front of him. He may not succeed in reaching the top, but only a meticulous and careful step-by-step approach will ensure that he gets as far as is humanly possible in the circumstances.

Discipline

This may sound like a severe and inappropriate subject for discussion in relation to handicapped children, but it is not. Handicapped children must develop socially appropriate behaviour like everybody else, and they must learn that inconsiderate behaviour causes social disapproval. Even severely mentally handicapped people can learn to behave normally in social situations, because the learning of simple social behaviour requires little intelligence. It does, however, require consistent behaviour by the adults teaching the developing child, so that he is in no doubt as to what is expected of him. If the handicapped older child or adult still behaves in an infantile fashion, it is not because he couldn't learn to behave like an adult, but because he was taught to remain childish. Sitting still rather than running about; being quiet rather than noisy; leaving things alone rather than touching objects, pulling them down or knocking them over; cooperating with others rather than attacking or annoying them; playing with other children rather than stealing their toys: all of these are largely **learnt**, one way or another.

Discipline, or self-control, is learned gradually and begins early. Try not to think, 'He can't understand', but instead say to yourself, 'He's got to learn like other children'. Right from the start the infant will begin to form that all-important relationship with you which leads him to seek your approval and to avoid your disapproval. This is all that is required for the infant to learn which behaviour is acceptable and which is non-acceptable. Disapproval shown by a frown or scowl, and a more severe voice, should be enough to produce inhibition of the forbidden behaviour, and a desire to be restored to a position of friendship. Thus distraction into a more desirable activity is readily achieved, with encouragement facilitating the change. Needless to say, consistency is essential.

This process is, of course, used by most parents, but it can easily appear to fail, usually because it is not being properly applied. It only works if the proportion of approval to disapproval is high, so that the child can form a satisfying relationship on the basis of many mutually enjoyed activities. He then knows he is loved, and in turn he loves you – you both wish to please each other as much as possible. He will therefore, at least most of the time, try to avoid doing what displeases you. If, however, he feels that he is always, or very frequently, displeasing you, so that every time you see him move or hear him call out you disapprove, the relationship will clearly be mutually painful and disturbing. He will feel unwanted and unloved. Constant criticism and disapproval will cause retaliation, or withdrawal, or both.

He may therefore become increasingly naughty, and enjoy upsetting and annoying you, or he may take avoiding action in a fearful, timid way. In either case useful social learning will not be possible, and the situation may deteriorate eventually to the point where the child cannot be tolerated in the family at all.

On the other hand, a child who receives approval for say 95% of his actions, and disapproval or no response for 5%, has the opportunity to be able to discriminate right from wrong, while still feeling secure. If the disapproval is **consistently** and **firmly** given in relation to particular acts or behaviour, these acts will tend to be avoided. Consistency means that **both** parents must disapprove of the same behaviour, and the disapproval must be firm and unchanging. It is obviously confusing at best, and totally ineffectual or even cruel at worst, if verbal or other mild disapproval is followed by smiling or other encouragement, or if one parent is treating the child's behaviour in a contradictory way.

It is not always easy to realize that one may be encouraging behaviour which is naughty, unrestrained, inconsiderate or socially inappropriate. It is also easy not to realize that behaviour which is appropriate to one developmental stage is being prolonged inappropriately into a later age by continuing encouragement, when the normal process would entail a gradual cessation of encouragement, followed by the slow development of actual disapproval. Children cannot develop normally unless their parents develop, by which I mean that the parents' behaviour must 'grow up' with the child. In fact, the difficulty faced by the parents of a handicapped child can be summarized by saying that **the child appears not to be developing, and so the parents may not develop**, and if the parents don't develop, the handicapped child cannot move forward.

It is therefore very important indeed not to stand still in your mutual development with your handicapped child, so that you both remain locked firmly in the earliest infant–parent relationship, with no changes occurring. Behaviour such as scratching your face with his fingers, and pulling your hair, may be attractive in an infant. Its encouragement at first by parental smiling and gentle vocal response is appropriate for the development of the social bond between parent and infant, and essential for the acquisition of movement skills and for the learning of body awareness. At a later stage, however, the infant should learn to be gentle as he grows in strength, because he needs to become aware of other people's feelings, and he should be moving on to the exploration of toys, objects and his physical environment. This change is achieved by parental encouragement of these object-centred activities, and disapproval of the unwanted behaviour.

However, it must be heavily emphasized that it is **not disapproval** which is the most effective means of training social behaviour. It is far more effective to continue to encourage, and to 'move on' in a gradually unfolding sequence, so that the child is not allowed to stand still in his development. The introduction of a toy to an infant, who has previously enjoyed only physical contact games between himself and the adult, immediately changes the relationship into a triangular one, in which part of his attention switches to the toy. Encouragement of his interest in the toy, and his manipulation of it, causes him to move on in his development, so that he does not get stuck at the person-to-person relationship stage. Although he still needs adult encouragement, he does not now demand one's full-time undivided attention, because he now finds the manipulation of the toy rewarding in itself. The parent is rewarded by observing a gradually developing independence, and an unfolding personality which can adapt to other people and other social situations.

Obstinacy and tantrums

The tendency to carry on letting the child have his own way is likely to result in an excessively self-willed child. Eventually the parent may come to feel that the child should behave better, and then suddenly decide to change their demands. This abrupt, as opposed to a very gradual change, presents the child with an unpleasant and frustrating situation. He is suddenly expected to give up some

behaviour which he has for a long time performed without correction. It is hardly surprising if he now objects and gives a show of infantile anger, such as screaming or thrashing his legs about on the floor. If this tantrum meets with success, that is if the parent changes her mind and gives in for fear of upsetting the child, then tantrums may be used by the child to get his own way in continuing the form of behaviour. Prevention requires a gradual expectation of changing behaviour as the child develops, and a calm firmness on insisting that he conforms with reasonable requests.

If tantrums are already established, they may be difficult to control. It is best to ignore the tantrum and to withdraw from the child to another room or, if a group of people is present, to remove the child to another room for a few minutes until he has settled. On return to the group the child should not be comforted because of his tears of anger, but diverted to a constructive activity he enjoys, and then encouraged immediately by smiling and talking to him when he is cooperating. If the child is relatively helpless physically, it is often enough to withdraw attention while he is screaming by looking away, and then to restore your interest as soon as he has quietened.

It must be pointed out, however, that if tantrums are well established, the child will go through a period at first when he seems to get worse if a programme of control is started. This is because tantrums have worked previously in getting his way, and it is natural for him to increase his efforts using the hitherto successful method. He may therefore scream louder, and thrash about more fiercely and for longer, at the beginning of your efforts to control him. It is essential, therefore, to resolve that one is going through this period in order to achieve improvement later. If you give in again after a prolonged struggle, the situation will be worse, because the child now knows that even in the difficult circumstances when the parents are trying to hold out, he can win if he goes on long enough.

It is also important that one chooses the time and place carefully to start such a programme. Don't start it while out shopping: it is very embarrassing to try ignoring a tantrum in a crowded shop or public place! Begin at home and avoid public situations until some improvement has occurred.

It must be emphasized that this rather fierce method, in which one seems to be exerting a harsh external control over a more helpless person, can be avoided by the gradual teaching of self-control from infancy, in the expectation that the child should behave normally from the beginning. Ignoring tantrums (if they have become a regular feature of behaviour), coupled with placing the child away from social contact if the tantrums become fierce or prolonged, is still far preferable to smacking or physical punishment. The latter is not only more likely to destroy a satisfactory relationship with the child – it also teaches the child to be aggressive, as he will model himself on you. This may well lead to later fighting and spitefulness towards siblings or other children. Nothing is more irrational than a parent threatening a child with: 'If you hit him, I shall hit you!' This teaches the child that aggression is acceptable, but the bigger and stronger person wins.

Obstinacy of the kind where 'passive resistance' is used should be dealt with differently. This is often due to the child having been under pressure to achieve, accompanied by much criticism. In other words, if the child is often criticized for being too stupid or too slow, or for not trying, and the adult is impatient, irritable and frustrated by his fumbling efforts, the relationship will be unpleasant for both, and learning situations particularly painful. Refusal to try is a natural avoidance response, and at its worst is shown by muteness, a bowed head, averted or closed eyes, and clenched hands. Only by avoiding impatient, demanding pressure to achieve, and replacing it with gentle, patient encouragement of constructive effort, can this situation be remedied. It often requires the intervention of a teacher, or some other less emotionally involved person, so that the child can more easily start a new teaching relationship free from past painful experiences.

Food fads, toilet training, negativism

The more fiercely a parent holds to the belief that meat, fish, protein, or whatever, must be eaten each day to ensure health, brain growth or intelligence, the more likely it is that the child will refuse to eat it. The pressure to which the child is subjected makes him rebel. The rebellion upsets the parent and battle commences – a battle which the parent cannot win. You cannot force a child to eat and retain food; if you try he may well vomit it all up immediately afterwards. If the pressure is dropped the battle ceases, and in time the child may well feel that he wants what everyone else is having. He has lost the motivation for refusal, namely to upset you, which is obviously very easy if you are overconcerned with the need to give him certain foods.

A similar situation arises when there is pressure to eat more. The child who has had enough will start to play with his food, and make a mess. If pressure is exerted to make him eat more or quicker, he may rebel in order to upset his parent. If, on the other hand, he is treated as an individual who knows what he needs, playing can be taken as a signal that he has had enough. The uneaten food should then be calmly removed, with no retreat from this position, even if he protests, so that he goes without until the next normal mealtime. If he doesn't protest, then he didn't need any more; if he does protest, then he will quickly learn to eat what he wants without playing about.

For similar reasons toilet training is another common battleground. It may seem so important to a parent that pressure is exerted on the child to oblige, and he soon realizes that he is in control, and can therefore easily upset the parent. A child who refuses to use his pot, or who sits on it for 10 minutes and then soils his nappy just after it has been put on, may well have achieved full bowel control – but is using it for his own purpose!

Both the above behavioural problems are forms of negativism, or refusal to cooperate with a too-demanding parent. If you are easily upset by his disobedience, he will enjoy disobeying. If you keep pressing him to do something, such as eating protein, using his pot or tidying his toys away, he may refuse to cooperate and prefer to be negativistic. He has a will of his own which he wishes to assert, and if you try to dominate him, he will try to dominate you, and he may well succeed. In certain circumstances he has a right to say 'no' (many infants acquire this word before any other!), and he will if you keep pushing him to conform to an unreasonable demand.

Other behavioural problems

In a clinic, children are occasionally seen who exhibit severe behavioural problems such as screaming at night, head-banging, hand-biting, rocking or overactivity. Such problems need medical investigation as they may indicate an underlying medical condition, but often nothing is found which can be remedied. In that case we must attempt to help the child with educational methods.

The child who receives little attention, stimulation or social contact will tend to occupy himself with body-manipulation, especially if he has partial or complete loss of vision or hearing, or is severely mentally handicapped. Many stereotyped, repetitive behaviours such as body-rocking, head-rolling, tongue-stroking and complicated movements of the fingers appear sometimes to be substitutes for external stimulation and manipulation. They also seem to comfort the child, who may therefore use them for this purpose, particularly if distressed. These mannerisms are certainly difficult to eliminate once they are firmly established, because the child becomes absorbed in his self-stimulation, and is at the same time relatively unresponsive to social contact.

Trying to stop the mannerisms by a direct disapproving approach alone is bound to fail, so it is necessary to substitute something more interesting and pleasurable. Once these mannerisms are established, only a long, patient, gentle approach to the child by one or two people, who try to join in the child's world rather than forcing other activities onto him, is likely to succeed in establishing more social responsiveness and interest in the environment. From simple physical person-to-person contact games, progress can be made to physical games using apparatus (such as swings and roundabouts), and from there to simple object-centred play such as catching balls or rolling toy cars.

Physically handicapped children seem less liable to develop these manneristic behaviours or to become withdrawn, but if they do appear, or you feel your baby is unresponsive to you, it is wise to seek expert help early, so that vision and hearing can be checked (or rechecked), and advice given regarding play and stimulation.

Other disturbing types of behaviour, such as disruptive rushing about and touching forbidden household objects, are often a means of attracting attention. Mute children, in particular, are likely to develop some disturbing types of behaviour in order to attract the attention of adults, and if the child is physically helpless he may be forced to use screaming. It is common to believe that talking to, picking up, caressing or taking the child into one's own bed are comforting to the child who is distressed. This is certainly true in infancy, but the child may quickly learn to use screaming as a signal that he wants the social contact. As time goes by, parents may get worn out with the noise, and having to respond to the child's demands, which may even become incessant. They may try to break the pattern by ignoring the screams, but the child often then responds by redoubling his efforts. He therefore screams louder and longer, and the parents may then give in, or smack him in irritable bad temper. In the latter case they will then probably feel guilty at having caused more distress, and will then comfort him again.

A normal young child obviously needs frequent social contact with an adult, and even casual observation reveals that he signals to the adult every few minutes by vocalization, eye contact (looking at the adult's face) and physical contact (touching the adult's arm or climbing onto a knee), and that he gets a response from the adult. Unfortunately, the physically handicapped child, who has the same social needs, is often less able to signal effectively by these normal methods. If he cannot move, cannot vocalize, cannot turn his head, and sometimes not even his eyes, what is he to do? He does the only thing possible – he cries. If this works, he goes on using crying as a signal for attention. If he gets little response, he may eventually become withdrawn and apathetic.

The remedy may be obvious to some, but is certainly not easy. The parent needs to make a very special effort to keep the infant near her at first, and in a position where he or she can establish frequent vocal contact, eye-to-eye contact and physical contact. It sounds easy, but it is not. **You** have to make all the effort, because **he** is not able to signal his needs in the normal way. You also have to keep this up for many more months, and in some cases years, than you would with a normal child. This will need great persistence and patience, because there is less reward for your effort.

Another very important point is that you need to be very observant in order to detect the tiny signals which your baby, unless he is very grievously handicapped, will soon start to make. If he does look at you, you must at once look back. Of course, you cannot sit watching him all the time, so listen carefully for little vocal sounds, and respond with your voice and interest to these, so that he quickly learns to 'call' you. If you don't respond to these quieter sounds, he will be forced to use louder and less desirable ones. Try to remember how frequently a normal infant or young child keeps on contacting its parent, and that the handicapped child has the **same** needs. It is tiring – yes; mothers frequently and justifiably complain of the strain of responding to the demands of normal children, but nevertheless we have to recognize the importance of this social contact for the development of children.

The adult's response will therefore determine which signals the baby comes to use by habit, to obtain the attention which he needs for his social development. If he is using screaming, this indicates that his need for social stimulation is probably being insufficiently recognized when he is quiet, or when he makes the early signals of eye contact and gentle vocalization. He **may not** need **more** stimulation than you are giving already in response to the screaming, but he may be having to 'shout' loudly before he is heard. In other words, it is possible that he is being ignored unless he screams, and **then** he gets what he wants! What is needed is the **social stimulation** (or your response) to be given **before** he screams. Ideally this is achieved by your heightened sensitivity to the gentle signals which the baby is giving. It may also be true that the **quality** of the social stimula-

tion in inadequate. The response to screaming is often just a comforting, kissing, cuddling, caressing or rocking. What is really needed, certainly after the first few weeks, is the introduction of play activities, and therefore 'peek-a-boo' type games should be introduced as soon as possible, followed by the use of rattles, paper and other toys and materials, in order to encourage interest in the environment.

The child who is **less** physically handicapped, may, because of the same causes, develop head-banging, hand-biting or disruptive overactivity and other disturbing types of behaviour. The more severe and disturbing the behaviour, the more certain it is that it will effectively 'switch on' the adults in the environment to pay attention to the child. The adult therefore tries to stop the child carrying out the disturbing activity, and in doing so provides him with the rewarding social contact he needs, and which he is almost certainly not getting at other times. Again one must **ignore** the disturbing behaviour as much as possible and, most importantly, provide him with more satisfying and interesting stimulation **at other times**. It is surprisingly difficult for some adults to be interested in children when they are quiet and constructively occupied, rather than when they are noisy or disruptive. You must be **positive** in your relationship, like a teacher. You must go to the child to interest him, encourage him, and play with him, because **you** want him to **learn**; not chase him to stop him doing things you don't like, nor go to him only when he seems to need comforting. Ask yourself: 'When do I talk to him? When do I touch him? When do we play together?' If the answer is, usually **after** he screams or throws ornaments on the floor, or bangs his head, then you are teaching him to do these very things in order to obtain your interest.

Over-attachment

The child who is dependent for a longer-than-normal time is in danger of over-attachment, especially if only one person cares for him for most of the time. Not only may this make it difficult for him to adjust later to playgroup, nursery or school, but it may leave him very vulnerable if you become ill and have to go into hospital, or if you die, or if he has to go into hospital for a period. It is important that both parents, and his brothers and sisters, should play a full part in the first year of his life, and that other people should be in some contact with him from time to time.

Being handled by other people should be as routine a part of his life as for any normal child of the same age, so that social contact is pleasurable and not frightening. After 2 years of age these contacts will become more important, and should result in a gradual widening of the child's acquaintances, so that nursery activities are enjoyed at age 3–4 years without any trouble or separation-anxiety. If the child has been overprotected, and has therefore become over-attached to the mother or to both parents, the introduction to a nursery group will be painful and distressing to both, and this will further convince the parents that the child is too young to leave them, even for a few hours. He may therefore still stay at home, and the longer this occurs the more over-attached he (and the parents) will become. Again these processes of social development must be **gradual**, so that the child feels secure within the family at first, and then slowly generalizes this feeling to more and more people and relationships. An overprotective parent does not produce a happy, secure child, but one who is anxious, dependent and frightened of the rest of the world. Remember that your child, like your other children, cannot belong totally to you: he has a right to grow away from you and towards others, who must be allowed, and encouraged, to share his care and happiness.

Brothers and sisters

It is easy to forget the brothers and sisters (siblings) of a handicapped child, but they need special attention in their own right. The birth of a new baby can easily cause jealousy in a toddler, especially if all attention switches suddenly to the newcomer. This is even more likely to happen if the new baby has medical problems, which worry the parents and are time consuming to deal with. A special effort therefore needs to be made to continue to give time and attention to older siblings, in order to satisfy their needs for play, attention and affection. They must not be allowed to feel forgotten, or even resentful.

It is possible, and helpful, to involve older siblings in the care of a handicapped child, thus giving your attention to the needs of both. If you praise the helping child, he or she will enjoy being useful and develop a caring and loving relationship with the handicapped one. Later, questions will be asked about the handicapped child's slowness to progress, or inability to sit, talk or walk. These should always be answered truthfully, at a level that the child can understand.

Siblings in their teens may feel embarrassed by a handicapped brother or sister, especially when opposite sex friends are brought home. However, if the parents have always answered questions truthfully and without embarrassment, and generally involved their friends and neighbours in an open and cheerful fashion, it is likely that siblings will also be able to act naturally and with minimal embarrassment.

An important lifelong parental anxiety concerns the care of the handicapped child when the parents are themselves old or dead. In the past, siblings were often pressurized by parents to take over the care, sometimes even being forced to promise this at the parent's deathbed. This action often stemmed from a fear of old-fashioned institutional care, but with the development of modern, high-quality residential care such severe parental anxieties should now be rare. Handicapped children, as they grow into their teens, should be able to experience periods of short-term residential care in modern small homes close to their family home, and the parents' observation of the child's enjoyment of such stays should do much to reassure them, and help them to foster eventual independence.

Most handicapped young adults today (in the UK) are therefore familiar with short-term care, and increasingly they have the opportunity to move out of the parental home when the family feels this is right. As young adults they should have their own home if they wish, with whatever degree of care and supervision is necessary, and their parents should have the normal right to expect a relatively care-free middle age and retirement. Similarly their siblings should expect to form their own new families without having to care full time for a brother or sister (unless they wish to), although of course many continue to keep in touch.

Social behaviour

Parents naturally want their physically and possibly mentally handicapped child to be able to read, write, count and to make further progress in formal education. But **social** behaviour is much more important than intellectual achievement, whether for normal or handicapped people. For the mentally handicapped in particular, with limited abstract learning ability, it is essential to concentrate on the fundamentals for social adaptation – the acquisition of basic self-help skills (feeding, walking, continence, dressing, speaking) and the development of a likeable personality, so that behaviour immediately evokes from others a friendly and helpful response. One of the most valuable, and relatively sophisticated, social skills is the ability to put others at ease and to get them to help us or cooperate with us. To be able to approach people in a friendly, outgoing and charming way in order to ask for help, or to offer it, is a great asset. Timidity, awkwardness, or fumbling, incoherent approaches on the other hand may be met by rejection, rebuff or humiliating amusement. This in turn is hurtful, and increases the handicapped person's social anxiety, clumsiness and misery.

This brings us to the importance of allowing, and encouraging, the handicapped person to help others. Full community recognition as valuable members is accorded to those who are seen to be making a valuable contribution to society. The active helpers and doers, 'the pillars of society', have the highest status, while those who are dependent and helpless – 'a burden on society' – have the lowest. It may seem strange to try to encourage handicapped people to help others, but it can often be done. There are many mildly handicapped adults who enjoy looking after severely handicapped infants and children, and who give them devoted care. In turn, the severely handicapped child may give the adult a loving relationship which they might otherwise never have. Both parties in such a relationship are able to help each other in a way which *we* may be unable to do for either.

Generally then, the handicapped person who might spend most of his life being helped by caring people at home, at school or in a sheltered workshop or residential home should be encouraged to give direct personal services to others. He should be involved in small responsibilities as soon as possible – for you at home, for his brothers and sisters, for neighbours and friends. There is no reason why the mildly handicapped person should not enjoy helping old people, for example, either at the neighbourhood level or by taking part in organized community projects. We must not only aim at encouraging handicapped persons to make their own decisions, to exercise choices, to feel the satisfaction of recognized achievement, and to enjoy the same variety of opportunity as the rest of us: we must allow them to step into the helping, caring role that we have in the past carefully reserved for ourselves. Only in this way will they really feel part of the adult community.

Conclusion

It is a difficult task to write a helpful chapter for the many different parents of children of different ages with different disabilities. Some problems have been left out, while on the other hand some parents may well feel daunted by the many difficulties which have been presented. It is better, however, to have a quick look at the country ahead, with all its hazards, before setting off on a journey, provided that one is then determined to plan well in order to avoid the worst pitfalls. Being a parent is never an easy job, and none of us is perfect. Luckily children are very resilient, and most parents make a good job of their children's upbringing without instruction or much help. I hope, therefore, that after having skimmed rapidly through this chapter, parents will turn back to those parts most applicable to their situation, and then read them more carefully and frequently. If you still have difficulties which do not seem to be easily resolved, and particularly if you remain distressed, anxious or depressed, you should seek additional help. It may be that other parents will be able to help you, either directly from their own experience, or because they know better than anybody the best source of professional help in your locality. Whatever you do – don't try to press on in misery and hopelessness by yourself.

Chapter 4

Psychological guidance

Mary Gardner

- Learning in the child with cerebral palsy
- Importance of parental expectations and encouragement
- Sensory and perceptual difficulties
- Emotional aspects

Asking the right questions

If a young child is handicapped, it is natural that we should want to find out exactly what is holding him up, so that we can make plans for helping him, and seeing how far and in what ways we can reduce the difficulties. In the case of children with severe cerebral palsy, this process of finding out what is wrong can be quite complicated. This is because spasticity and other forms of cerebral palsy are due to some impairment in part of the brain. Since the brain is very complex, and controls most of our behaviour and learning, our speech and motor movements, our thinking and feeling, it is no simple matter to sort these things out, and to find out what is causing the difficulties, and then to present a remedy. The joint efforts of experts working in close partnership with you the parents are essential.

Sometimes such an array of experts (medical, psychological, therapeutic, educational and social work) seems very formidable to parents – but you should realize that these experts exist and have come together for only one purpose: to help the family and their child. The younger the child, the more important it is that help should be channelled through the parents; they are the child's first diagnosticians, therapists and teachers. Their influence is paramount and remains so throughout the early years of the child's life, and no matter how much professional help the family

is getting, it is the parents who really have to cope with the day-to-day problems that may arise.

Parents can get most help from experts if they know more about their work and the methods they use. The parents are then in a better position to ask the right questions. You shouldn't hesitate to ask questions, or worry that your queries might be viewed as criticism.

Most professional people really like answering questions; it reassures them of the importance of their work, and helps to reduce their tendency to look at problems purely from the point of view of their own expertise.

In this chapter we will discuss the work of one of these experts – the child psychologist – and her part in supporting the parents and the child with a disability.

Psychologists are chiefly interested in the processes by which children learn and in their emotional response to the world around them. The more we know about how children learn, the better chance we have of helping a child who has difficulties in learning.

How children learn

Babies start learning **right from birth**; for example, a small baby (or any young creature) makes a variety of uncoordinated movements. By chance, some of these movements result in a sensation that he finds enjoyable. The baby's waving arms, while he is lying in his cot, may for instance encounter a dangling ring, which he may hold on to with a primitive hand grasp.

His reactions are too disorganized to grip the ring intentionally, but gradually over days and weeks of repeating this same movement, the developing brain discerns a pattern which finally results (by around 6 months) in the baby being instantly able to grasp the ring whenever it is in view. From this example, we can see that as the infant's nervous system matures, he learns, by means of repetition, to coordinate hand and eye movements.

In more complex situations, **repetition and practice** may also be just as important. For example, we have all observed and wondered at the apparently purposeless dropping of toys over the side of a high chair or cot. When the child repeatedly cries for the toy to be picked up, we might be justified in thinking that he is doing it merely to annoy. This may be so in an older child, but in a young baby who has recently learnt to sit up, the action shows that he is beginning to have the first glimmerings of an idea that objects continue to exist even though they have disappeared from sight.

This is such a novel and fascinating insight for the child that he feels the need to drop the toy, over and over again, to see if the same thing happens each time. By means of these simple actions, he is beginning to appreciate quite complicated ideas of cause and effect and the influence of gravity, of which he needs to be aware before tackling more advanced activities, such as climbing or building with bricks.

A baby also learns about the world by **experimenting** and trying things out for himself. Telling a child constantly 'not to touch' is depriving him of a necessary sensory experience, in much the same way as shutting him in a darkened room. The child learns about the characteristics of things around him by comparing what his eyes and ears tell him, with what he can feel with his hands and mouth.

Another important way that a child learns is by **imitation**. One of the earliest imitative behaviours is connected with making sounds. A baby babbles spontaneously during the earliest months, but by about 12 months many babies will attempt to make the same sounds as the adult who is playing with him. When he is alone, he practises these sounds, listening to himself doing so and gradually widening his repertoire. A cross-cultural study has shown that by the age of 18 months babies are beginning to 'specialize', when they babble, in those sounds which are most common in their native language. We can see from this that imitation starts very early in a child's life.

These simple examples show the way in which babies begin to make sense out of the mass of impressions that bombard them from all sides. They are starting to make sense out of the sounds and sights and the feel of objects around them; moving and manipulating things, vocalizing and talking; gradually increasing their understanding and control of their surroundings.

How does a child with severe cerebral palsy learn?

The fundamentals for effective learning are the same for the handicapped as for all children; with, of course, some important differences of emphasis and timing, depending on the severity of the problems.

In considering the learning process, we note that learning involves **eagerness** and **striving to achieve,** the drive to explore and seek new experiences, plus the confidence to do so.

Confidence is vitally important for learning. Although the drive and eagerness to learn may not be so clearly evident in some children with severe cerebral palsy, for the vast majority the urge to learn is there, but may be reduced by frustration and failure. This is likely to occur when the stimulation given to a child and the activities expected of him are either too difficult and upsetting or, at the other extreme, too simple and boring – both of which provide the child with little sense of achievement. He may therefore fail to develop a view of himself as a competent and managing person.

Confidence is increased by parents' encouragement and praise for their child's efforts, rather than by constantly drawing attention to his inadequacies.

Parents' expectations

Sometimes a child's failures are not really failures, but simply a matter of setting standards that are too high. Parents' **expectations** about their child's rate of learning are very important. These expectations must be realistic, and the goals they expect their child to reach, in walking, handling objects, using speech and reasoning things out, must be related to the severity of the child's handicaps – physically, intellectually and emotionally.

It is here that the help of the professional team can be useful, in setting reasonable expectations and reasonable targets. Otherwise, parents may be expecting either too much or too little of their child. He may then become quite discouraged and show less eagerness when tackling new tasks.

How can we assess learning ability?

Parents, quite naturally, when looking at signs of their child's progress, compare him with his brothers and sisters, or with friends' children. Making allowances for differences in age, they notice how 'quick on the uptake' certain children are, compared with others, in their daily life and in their play with bricks, toys, books, etc.

The psychologist makes the same sort of comparison, only in a more systematic way, and with the help of intelligence tests that have been carefully worked out over many years. These tests give us a fairly accurate idea of what abilities are to be expected of the average 2- or 3-year-old child and so on. For example, if a child aged 2 years completes the set of simple tasks which are suitable for his age group (such as building with bricks, naming a certain number of toys and pictures, picking out a particular toy on request), it suggests that he has a mental age in the region of 2 years. Since this mental age corresponds exactly with his actual age of 2 years, we can say that he is of average intelligence. Another way of expressing this is to say that he has an intelligence quotient (or IQ) of 100.

There is nothing magical about the IQ figure. It is simply a convenient way of expressing the degree to which the mental age corresponds to the chronological age of the child. The IQ figure is calculated by dividing the mental age by the actual age, and multiplying by 100. In the case of a 4-year-old child who succeeds in the test at a level appropriate to a child of around 3 years, we can say that he has a mental age of 3 years, and therefore an IQ of about 75, which is at the lower end of the normal range of intelligence.

Parents may consider that this kind of measurement might be all right for the average youngster; but those with a child with cerebral palsy might well ask: 'How can you expect my child to show his intelligence, when he cannot use his hands, or speak clearly, and has had very little experience with these kinds of activities?' This is where the skill of the child psychologist comes in. It is her job to get through to the child's intellectual abilities, although these may be hidden by the presence of severe physical and speech handicaps.

The psychologist makes careful observations of the child playing spontaneously, noting what catches his interest and how he interacts with his family. The degree of interest and concentration he shows, when presented with specific tasks, are important indicators of his level of development.

We are also interested in assessing a child's **intentions**, rather than his actual performance in the tests. His attempts, however clumsy, to build a tower of graduated bricks, for example, are carefully observed and can provide quite convincing evidence that he has grasped ideas of size and sequence; the fact that his tower bricks may keep falling down is not important for this purpose. Most children with cerebral palsy have sufficient motor control to give a reliable indication of their intentions and their understanding.

For those children with only very little hand control, however, some specialized tests are available that require practically no motor control or speech – the child merely has to point in the right direction with his eyes or hands, in response to a series of questions. Or simply give some sign, to indicate 'yes' or 'no'. For example, in multiple choice tests, given a series of pictures, the psychologist will point to each one in turn, asking the child (after letting him practise if necessary) to give some sort of indication when the picture is reached which represents, say, 'the bed', or 'the one we sleep in' or 'the one with four legs'.

On the whole, intelligence tests are not as reliable for children with handicaps as they are with the average child, but in the hands of a psychologist, who is experienced with handicap and aware of the strengths and limitations of the tests, useful guidelines can be obtained.

The need for guidelines

The chief purpose of these formal assessments of learning abilities is to provide guidelines. They tell us, at least approximately, how far a child has reached in his learning, and how much progress may reasonably be expected over the next few years.

We mentioned earlier the importance of adult 'expectations' about what a child may or may not be achieving at certain stages in his life. If we expect a 5-year-old child, whose present reasoning level is around 2 years, to begin reading and number work, then disappointment is bound to ensue. Both the child and his parents are likely to become extremely frustrated. Alternatively, if we expect too little, we may miss the chance of encouraging a child's efforts, at a stage when he is receptive and ready to learn.

Numerous studies have indicated that approximately half of children with cerebral palsy function within the average or above average range of intelligence; about a quarter are within the moderately slow learning range, with the remaining quarter being very slow learning (this means that their intellectual level is rather below that of an average child of half their age). It is these very slow-learning children, who often also have severe physical and speech impairments, who need a great deal of expert educational and therapeutic help.

Encouraging your child's interest in learning

Some people might question the point of trying to improve the performance of a severely handi-

capped child. They might argue that his skills are so limited that the time and effort are scarcely worthwhile. Any parent after a tiring day may expect to feel the same, on many occasions!

However, anyone who has watched a child struggling with determination and persistence to master some task that they have observed others doing, and has seen the delight which accompanies success, will realize that achievement is as important to the handicapped as it is to any child. Indeed, one might argue that the smallest steps towards self-help in dressing, feeding and moving around, take on a greater significance in the life of a child with severe cerebral palsy whose horizons are necessarily so limited. The parents' aim should be to encourage the child's efforts in self-help skills, ensuring that any task is **almost** within the child's reach, so that continued disappointment does not dampen his eagerness. **Teaching a new skill is a subtle compromise between you doing too much of what he could manage himself, and setting so hard a task that failure is bound to ensue.**

We can summarize the most effective ways of encouraging learning, as follows:

- **Interesting tasks.** Some severely handicapped children do not, in the early years, seem to show much curiosity, or eagerness to learn. The parent must therefore work towards stimulating his interest, by using large bright toys and materials, including something different each week that he has not seen before, or has not seen for some time, so that an element of curiosity is maintained.
- **Short sessions.** Set aside one or two periods of say 10 to 15 minutes each day, for carrying out some fairly concentrated learning. This is better than trying to carry on for hours at a time – children can concentrate and achieve quite a lot, in fairly short spurts, with rest and relaxation in between.
- **Set a target.** It helps both parents and child to aim at a goal; it enables us to be aware of progress, and to get satisfaction from knowing when we reach a certain goal, or nearly do so. These goals can be very simple activities in building with bricks, or putting objects in and

out of containers, to matching shapes or coloured cards, completing form boards, and so on.

● **Small steps.** Choose simple activities and break them down into manageable steps. For example, with a game like 'Picture Lotto', the matching of pictures can start with a few obviously different pictures, moving gradually to matching those in which differences between them are more subtle. Give plenty of opportunities for practice.

● **Encouragement.** Give plenty of praise for success – praising for effort, as well as for actual accomplishment. Play down failure, as much as possible, without showing surprise or irritation.

If these general principles are kept in mind, the mastering of the simplest skill will bring with it much satisfaction to the child. Learning can be enjoyable!

Learning in the child with additional impairments

Visual problems

There are some children with cerebral palsy who have visual as well as movement problems. The baby with poor vision, because he does not see his parents' faces so clearly, will need more in the way of touching and cuddling and singing than the average baby. He will become aware of affection by the way he is handled and by the tone of the adult's voice; and will gradually be able to recognize familiar people by these means, as well as by the texture and smell of their clothes. He will begin to learn about his world by touching and exploring with his fingers, and with his mouth, and will gradually come to appreciate feelings, through the sound of laughter, or the tone of disapproval in his parents voice.

But most of all, the child with a visual problem will learn by listening – to all the wide variety of sounds around him, as well as to people talking. Being talked to is of vital importance to the visually impaired child. For instance, it is especially helpful if the parent provides a running commentary, while preparing a meal, so that the child will begin to associate the sounds and smell of a meal preparation with the feel and taste of the different foods. Similarly with the preparations for a bath or an outing.

Children with limited vision obviously enjoy musical toys and those that make a noise, including saucepans with lids, trays to bang with a spoon, or friction-drive cars. They may need more than usual encouragement to explore their surroundings, whether by rolling or crawling, since they may be understandably timid until accustomed to a familiar room and to avoiding obstacles in it. Toys that make a noise, such as a ball with a bell inside it, will tempt a child to go after it, whether by rolling or crawling.

As for the child with **milder visual problems**, it is perhaps more difficult for us to imagine what it must be like to have only a rather vague impression of other people's faces; to be not quite sure whether we are seeing a frown, or a grin. So, as with the more severely impaired child, it is the adult's tone of voice that becomes all important, and we need to give a clear message, for instance, about future activities.

Even with quite minor visual problems, a child may not be able to make out distant objects; to know, for instance, which is his own coat, until he gets near enough to feel the texture. Tidiness and routine play a major part in the lives of these children, and it helps if the household is well organized! Otherwise he will trip over things left lying about, or get very frustrated at not finding things in the expected places.

When we are outside the house, knowing where we are depends on recognizing a series of familiar landmarks, which we 'tick off' in our minds, so to speak, as we go along. For a child with poor vision, who is being taken out in a buggy or wheelchair, it is especially helpful if he can sometimes be allowed to touch the hedge or fence as you pass, so that he can recognize where you have got to, along a familiar route. Also it is obviously helpful if the adult can talk about the interesting buildings or vehicles they are passing, and the reasons for stopping at a particular crossing point. By doing this the visually handicapped child will quickly build up a series of clues into an auditory and tactile 'map' of his local neigh-bourhood. You will thus be able to supplement whatever visual impressions he is able to receive, and enhance his understanding of the world around him.

Playgroups and schooling

Once the child is 2 or 3 years old he may need wider opportunities to learn and to engage in exploratory play than can be provided at home. Provision varies: in some areas, a child with visual and motor problems may attend a local nursery group where visiting specialists can advise staff and parents. The ordinary bustling nursery envir-onment may need some adaptation, with attention being given to lighting levels, and the various hazards provided by wheelchairs and walking frames, for instance. A very gradual introduction with a parent present is usually needed, so that the child can get used to the noise and excitement of group activity; something which they usually soon learn to love, and look forward to as the highlight of their week.

Although in some countries separate units have been set up for the visually handicapped, the more recent emphasis is for pupils to be integrated into schools most appropriate for their intellectual level. When children attend neighbourhood schools, supportive services of visiting teachers are necessary to give advice about teaching meth-ods and any auxiliary aids to learning. Special aids can range from simple whole-page magnifying lenses, special slow-speed tape recorders and closed-circuit TV magnifiers. Tape recordings and radio programmes also clearly play a very important part.

Hearing problems

Nearly everybody has occasional hearing prob-lems, due to ear blockages and infections, espe-cially after a common cold. These can cause a mild temporary hearing loss, known as a 'conduc-tive loss', which usually responds well to medical treatment. A very small percentage of children with cerebral palsy have hearing losses which are not due to blockages, but to a defect in the nerve fibres, either within the inner section of the ear or in the nerve pathways to the brain. This is known as a 'nerve' or 'sensorineural' hearing loss, which can range from mild to severe, sometimes affect-ing the hearing of higher rather than lower tones.

The parents are often the first to notice a hear-ing difficulty, comparing their child's responses to their own responses (and those of other children) to everyday sounds such as the doorbell, radio or telephone, in situations where their child's atten-tion is not fully engaged in some other activity that completely absorbs him.

If a hearing loss is suspected, then prompt expert testing is essential, so that if a loss is con-firmed, we can determine its causes and extent, and plan treatment and remedial action. As we have mentioned, conductive losses can nearly always be treated effectively. For 'nerve' deafness there is no medical or surgical treatment that can cure it – given our present state of knowledge – but there is a great deal that can be accomplished through specialized teaching, combined with hearing and other communication aids, particu-larly by parents in the natural everday situation of their family life.

The main effect of a significant and permanent hearing loss is to delay a child's language, com-munication and social skills, so early advice on training and equipment is very important. In the UK, such advice is obtainable from local Audi-ology Units, working in conjunction with medical and educational services.

Hearing aids can help a great deal, amplifying sounds without distorting them too much; and radio aids, through which the speaker uses a microphone and a transmitter, are even better.

Lip reading and gestures and sign language (such as the Makaton) should also be encouraged in children with severe hearing losses, using visual cues to compensate for their impaired hearing.

It is particularly important for children with physical handicaps to be properly positioned for good communication, e.g. head and trunk well supported, facing the speaker in a good light; ear-pieces (for the hearing aid) fitting properly and not too much disturbed by movements which would cause unwanted noises through the hearing aid. We cannot hope to maintain these proper conditions for good communication all day and every day, but we can maintain them for some periods during each day. This is important to ensure that simple language is going in, vocabulary is building up, sentence formation is gradually growing, and from this input, communication from the child will follow; through speech, or signing, or by using electronic equipment, including word processors when the child is older.

Help from a teacher of the hearing impaired will be very important in furthering your child's language and communication skills, on which a great deal of his social skills will depend. It is difficult to relate to people if you cannot fully understand what they mean. This help, during the early formative years, will ensure that a child is well prepared for nursery and primary schooling. In the UK, most schools have the services of a visiting teacher of the hearing impaired, and some have special units for children with severe hearing losses who require concentrated help within small groups.

Subtle learning difficulties

Some children with cerebral palsy, who possess adequate intelligence and vision, and relatively minor physical problems, may nevertheless have very unevenly developed learning abilities. For example, they may be very good with words, conversing readily, using sentences well at an early age, but may be extremely poor at practical things, such as handling constructional toys, or dressing. These children have quite subtle difficulties in their perception of the world around them.

Visual perception is the ability to recognize and distinguish between shapes, such as a circle and a square, to distinguish between the outline of a drawing and its surrounding background, and to recognize different directions in space (left and right, up and down, etc.), especially in relation to our own body. Some children are easily confused about which direction to take, and how to get their bodies past obstacles, their arms into sleeves, and so on. They may also have difficulty in relating what they see to what they hear and to

what they touch. In other words, their different senses do not hang together very well. For example, most babies, by 6 months of age, not only hear a sound, but will usually turn their head and look inquiringly round, attempting to identify what might be making the noise. Hearing, vision, motor control and intelligence have, over the months, worked together to accomplish this, whereas a child having perceptual handicaps (although the separate senses of hearing, vision and touch might all be all right in themselves) cannot link these up, or rather may be very slow in learning to do so.

This linking-up of visual and motor performance is very important, since we use our visual perception a great deal in everyday life. Indeed, much of the information we receive from our surroundings comes through the eyes, and is then interpreted by the brain. We may act on the information we have gained, and make some sort of motor or vocal response. In short, we integrate vision with movement. The baby starts to do this during the first months of life; for example, in watching his own hand movements, or reaching for a toy.

How to help the child with poor visual perception

In helping the child with perceptual problems, we need (as is often the case with handicapped children) to encourage and teach things that come more or less automatically to the ordinary child. Otherwise they may tend to shy away from what they find difficult – visual judgement in this case – and 'overdevelop' (sometimes rather superficially) what might come more easily, such as speech and appreciation of language. In short, they become great talkers and poor doers.

Therefore, lots of encouragement and opportunities are needed to help bring on a child's appreciation of shape and pattern, and to link up these perceptions with the use of his hands. There is plenty of material available for this, described in Chapter 13 on play, such as simple form boards, posting boxes, graduated beakers and boxes of bricks. As we have emphasized before, try to start off with some measure of success, by using the simplest posting box or form board, with just a few shapes in it. At first, encourage the child to place just one or two shapes, a circle or square, for instance, while you help with the rest. If you start in this gradual way he will be pleased that he is succeeding and will want to tackle the whole task himself, as soon as he is confident that he has a chance of succeeding.

Modern form boards are often in bright colours thought to be attractive to younger children (they certainly are helpful to those with a visual problem). However, whether plain or highly coloured is not of particular significance. It is the act of selecting the shape, looking at it carefully and comparing it with the hole that is the important thing. The child is discovering that by scanning the alternatives, before making a choice, he will gain more success than trying the first piece that comes to hand. An important lesson is being learnt here, especially for children who tend to be impulsive and have difficulty in controlling hand and arm movements.

If a child is good with words, use this to help his visual judgement, for example by naming a circle and pointing out its similarity to a football, thus helping him distinguish between a round and an oval shape. One formboard inset could be described as 'like a roof', another 'like a tunnel'.

These early experiences with shapes form the basis for later attempts at reading, which is basically a process of distinguishing one only slightly different shape from another.

How to help the child with attention problems

Some children show a short attention span and are easily distracted from the task in hand by any extraneous sound, such as a lorry passing, or the sight of a curtain swaying in the wind. With children who are so easily diverted, a helpful move is to cut down the amount of distraction around them.

Therefore, for our teaching and training periods, we should use a quiet corner of the room and keep it fairly plain and bare, tidying other toys out of sight and presenting the child with only a few pieces of equipment at a time. This helps him to focus his attention and eventually to get more satisfaction from what he is doing (one learns very little if one is flitting from one thing to another), so that eventually, as he becomes older, he can cope with ordinary surroundings and distractions.

Most psychologists regard these perceptual and attention handicaps as a kind of time-lag in a child's development, rather than a permanent impairment; that is, the attention and perception of the handicapped child is often at a level appropriate to a younger child. The techniques we have briefly described may help to focus and extend concentration.

Alternative forms of communication

We have been considering various factors to do with the way a child learns – the input of impression through his various senses, and the intelligence, perception and attention that enable him to organize and make sense of these impressions. We will now mention the 'output', as it were, from the child; his means of expression through speech, hand control, gesture, etc.

Careful consideration needs to be given to those children whose communication difficulties are such that they cannot properly express their thoughts and ideas (either through speech or hand movement), if constant frustration is to be reduced. We have already mentioned some of the ways in which the psychologist communicates with severely handicapped children, such as by providing toys and test situations in which the adult can do the talking and movements, and the child merely has to signal 'yes' or 'no' at the right time.

Parents can practise this sort of communication with their child. For example, a 3- or 4-year-old child, without speech or very much hand control, can gain stimulation and enjoyment from a simple picture – say of a street scene. The parent can talk about it and then ask questions, 'Is this the policeman?' 'Is this the ice cream van?', pointing to various parts of the picture in turn, and waiting for the child to give some sign for 'yes' when the correct part is reached.

These signs for 'yes' and 'no' are extremely important; any sign will do, such as nodding the head, looking at the speaker to indicate 'yes', looking to one side or grimacing to indicate 'no'. When reliable signs of this kind are established, a child can begin to express his ideas and preferences, in spite of severe speech and hand control difficulties.

Some equipment can be provided to extend this expression; a head pointer can be used if hand control is too weak, or better still, an electronically operated indicator, with the child using a very simple switch, that allows him to control a moving light to express his choice.

Signing is a wider ranging alternative to speech, through hand movements and gestures (as used by people who are deaf) to indicate words, such as the Paget–Gorman system and its simplified form, known as Makaton, for younger children. Makaton signs are also available in the form of symbol boards, which can be operated electronically, for children with severely limited hand control.

For children with a mental age of 5 years plus, who are beginning to learn simple reading and spelling, some form of electronic typing is the most advanced form of expression for those with limited speech and hand control; a wide range of computer-based communication aids is available in many countries. Keyboards can be in expanded forms, or activated by foot controls, vocalizations, or even eye movements. Output can be on a video screen, on paper, or through a voice synthesizer.

Expert advice and proper training in the use of such equipment is essential (such as, in the UK, through the Regional Communication Aid Centres). Then such communication aids can be of enormous value. They do not, in our experience, interfere with the child's efforts to develop his own more natural ways of communication (see Chapter 11 on communication and technology).

Educational groups

Education, in the broadest sense, begins at home with the family. The family can benefit from professional expertise, but nothing can substitute for its unconditional love and care during the early impressionable years.

Playgroups and schools provide the child with wider horizons, new challenges and stimulation; learning to become accustomed to other adults and children outside the family nest, and how to cope with new demands.

The majority of children with cerebral palsy can benefit by early admission, a few hours each week, initially, to an ordinary neighbourhood playgroup or nursery, provided that the staff are alerted well in advance, through the parents and their professional advisers, concerning the child's special needs, such as in seating, mobility, feeding, toileting and communication arrangements.

Some parents will find that these arrangements are not so complete as they would wish. This is partly because the playgroup staff's time and energy has to be shared among several children. This sharing and 'turn-taking' is an important part of the group's purpose – to help the child to mature socially. Regular contact between staff and parents helps to resolve these issues.

Much depends on the degree of handicap. Children with severe physical, communication and learning difficulties are likely to need 'special' rather than ordinary nursery groups, which have the advantage of providing a wide range of teaching and therapy and care facilities 'under one roof'.

More formal education at school, around age 5 years, is the rule in the UK, for which assessment teams of psychologists, doctors, therapists and educationists provide expert advice on educational facilities, ranging from mainstream schooling with various degrees of extra help, special units attached to ordinary schools, to specialized schools for children with multiple handicaps.

Since parents' commitment to their child's education, from birth onwards, is usually so strong, their part in the assessment team's deliberations is crucial.

Formal educational provision

When considering schooling for pupils with any type of handicap, the emphasis has changed, in

Britain, since the Education Acts of the 1980s came into force. Before the Warnock Committee's report, children were categorized according to their disability, and then allocated to schools accordingly. The emphasis now is on the assessment of the educational needs of each child who may have a handicap; and the local education authority, along with the parents, may make a formal Statement of Special Educational Need. The aim is to provide an appropriate teaching environment that will cater for each child's particular brand of abilities and difficulties. This may be in a specialized school or unit, or in the ordinary classroom, with extra support if necessary.

When planning the style of education best suited for a child, those professionals already involved will discuss the various alternatives with the parents, and together they will work out what seems most appropriate at each stage in the child's school life. The type of schooling decided upon will, of course, depend on local circumstances, with such practical matters as distance, transport facilities and amount of awkward stairs within the school being taken into account.

Another factor that needs to be considered is the unique qualities of each child: his temperament and his intellectual capabilities, as well as his physical difficulties. For instance, two children with moderate cerebral palsy, who need to make use of a wheelchair for part of the school day, might have quite different requirements. One may be an outgoing child, easily bored with his own company and inspired to succeed by the competition of other children – he may thrive in an ordinary classroom with some additional support. By contrast, a child with similar physical difficulties who is hypersensitive to noise, and agitated by stimulation and bustle, may respond best in a small unit with a protective and encouraging atmosphere. Small specialized classes within the ordinary neighbourhood school are ideal for these sensitive and sometimes timid children; they gradually become accustomed to larger groups, joining the mainstream class, on occasion, for story or music sessions.

Many countries are at the planning stage of setting up special facilities for pupils with varying handicaps; and it is this variety of provision that

is important, since it gives families a range of options. An option which is favoured in the UK is the setting up of small units, staffed by specially trained teachers, attached to mainstream schools, so that those with a disability can integrate as appropriate, making use of equipment – such as computers, typewriters, science apparatus – that is available for the whole school. In this way pupils can feel part of the larger school community and not isolated in a protective environment, which perhaps does not have much contact with the wider life beyond school.

Striking the right balance – emotional factors

We have concentrated, in the first part of this chapter, on considering how children learn, including learning in those children with sensory and perceptual problems.

We have stressed how much a child's development involves his curiosity about the world and his eagerness to master new tasks; this means that he will have learnt a great deal before he reaches school age. However, when this striving to explore and gain some mastery of his environment is held up by physical incapacity, then it is understandable that the child should seek other means of exercising some control – and he may focus instead on controlling his parents and carers!

Being denied the opportunity to satisfy his wish to investigate his surroundings by opening every cupboard, as a toddler loves to do, the very young child with cerebral palsy is particularly prone to boredom.

Relative immobility means that he comes to rely on his parents, and brothers and sisters, being close at hand to provide entertainment, to make up for the limited range of things that he can do for himself. In the early months, especially if the baby is very premature and delicate, the mother may carry him around in a sling most of the time. It does sometimes happen that the baby wants this to continue for 24 hours a day, so that her own needs to have a bath, to wash her hair, or even to get dressed, are resented by the infant, and a screaming bout may ensue. This is clearly upsetting for all the family, often leading to a build-up of irritation, as well as exhaustion.

Even the most patient parent experiences resentment (mixed in with love) at the seemingly overwhelming demands of a young infant. However, these feelings are often exaggerated when a baby is slow to develop, partly because he cannot so easily occupy himself, and partly because of the family's understandable mixture of emotions – of sadness, protectiveness or uncertainty as to how to act for the best.

Sharing the care

This situation – of the baby becoming extremely dependent on his mother's presence – is clearly most likely to occur in a single parent family, or where the mother is on her own for much of the day. In this case it is important to seek suggestions and support about sharing your baby's care with some knowledgable person, either from your physiotherapist, health visitor or social work department. Friends, or members of neighbourhood or church groups, usually want to be helpful, but may be hesitant if they doubt their capacity to cope with an infant who seems so vulnerable.

You might need to pluck up your courage to ask for support but when you do, you will find that other people are eager to help, once you explain the situation. You will also need to build up **their** confidence, by demonstrating the type of handling methods that you have discussed with your therapist. Begin with very brief periods away from your child (otherwise you may become anxious!) – at first, maybe, only for as long as it takes to write an important letter, or make a phone call. Once you and your helper are confident that your baby is in good hands, then longer outings could be attempted.

These brief respites give you a chance to consider your own needs and recharge your emotional batteries. Sharing the caring with relatives, friends and voluntary, as well as professional helpers very often brings great benefit to the child as well as the parents. Children need some changes of routine too!

Part II
Basic information

Chapter 5

Understanding movement and development

- Understanding movement
- Primitive reactions and automatic movements
- Basic differences between normal and abnormal sequences of movement
- Normal sensorimotor development – the early stages

This first section is intended to help the reader understand how we move and the difficulties experienced by the child with cerebral palsy. In order to reach this understanding it is important to know how we develop from being a relatively defenceless creature at birth – our movements characterized as spontaneous and random with involuntary reflex activity sometimes interfering – to an adult capable of performing complex voluntary and purposeful tasks.

In order to help the child with cerebral palsy reach his full potential in functional activities, we must modify and modulate his responses by our handling. The information provided in this section is intended as a background to understanding the difficulties children with cerebral palsy experience in maintaining postural control against gravity in different positions, how this varies according to the distribution and type of abnormal postural tone present and the position the child is in, interfering with his ability to move in and away from one position to another. It is also intended to make Part IV on handling during routine activities more meaningful.

Movement

If we are to be competent in appreciating and understanding the changing problems in the phy-

sical development of the child with cerebral palsy, it is essential that we first know something of the physical development of the normal child, including these most important basic patterns of movement underlying future activities. It is also helpful to observe and understand how **we** move, thus making it easier to assess why the child with cerebral palsy moves in a particular way and what is interfering with his movements.

Our muscles work in patterns, and the brain responds to our intention by making groups of muscles, not single muscles, work. As adults we never consciously think which component of a movement is going to occur first or which muscles do the work. The highly complex centres in our brain are constantly working to coordinate the vast amount of information arriving by sensory pathways that provide information on, among other things, where we are in space, the position of our limbs and trunk, and the state of readiness of our muscles. Our eyes and ears provide us with additional sensory information.

The centres in our brain filter the information and constantly update the control centre which in turn sends out messages (neural signals) along motor pathways to the muscles of our body to make the fine adjustments necessary to maintain our position. When we signal our brain of the intention to perform a particular activity, the control centre instantaneously computes which joints need to move, in which order and sequence, and by how much, at the same time, of course, making all the other adjustments necessary to maintain our body in balance.

If you consider another type of activity, such as drinking a cup of tea, you will realize that not only are you able to pick up the cup and take it to your mouth without spilling the contents, but as you drink, and reduce the weight of the cup, you are still able to move the cup in a smooth coordinated way. This achievement is in part due to the mechanisms already described, but in addition there is the muscle or force factor. The sole purpose of muscles is to generate force. The extent to which the force is generated and released is again controlled by the centres in the brain.

Types of muscle activity

To complete this simple introduction to understanding movement it is necessary to explain briefly about different types of muscle work. Consider the everyday task of writing. Once the pen is held between your fingers and thumb, small bending (flexion) and stretching (extending) movements of your fingers enable you to form the letters. These controlled but fluid movements are only possible because your wrist is extended and firm and your elbow and shoulder stable. It becomes obvious that in order for your fingers to bend, the muscles on the palm side must contract, becoming shorter and those over the back of your fingers, the extensors, becoming longer. The balance is perfect, and we refer to the active, shortening muscles as the agonist and those muscles that oppose the movement, in this case the extensors, as the antagonist. The muscles at the wrist, however, are working in synergy to provide stability: the flexors and extensors are co-contracting at different lengths but with equal force.

Muscles are composed of bundles of fibres, each of which is a cell, and the number of fibres is determined at birth. During muscle activity these fibres or at least the structures within them slide on each other to effect the shortening or lengthening. The bundles of fibres are bound together and finally a sheath surrounds the whole muscle and this sheath is extended to become the muscle tendon, which is the specialized fibrous tissue that connects the muscle to the

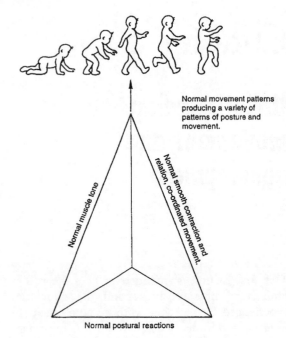

Normal movement patterns producing a variety of patterns of posture and movement.

Normal muscle tone

Normal smooth contraction and relation, co-ordinated movement.

Normal postural reactions

Figure 5.1   (a) Illustrates the background of normal muscle tone, postural reactions, etc., necessary for normal movement patterns, producing a variety of patterns of posture and movement

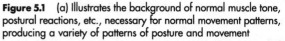

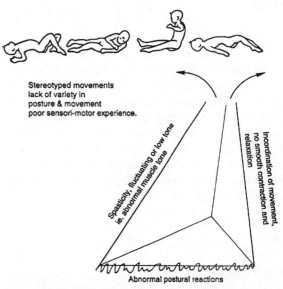

Stereotyped movements lack of variety in posture & movement poor sensori-motor experience.

Spasticity, fluctuating or low tone ie. abnormal muscle tone

Incoordination of movement, no smooth contraction and relaxation

Abnormal postural reactions

Figure 5.1   (b) Shows how, with an abnormal background of muscle tone and postural reactions, etc., movements will be stereotyped and lack variety

skeletal bone. An example of this is the large tendon at your heel, the tendo Achilles, that connects the big, powerful muscles of your calf to your foot.

By now, I hope you will be as much in awe, as I remain, with the complexity and precision of the underlying systems that allow us voluntarily to conceive and execute a highly complex task smoothly and in a coordinated manner, all without conscious thought.

The child with cerebral palsy

In the child with cerebral palsy the early insult to the developing nervous system has damaged different parts of the centres and pathways described. The exact manifestation of the lesion will depend on many factors, some of which are:

- when the insult occurred before, during or immediately after birth
- the size of the lesion
- what type of lesion it was – haemorrhagic (bleeding), anoxic (lacking oxygen)
- the location in the brain – which structures were damaged.

These factors will determine whether the child is described as having **hemiplegia, diplegia** or **total involvement (quadriplegia)** and further whether there is increased postural tone (spasticity), decreased postural tone (hypotonia) or fluctuating tone (athetosis) or a mixture of these. The expression of these lesions will mean that the child with cerebral palsy exhibits abnormal patterns of posture and movement. The exact presentation will also be influenced by the extent to which normal maturation and development has been arrested or delayed.

The child with cerebral palsy, in common with other children, learns a movement by 'feeling' it and trying it out. Whereas the normal child has a natural or built-in ability for adapting his movements to his own satisfaction, the child with cerebral palsy is limited to a varying extent to a few and inadequate patterns of movements, that become stereotyped and on which he will base whatever skills he may acquire later. If a child is unable to initiate movements by first changing his posture and is limited in the variety of postural patterns that accompany normal movements, there is always the possibility that contractures may develop. That is why the objective of early handling is to moderate unwanted patterns of movement, establish postural control, and at the same time encourage and facilitate more normal patterns of movement – in this way, giving the child a wider choice of movements before compensatory patterns of movement are established.

The background or matrix of early infantile reactions (primitive reactions) which serve as a platform for the development of movement are given next.

Primitive reactions (early infantile reactions)

In this section we will describe a few of the early primitive reactions, also known as infantile reactions, present at birth and the normal automatic postural reactions which are essential for the development of coordinated patterns of movement and that underlie all our voluntary activities.

A baby is born with a number of immature patterns of responses which take place against a background of normal postural tone. These responses are evoked automatically following a specific stimulus or experience and are called '**primitive reactions**'. Some of these primitive reactions, such as rooting, hand grasp and Moro, disappear completely during maturation, whereas others are modified, a few remaining with us for life.

I think it is important that the reader is aware that there is a **difference** between the immature primitive reactions of a normal baby, and the **persistent** pathological primitive reactions of children with cerebral palsy.

When these primitive reactions are elicited in the immature baby they are **spontaneous** and **variable**, but when present in the child with cerebral palsy, although the response is similar, it is a pathological and obligatory response against a background of **abnormal** postural tone, a pathological response, that is repeated in the **same way** each time (stereotyped).

A few of these primitive reactions, with the stimulus that causes them to happen, and the baby's response are shown in Table 5.1.

Normal postural tone

Normal postural tone provides the background on which movement is based, high enough to withstand gravity, but low enough for easy movement.

Both posture and movement are dynamic and interact to such an extent that they cannot be separated. Postural changes are part of every movement, and movements themselves are, in effect, changes in posture.

During the first year of life on a background of **normal postural tone** the primitive reactions gradually become moderated and integrated into the baby's voluntary coordinated patterns of movement, enabling a group of mature reactions to develop. These are called **postural reactions** and remain with us throughout life. As gravity affects all our movements from birth onwards, these reactions help the baby to master gravity in conjunction with increasingly organized and coor-

dinated patterns of purposeful movements seen during the child's early years. These reactions help him to master gravity, enabling him eventually to stand up and walk.

Postural reactions (also known as automatic reactions)

Postural reactions provide the baby with a **stable postural base** so that he can maintain and adapt his body position against gravity, and have his body in alignment, weight evenly distributed, with sufficient stability at his shoulder and pelvic girdles to move his limbs independently. This **truncal stability** also enables him to shift his body weight against gravity.

Righting reactions

These reactions form the basis of future coordinated patterns of movement. When a baby is moved or moves himself, they maintain the normal position of his head in space, and in relation to his body, trunk and limbs. They underlie all a child's activities, such as rolling, sitting up, getting on hands and knees, and kneeling – all sequences

Table 5.1 Some primitive reactions, their stimuli and the baby's responses

Name of reaction	Stimulus	Response
Rooting	The side of the mouth or cheek is lightly brushed with a finger	The bottom lip goes forward to that side, the tongue moving towards the stimulus
Moro	Held at an angle of 45° from the support, the head is allowed suddenly to fall back a short way	The arms are extended away from the body, with open hands, followed by the arms coming in towards the body in an 'embrace'
Asymmetrical tonic neck reaction	The head is turned passively to one side	Extension of arm and leg on face side; flexion of arm and leg on skull side
Hand grasp	An object or finger is introduced into the palm of the hand from the ulnar side (by the little finger)	The fingers flex and grasp (release is not possible)
Foot grasp	A finger is pressed against the ball of the foot (behind the toes)	The toes grasp (curl) around the finger
Placing the lower limbs	The front of the shin and foot is brought up against the edge of the table	The leg bends and the baby takes a step; the foot is placed flat on the table
Placing the upper limbs	The front of the forearm and back of the hand are brought up against the edge of the table	The arm is raised and the hand is placed on the table
Automatic walking	Supported under the arms, hands coming around the chest, the baby is tilted forwards	Automatic stepping follows, the foot coming down flat on the support
Neck righting	Lying in the supine position, the head is rotated passively or turns actively to one side	The body turns 'as a whole' in the direction of the head

of movement that will eventually enable him to stand.

These reactions later become integrated with the balance (equilibrium) reactions.

Equilibrium reactions (balance)

Their function is an automatic rapid response to loss of balance, helping us to both maintain and regain our balance, thus making free and independent movements of the head and limbs possible in all positions.

Saving reactions

Very sudden or unexpected loss of balance elicit saving reactions. Their purpose is to protect our face if we should lose our balance or fall, by thrusting out our arms with straight elbows to place our open hand on the supporting surface.

In the child with cerebral palsy, because of abnormal postural tone and abnormal movement patterns these mature automatic postural reactions will either be absent, incomplete or exaggerated.

Some basic differences between normal and abnormal sequences of movement

In this section we will discuss the sequences of movement that enable us when lying in the supine position (on the back) and the prone position (on the front) to move away from these positions in a smooth, coordinated manner, with a brief reference to rolling, standing and walking, and the reasons why the child with cerebral palsy either cannot or has difficulty in both initiating and carrying out these sequences of movements.

Sitting up from the supine position

Before we sit up, the first thing we do is automatically adjust our position so that we are lying symmetrically, our head, trunk and pelvis in alignment, our limbs lying in a symmetrical and relaxed position.

Our body weight would be evenly distributed, so if, for example, someone tried to put their hands under our shoulders or our bottom, they would not be able to do so as both would be in contact with the supporting surface.

The way we come up to sitting will depend on how fit we are and the strength of our abdominal muscles. Assuming we had good abdominal muscles, we would sit up by lifting and bending our head forward, chin tucked in, **at the same time** rounding our spine, bring our shoulders and arms forwards, hips flexing as our body moves over our legs. Depending on the strength of our abdominal muscles, our legs would either remain on the supporting surface throughout the movement, or be slightly bent, straightening just before we arrive in the sitting position (Figure 5.2a,b).

If you should be thinking that this is not what I do when I sit up, I suggest you try the following: **lie on your back and lift your head, wait a second, and then lift your arms. Now try and sit up.** I hope this proves the point!

Let us now look at the difficulties that confront the child with cerebral palsy. First, a child with severe spasticity and secondly a child with moderate spasticity.

Sitting up from the supine position

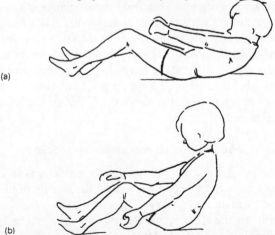

(a)

(b)

Figure 5.2 (a) A normal child sitting up from lying on the floor, raising her head forwards and at the same time bringing her arms and shoulders forward, hips and knees bent. (b) Stage two, sitting up from lying on the floor

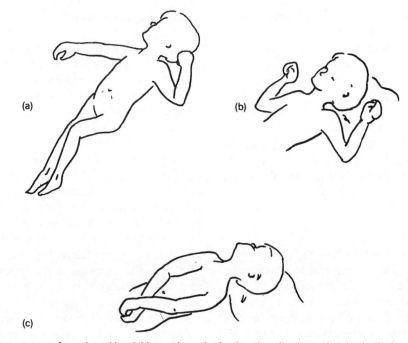

Figure 5.3   (a,b) A position often adopted by children with cerebral palsy when they lie on their back. The head, shoulders and arms pushing back make it difficult or nearly impossible to move in or away from this position. The position of the arms increases the **extension of the hips and legs**

(c) The head pushes back, the shoulders forward (protracted), internally rotated and extended – the adduction (drawing in to the middle of the body) and inward rotation of the arms increasing adduction and inward rotation of the legs

The child with severe spasticity

The child with severe spasticity is at his most vulnerable when lying on his back, as the pathological reflex activity and abnormal motor patterns present are at their strongest in this position. Lacking anti-gravity flexor tone and unable to make the necessary postural adjustments to get his body in alignment, the child is either unable or limited in his ability to sit up, i.e. to lift his head and trunk against gravity at the same time flexing his hips (Figure 5.3).

The child with moderate spasticity

Although the child with moderate spasticity is able to sit up, the way he does so and the quality of his performance may vary. These variations may be due to the developmental level he has reached, distribution of abnormal postural tone, and absence of postural reactions. And whether his arms are more involved than his legs or vice versa, or, in the case of some children, if their muscle tone increases on effort.

We will take as our example a child with a hemiplegia. The child's posture is asymmetrical and unstable, when lying on his back with all his weight taken on his **unaffected side,** so that the only way he can sit up is by pushing on the hand on that side. The effort involved in doing so increases the tone in both the arm and leg on the **affected** side (Figure 5.4).

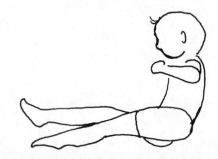

Figure 5.4   A child with a left-sided hemiplegia weight taken on the *unaffected* side. The effort involved increasing the tone in both the arm and leg on the *affected* side

Getting into sitting from the prone position

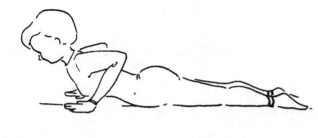 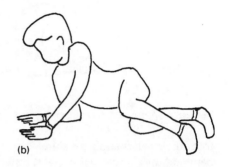

Figure 5.5   A *normal* sequence

Getting into sitting from the prone position

Starting from a symmetrical stable position, we lift our head extending our spine and hips as we bring our arms towards our body, pushing on our hands at the same time turning our body as we move into sitting, i.e. movement taking place between pelvic and shoulder girdles (Figure 5.5a,b).

The child with severe spasticity

Figure 5.6(a,b) illustrates a typical posture adopted by a young child in the prone position who because of his abnormal postural tone, asymmetrical unstable posture and lack of anti-gravity extensor tone is **unable to move in or away from this position**.

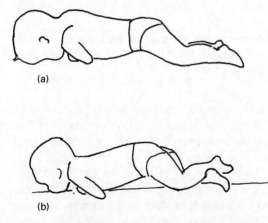

Figure 5.6   (a) An *abnormal* posture adopted by a child with severe spasticity in the prone position. (b) Attempts at extension resulting in hips flexing, weight forward, arms retracted

The child with moderate spasticity

The majority of these children are able to get from prone to sitting. We will take as our example a child with good head control whose legs are more affected than his arms, limbs on one side more affected than the other, i.e. a child with spastic diplegia. These children often present with asymmetry of flexion when lying in the prone position. One leg is more flexed than the other and the pelvis is raised on the side of the flexed leg, so that not only does the child lack stability/mobility at his pelvis but all his body weight is shifted to the one side. This will inevitably mean that any movement away from this position will be asymmetrical, and trunk rotation will not be possible or very limited. To overcome this problem, many children resort to pushing themselves back onto their knees, often ending up in a 'W' asymmetrical sitting posture with their bottom between their legs.

Rolling from supine to prone

The way we roll over can be influenced either by our muscle power, habit, whether we have a bad back or sustained an injury to some part of our body. Rolling, I have always found, is a movement where there seems to be endless variations. We all start from a symmetrical stable position and initiate the movement by lifting our head and shoulders off the support with varying degrees of trunk rotation, but here the similarity ends. Some people lead from their head and shoulders, others

Rolling from supine to prone

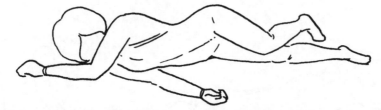

Figure 5.7   A *normal* sequence, movement taking place between pelvic and shoulder girdles i.e. rotation

from their pelvis and legs; some keep their top leg bent and their under-leg straight, others keep both legs straight. The position of our arms as we roll over will also vary. Figure 5.7 illustrates one of the ways in which the majority of adults roll over.

The child with moderate spasticity

The child with cerebral palsy also rolls in a number of different ways, but in his case the manner in which he rolls will again be dictated by how badly he is affected, his abnormal postural tone, his absence of postural reactions and it may even in some cases be modified because of the presence of contractures or deformities. Most children, because of a certain amount of asymmetry, will roll to a preferred side and rotation will be absent.

The child with moderate spasticity, i.e. spastic diplegia, usually initiates rolling by using a pattern of total flexion of his head, upper trunk and arms. This pattern of excessive flexion of the upper trunk often results in his under-arm becoming trapped beneath his body (Figure 5.8).

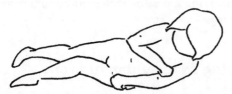

Figure 5.8   A child with a spastic diplegia – illustrates the effect on the pelvis and lower limbs when rolling is initiated with excessive flexion of the head, upper limbs and trunk

The child with fluctuating tone and involuntary movements

The child with fluctuating tone and involuntary movements initiates rolling from his hips and legs which increases the extension of his head and trunk, retraction of the shoulders and the outward rotation of his arms (Figure 5.9).

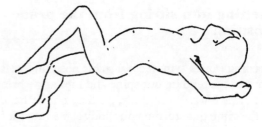

Figure 5.9   A child with fluctuating tone and involuntary movements – illustrates the increased extension of the head, upper limbs and trunk when the child initiates the movement from the pelvis and lower limbs

The child with low truncal tone

The child with low truncal tone will roll in a primitive manner, by using a pattern of total extension, a minimal amount of movement taking place between his shoulder and pelvis.

Movements possible but abnormally performed by the child with cerebral palsy

These are movements which if continually repeated will affect a child's ability to develop smooth, well-coordinated patterns of movement, and fine motor skills at a later stage. While obviously we need to do all we can to encourage a child with cerebral palsy to move independently, and the fact that he does so is a great achievement, we should try to avoid encouraging him to move in a way that in time may lead to contracture and deformity developing and may create a block to the acquisition of other skills and function.

Bridging and pushing himself backwards along the floor

At around 5 months a baby will often be seen practising a movement that we call '**bridging**'. Keeping his head on the support with his **chin tucked in, he shifts his weight back onto his shoulders**, bends his knees and by pushing his feet against the floor lifts and holds his bottom in the air. At times, he shifts his weight from one foot to the other. Later, using the same sequence of movement, he is able to push himself backwards along the floor (Figure 5.10).

Bridging and pushing himself backwards along the floor

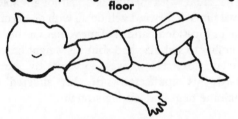

Figure 5.10   A *normal* sequence. Head on support. Chin tucked in, pelvis stable, weight taken on back, shoulders and feet

The child with severe spasticity

A child with severe spasticity because of his abnormally extended/adducted legs, lack of pelvic stability or mobility and his inability to isolate movements at his knees and feet is unable to either bridge or push himself backwards. He will however sometimes try to, and does so by pushing against a solid object, for example a wall or the end of his bath. This should **not** be encouraged, as not only does it increase abnormal extensor tone, but also blocks the development of pelvic and hip mobility (Figure 5.11a).

The child with moderate spasticity

A child with mild or moderate spasticity, associated with the hemiplegic or diplegic type of cerebral palsy, will have sufficient abdominal, trunk/pelvic control to manage a semi 'bridge'. This means that as they push themselves backwards, they do so asymmetrically. This should not be encouraged, as it will only reinforce an asymmetrical method of weight-bearing.

The child with fluctuating tone and involuntary movements

The child with fluctuating tone and involuntary movements lies on his back with his head extended, chin up and shoulders retracted. His hips and legs are flexed, abducted and outwardly rotated (Figure 5.11b) – a position that makes it impossible for him to actively extend and bridge. Because it is difficult for him to take weight on his arms and creep, pushing himself backwards is a form of locomotion he will often choose. Lacking extension and stability at his hips, as he pushes his feet against the floor he reinforces the extension of his head, trunk and the retraction of his arms. It is therefore important to encourage other means of locomotion with these children.

Creeping

Once a baby has sufficient head control, trunk extension and stability at his shoulder and pelvic

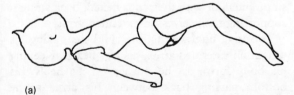

(a)

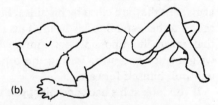

(b)

Figure 5.11   (a) A child with *severe spasticity*. Excessive extension is increased as he pushes himself backwards with his toes.
(b) *A child with fluctuating tone and involuntary movements*. (Head extended, 'chin up', shoulders retracted, no pelvic stability, pushes himself asymmetrically

Creeping

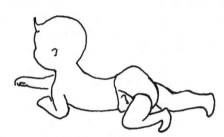

Figure 5.12   A *normal* creeping pattern

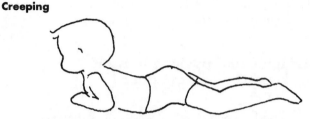

Figure 5.13   *A child with moderate spasticity.* His abnormal posture prevents the child from taking weight on his forearms or shifting his weight to enable him to move forwards

girdles to shift his weight from side to side in the prone position, he will often propel himself by **creeping** on his tummy. He does this by shifting his weight onto his chest (upper trunk) and forearm as he reaches forward with the other hand to pull himself forward. At the same time, he shifts his weight in the lower part of his body (lower trunk), his pelvis rotating on the opposite side, so that he can flex his leg and push himself forward. In this way, a diagonal movement takes place between his shoulder and pelvic girdles with trunk rotation (Figure 5.12).

The child with moderate spasticity

This group of children, although they are able to propel themselves forward, cannot do so by creeping, as described above. To understand the reasons for this, let us first look at the method of moving used by the child whose arms are less affected than his legs, i.e. a spastic diplegia, then with a child whose arm and leg are involved on one side only, i.e. a spastic hemiplegia.

If you look at the illustration in Figure 5.13, you will see that although the child can lift his head up, his neck is hyperextended and his chin is in the air, jaw pushed forward. He props himself on his arms, but they are close by his sides, his shoulders raised to help stabilize his head. This is a position that makes it impossible for him to transfer his weight onto one arm, freeing the other to reach and pull himself forward.

If you look at his back and hips, you will see that they are excessively extended, and adducted, his feet plantar flexed, pelvis tilted posteriorly. Lacking mobility at his hips, trunk and pelvis, disasso-

ciated movements at his hips cannot take place. Therefore, the only way he can move forward is by lifting and pulling both arms towards himself, his legs remaining straight. The effort of using his arms in this way increases the extension of his hips and legs.

The child with hemiplegia, although able to propel himself forward will do so with an asymmetrical or lop-sided pattern of movement as he lacks the ability to stabilize and shift his weight onto the affected side. He moves forward by turning towards his unaffected side, his affected arm remaining bent and his leg straight.

The child with fluctuating tone and involuntary movements

Although these children are able to extend against gravity, because their head control and trunk and pelvic stability are inadequate they dislike lying in the prone position. Unable to propel themselves forward, they resort to rolling or pushing themselves along on their backs as previously described (see Figure 5.11b).

Moving backwards and forwards in a sitting position is an effective means of locomotion for some of these children once they have learned to sit on the floor with their hips flexed, back straight supporting themselves on extended arms.

To move backwards, the child sits, taking his weight on extended arms, his legs flexed. Keeping his body forwards, he pushes on his heels, his bottom passing back between his arms as he straightens then bends his legs. **To move forwards**, the child sits, taking weight on extended arms keeping his trunk forwards. As his bottom

Moving in a sitting position

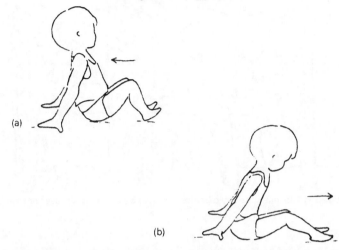

(a)

(b)

Figure 5.14   (a) *Pushing backwards*. Weight taken on extended arms, pushing with his heels as he pushes his bottom back and straightens his legs. (b) *Pushing forwards*. Weight taken on extended arms, moving his trunk forwards, with bent legs pushing his bottom forward as he straightens his legs

passes between his arms, he bends then straightens his legs (Figure 5.14a,b).

As soon as a child has good sitting balance he should be encouraged to get off the floor and use any form of mobility that provides him with a stable symmetrical sitting base (see Chapter 21 on aids to mobility).

'Bunny-hopping'

When playing on the floor many children prefer to **'bunny-hop'** from time to time, but unlike the child with cerebral palsy it will be one of many ways they have of moving around. They do so by tucking both legs under their bottom and often play sitting in this position.

The child with spasticity, on the other hand, sits and moves forward with his bottom **between** his legs which are **flexed and turned in at the hips (internally rotated)**, usually taking weight more on one leg than the other. This increases the spasticity of the muscles that flex the hip and knees and also the possibility of deformities developing in the feet. Moving in this way will also impede the development of balance reactions in sitting and the child's ability to move in and away from the sitting position.

The child with **fluctuating tone** and involuntary movements also sits with his bottom between his legs when 'bunny-hopping'. Lacking trunk and hip stability, he 'bunny-hops' by taking weight forward on his arms and extending his head, drawing both legs together towards his arms.

Standing, cruising and walking

Standing

There is considerable variation regarding the age at which a baby first pulls himself up to **stand**, cruise and walk, a number of babies preferring to 'bottom shuffle' or crawl, then one day just get on their feet, and a few days later walk.

It is important to note, that a baby pulls to stand before he has perfected his balance in sitting; cruises before he has perfected his balance in standing; walks before he has perfected his balance in standing. When the baby first pulls himself up to stand, he relies on his hands to stabilize himself to compensate for his lack of stability and control in trunk and pelvis. Activity in his lower limbs at this time is confined to bending and straightening his legs. Gradually, as he gains

Standing

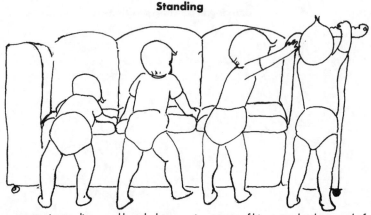

Figure 5.15   Illustrates **arm support** in standing, used by a baby at *various stages* of his *motor* development *before* he achieves standing balance

more control, he experiments with different methods of getting to standing, finally managing to do so through kneeling and later half-kneeling.

His method of **supporting himself** when standing also goes in stages. To begin with he takes his weight on his forearms, then on extended arms, and finally on one arm only (Figure 5.15).

Figure 5.16 illustrates the posture a baby adopts when he first starts to stand independently. To overcome his lack of trunk and pelvic stability and immature balance reactions in the upright position, the baby stands:

- legs wide apart, hips and knees bent
- pelvis tilted forwards (anteriorly) with a marked lordosis (hollow back)
- feet apt to splay outwards, with weight taken on the inner borders of the feet
- arms flexed and abducted.

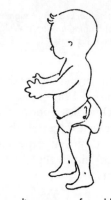

Figure 5.16   The standing posture of a toddler. Because his pelvis is unstable, he stands on a wide base. His lower spine is extended (lordosis) his pelvis tilted forwards (anteriorly), hips and knees slightly bent. He stabilizes his upper trunk by either having his arms in the position illustrated, or in a position of 'high guard', i.e. arms bent and held away from the body

Cruising

A baby first moves in an upright position by **cruising**, facing the direction in which he is going, only moving sideways as he becomes more adept at transferring his weight sideways from one leg to the other. As he becomes more adventurous, he cruises from one area to another, at times letting go, at first just 'plopping down' on his bottom, gradually learning to lower himself into a squatting position. At this stage he is able

to move at speed while cruising, but loses this ability when he starts walking forwards.

Walking

When a baby takes his first **walking** steps, he holds his arms abducted and flexed in a position we describe as **'high guard'**. Holding his arms in this position helps him to stabilize his trunk and enables him to have more mobility at his hips. He walks using excessive movements of his trunk, with a 'waddling' gait, one which always reminds me of the way a sailor walks when he first comes ashore after a long period at sea.

The child with cerebral palsy

Regardless of the severity of a child's handicap, **early weight-bearing should start as soon as possible**, even if the child has to be placed in the standing position. Whether some form of standing

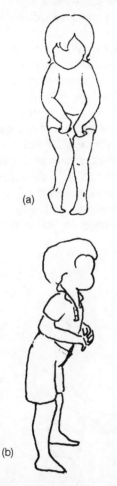

(a)

(b)

system is needed will, of course, vary according to the age of the child, as well as the severity and distribution of abnormal postural tone. The presence of early contractures and/or deformities will also be a factor.

The child with moderate spasticity

The postural abnormalities seen in both standing and walking of children with moderate spasticity are due to the adjustment that they have to make in their trunk and limbs to enable them to maintain their centre of gravity, i.e. to compensate for their lack of balance in the upright position.

Figure 5.17(a) illustrates one of the standing postures of a young child whose legs are more involved than the arms (spastic diplegia). Her posture is one of flexion, the child having to extend her neck, chin poked forward and up in an attempt to compensate for the lack of extension in her trunk, hips and knees. This is a posture that she adopts to stop herself falling forwards. The pelvis is tilted backwards (posteriorly), legs turned in at the hips (internally rotated) which are drawn together (adducted) and the weight taken on the inner borders of the feet (a valgus position).

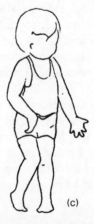

(c)

Figure 5.17   Two standing postures of a child with a spastic diplegia. In (a), the tight muscles that extend the child's hips pull the pelvis back (posteriorly), rounding the lower part of her spine. These children are usually able to take weight on one leg as illustrated, with the other leg turned in (internally rotated) at the hip and the foot plantar flexed. To compensate for lack of stability she juts her chin forward which rounds the upper part of her spine, her shoulders and lower arms slightly bent. In (b), because his legs are less affected, the child is able to keep his feet flat on the floor by flexing his hips, his legs hyperextended. He compensates in a similar way to prevent himself falling forwards.

(c) The posture of the child with a spastic hemiplegia when standing is asymmetrical, his weight taken on his unaffected leg. His affected arm is flexed and turned in at the shoulder which presses down, his trunk flexed on this side. His head may also be pulled over to this side. His leg is extended, turned in at the hip, his pelvis pulled up and back. The foot is plantar flexed, his ankle extended so that he takes weight on his toes and the ball of his foot

Often an attempt is made to help these children 'walk' by holding them under their armpits or by their hands while their arms remain flexed. Lacking balance and sufficient extensor tone against gravity, all they can do is fall forwards from one leg to the other, their weight falling more and more onto their toes. This results in the legs becoming stiffer and often crossing.

One might possibly be encouraged by the thought that in this way the child is beginning to walk. Unfortunately this is a false hope, as the abnormal pattern of movement involved in this so-called 'walking' will simply increase the difficulties of the child in his efforts to stand, and later walk.

Figure 5.17(b) illustrates a standing posture often adopted by those children whose arms show little involvement, who flex at their hips with hyperextended knees, pelvis tilted anteriorly. To overcome the flexion at their hips they extend their lower spine (lumbar lordosis).

Figure 5.17(c) illustrates the standing posture of a child where one side of the body is involved (spastic hemiplegia). The child's posture is asymmetrical, with all his weight being taken on the unaffected leg which he places in front. His pelvis on the affected side is pulled up and back, the leg turned in at the hip and extended, with the foot in an equinus position (turned in). His shoulder is pulled back, the arm flexed and forearm pronated wrist flexed. This pattern of his arm often becomes more pronounced when the child walks quickly or runs.

According to the severity of the spasticity present, he will take a step either by flexing his hip and hyperextending his knee to get his foot on the ground, or take his leg out to the side (abduct) and swing his leg forward, often with his toes contacting the ground first, with the foot turned in.

The child with fluctuating tone and involuntary movements

A child with fluctuating tone lacks postural control and stability, and therefore has difficulty in maintaining an upright posture. As his balance reactions are exaggerated, he is unable to shift his body weight from side to side or forwards.

When placed on his feet he has a tendency either to go into total extension and fall backwards, or total flexion and collapse. If one leg is lifted, the weight-bearing leg often flexes involuntarily and he falls. However, once he learns to extend both arms forward and maintain a sustained grasp he is able to have sufficient postural control to stabilize and flex his hips, which enables him to shift his weight both sideways and forward. Figure 5.18 illustrates one of the ways a child does this, by extending both arms forward and clasping his hands together.

If you turn back to Table 5.1, you will see automatic walking listed as a reaction present at birth. Possibly a more descriptive term would be 'high-stepping', for when the sole of one foot touches something solid one leg bends and the other extends, giving the appearance of walking.

If you 'walk' a young child with fluctuating tone and involuntary movements, their pattern of walking is very similar to this 'high-stepping' gait. We would therefore strongly advise you **not** to practise this type of walking, as it will delay the child developing the ability to stand with his weight

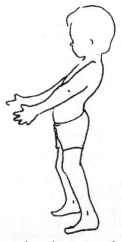

Figure 5.18 A typical standing posture of a child with involuntary movements and intermittent spasms. To compensate for his lack of postural control and lack of stability he often 'fixes' himself by clasping his hands together, 'gripping' with his toes to prevent himself falling backwards

evenly distributed on both feet, and later to shift his weight from one foot to the other – a prerequisite of future walking.

The child who has fairly good arms and can maintain a sustained grasp will be able to stand and 'walk independently' **if** he has some form of walking aid. It is important to remember that all a walking aid does is to compensate for lack of balance, it does **not** alter the child's underlying gait problem or enable him to walk normally. Those children with minimal involvement will, of course, be able to walk independently.

Normal sensorimotor development – the early stages

Since we emphasize, throughout the book, the importance of head control, symmetry, stability and sensory input during the early years when handling a baby and young child with cerebral palsy, I thought it might be helpful if we discussed briefly with the help of illustrations how this sensorimotor learning develops with a baby who has **normal postural tone and normal postural reactions**.

The stages chosen are approximately 4 and 6 months in the supine, prone and sitting positions. The reader should remember that within 'normal' is a naturally occurring wide spectrum of achievement, as no baby develops in accordance with a strictly stereotyped course. For further discussion on the early normal sensorimotor development, see Appendix II.

Sensorimotor development at 4 months (head control and mid-line orientation)

Postural control

Symmetry – keeps head, trunk, pelvis in alignment.

Postural stability – weight evenly distributed throughout body, i.e. head, trunk, pelvis.

Weight shift – starts to transfer weight to the side (laterally) in the trunk, enabling limbs to move independently of the trunk. Ability to move upper limbs in advance of lower limbs.

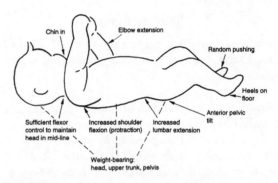

Figure 5.19

Muscle control

The increased control of the flexor muscles beginning to balance the strong anti-gravity extensor muscles. The baby also practises extension against gravity in prone. (Fig. 5.22)

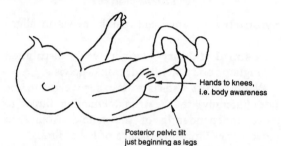

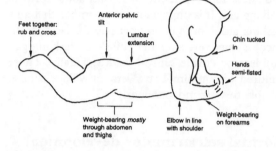

Figure 5.20

Posterior pelvic tilt just beginning as legs come closer together – done mainly with the pelvis on the support

Hands to knees, i.e. body awareness

Figure 5.21

Feet together: rub and cross

Anterior pelvic tilt

Lumbar extension

Chin tucked in

Hands semi-fisted

Weight-bearing *mostly* through abdomen and thighs

Elbow in line with shoulder

Weight-bearing on forearms

Sensory input

Head in mid-line chine tucked in – facilitates visual and auditory communication and social interaction.

Hands together in mid-line – provides further visual, tactile cues and information regarding the position of arms and hands in space.

Moving arms **independently** of the trunk – plus the ability to flex and extend the elbows – increases body awareness and exploration begins.

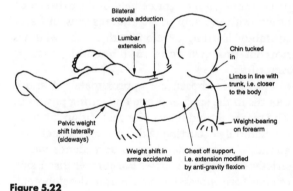

Figure 5.22

Bilateral scapula adduction

Lumbar extension

Chin tucked in

Limbs in line with trunk, i.e. closer to the body

Pelvic weight shift laterally (sideways)

Weight shift in arms accidental

Weight-bearing on forearm

Chest off support, i.e. extension modified by anti-gravity flexion

Gross patterns of movement

Provide additional sensory input through touch and pressure from skin, joints and muscles.

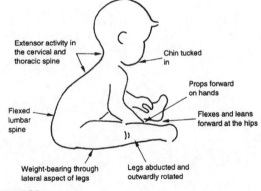

Extensor activity in the cervical and thoracic spine

Chin tucked in

Props forward on hands

Flexed lumbar spine

Flexes and leans forward at the hips

Weight-bearing through lateral aspect of legs

Legs abducted and outwardly rotated

In Sitting

The only balance between the flexor and extensor muscles in sitting at this stage are seen in the head, neck and upper spine. The supporting base is wide, the baby propping himself on his hands.

Figure 5.23

Sensorimotor development at 6 months (balance between flexor/extensor activity)

Postural control

Symmetry – able to readjust position if he gets out of alignment. Good head control against gravity in all positions.

Postural stability – in supine and prone takes weight evenly through head and shoulder and pelvic girdles or through trunk only.

Increased shoulder control so that weight-bearing on extended arms and protective extension now possible.

Good stability/mobility in the lumbar/pelvic region.

Weight shift – shifts weight anteriorly.

Posteriorly and laterally (sideways).

Muscle control

Good balance between flexor and extensor muscles. In supine and prone.

Sensory input

In both supine **and** prone, starts to integrate the sensory learning of previous months with purposeful movements.

Gross patterns of movement

In prone – extension predominates. Pushes back on extended arms, but when transferring weight onto one arm still weight-bears on a flexed arm for stability.

Equilibrium reactions starting in **supine**.

Rolls supine to prone and vice versa.

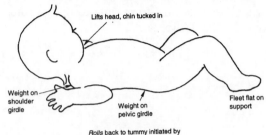

Lifts head, chin tucked in

Weight on shoulder girdle

Weight on pelvic girdle

Fleet flat on support

Rolls back to tummy initiated by flexed head or lower extremities

Figure 5.24

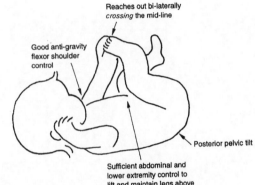

Reaches out bi-laterally *crossing* the mid-line

Good anti-gravity flexor shoulder control

Posterior pelvic tilt

Sufficient abdominal and lower extremity control to lift and maintain legs above body. Can do this also with straight legs

Figure 5.25

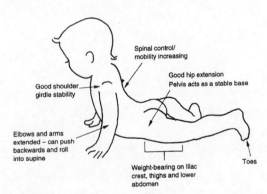

Spinal control/ mobility increasing

Good hip extension Pelvis acts as a stable base

Good shoulder girdle stability

Elbows and arms extended – can push backwards and roll into supine

Weight-bearing on Iliac crest, thighs and lower abdomen

Toes

Figure 5.26

In sitting – reaches forward to grasp and manipulate toys, rotates (turns trunk), but falls sideways and backwards if he moves out of his base.

Still rests with his hands on his knees or supports himself forward from time to time, protective extension forwards.

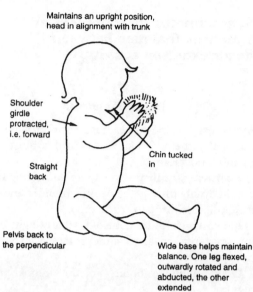

Maintains an upright position, head in alignment with trunk

Shoulder girdle protracted, i.e. forward

Chin tucked in

Straight back

Pelvis back to the perpendicular

Wide base helps maintain balance. One leg flexed, outwardly rotated and abducted, the other extended

Figure 5.27

Chapter 6

Basic principles of handling

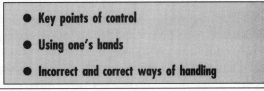

- Key points of control
- Using one's hands
- Incorrect and correct ways of handling

As discussed in Chapter 5, the child with cerebral palsy's abnormally coordinated patterns of posture and movement has his freedom and choice of purposeful skilled movements restricted. Due to the presence of **abnormal postural tone**, his movements are initiated from an **asymmetrical, unstable posture** disturbing the **alignment** of his head, neck and trunk, resulting in uneven weight distribution. Depending on the type and severity of the child's abnormal postural tone, the development of **automatic postural reactions**, such as balance, may be absent, delayed or exaggerated. Our aim, therefore, when handling the child is to stop any unwanted activity and establish more normal postural tone **at the same time** as we **facilitate** more normal postural reactions and guided voluntary movements, leading to active participation by the child himself.

We do this from '**key points of control**' which are mainly proximal. These are parts of the body where both normal and abnormal motor activity originates, i.e. the head, neck and spine. Other parts of the body are also used, such as the shoulder and pelvic girdles. Although similar 'key points of control' are used with the majority of children, handling techniques will vary.

How we handle a child at these 'key points of control' will be based on an assessment of postural tone, postural and movement patterns and functional abilities in relation to age.

If hypertonus, i.e. spasticity, is the underlying problem, we would **inhibit** abnormal reactions from the appropriate 'key points of control', help-ing the child adjust to changes in posture while **at the same time** facilitating more normal patterns of movement and automatic postural reactions.

If postural tone is low, or intermittent spasms and involuntary movements are present, we would give pressure at the appropriate 'key points of control', giving the child a point of stability (fixation), enabling him to maintain his posture against gravity and to organize, grade and improve the quality of his movements.

Using our hands

An important factor when handling the child with cerebral palsy, especially in the early years, is the ability to use our hands effectively and economically so that we become sensitive to the varying changes of tone under our hands.

To help you appreciate the differences in the 'feeling' and reactions to your handling of, for example, moving a limb that offers no resistance and one that does, try the following. Take a friend's arm and move it in different directions, then take away your support. You will find that the arm **feels light** as you move it and that there is **no resistance**. When you take away your support there is a momentary pause before their arm falls to their side. This happens because, even though you moved their arm passively, they were able to **follow** the movement **actively**, by controlling and making adjustments in their posture quickly and automatically to the movement.

Now move the arm of a child who has increased tone, i.e. spasticity, in the same way. You will find that his arm **feels heavy** and presses down against your hand, and as you move it there is **resistance**. When you take away your support, his arm immediately drops pressing against his side. The resistance offered by the child who has intermittent spasms and involuntary movements when his arm is moved will differ in that, while there will be an **initial resistance**, the arm then will suddenly 'give'. When you remove your support his arm will 'fly away' before dropping to his side.

A measure of a child's spasticity shows itself in resistance to both passive and active movements. For example, when trying to bring his arms forward in an attempt to sit him up, the degree of resistance that you feel will enable you to judge the difficulties with which the child is faced, and whether or not the movement is completely beyond his power. In other words, you will know how much cooperation you can really ask for and how much of the movement he can be expected to do on his own.

When handling a child we need **to take away our support as soon as possible**. Remember that when **you** are holding and moving your child, that **you** are doing the movement. The aim is to encourage the child to move actively without help and he can only do so if you take away your hand at the right moment and encourage him to move by himself. The importance of speed in handling and the gradual 'taking over' of a movement by the child himself will be taught to you by your therapist.

Learning to feel confident when using specific techniques of handling takes time. I would therefore strongly advise you to spend part of each therapy session handling your child under the supervision of his therapist. It is **not possible** to learn to use your hands **by just watching**.

There will obviously be some children who concentrate better when their parents are out of the room, but even so, whenever possible do spend at least part of each session in the room with your child and his therapist.

Figures 6.1 to 6.19 illustrate some correct and incorrect techniques of handling.

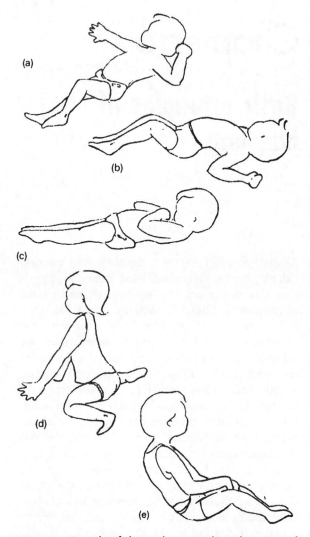

Figure 6.1 Examples of abnormal postures, due to the position of the head, which affect the whole body. These postures will result in abnormal patterns of movement, preventing the normal development of righting and balance reactions.

Note: These postures will be more permanent in the *spastic* child, intermittent in the *athetoid* child, and seen on the affected side only in the *hemiplegic* child.

(a) The child turns his head, which may also be bent to the side, and in the very severe child pulled back. The arm and leg towards which the face is turned are straight, the hand open; the arm and leg away from which the head is turned are bent and the hand is fisted. This pattern is seen most clearly when the child lies on his back or stands and is often present, but modified, when lying on his tummy or in sitting.

(b) The head and shoulders are pulled back and the back arches. The *athetoid* child's legs may remain bent, the *spastic* child's legs will be straight and stiff. If the child is as severely affected as shown here, he may even show the same pattern when he lies on his tummy.

(c) The head is pulled forward, the arms are bent and are pulled over the chest, the hips and legs stiffen. If the child shows this pattern while lying on his back, it will be even more accentuated when he lies on his tummy.

(d) Lifting the head up and back, as illustrated, results in the arms stiffly extending and the hips, legs and ankles bending. Sometimes, as shown in the sketch, the child will sit between his legs.

(e) Bending of the head has the opposite effect, i.e. the arms bend and the hips and knees extend. This pattern can also be seen when the child sits

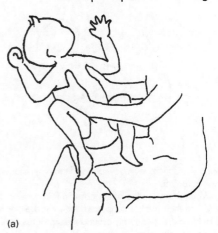

(a)

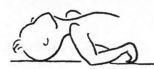

(a)

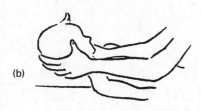

(b)

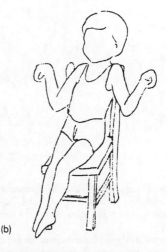

(b)

Figure 6.2 (a) Some children with cerebral palsy push their head back and at the same time bring their shoulders up and forward. Do not try to correct the position of the head by putting a hand on the back of the head, as this will only cause the child to push back more.

(b) Place your hands on each side of the head and push upwards giving the child a 'long neck'. As you do this, push the shoulders down with the forearms.

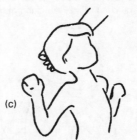

(c)

Figure 6.3 (a,b) When a young baby is held without adequate control, he continually pushes back when sitting as illustrated – although at this stage his legs are flexed and apart (a primitive pattern). If he continues to do this, in time his hips and legs will extend and become stiff, as in (b).

(c) Never try to stop a child pushing his head back by putting your hand on the back of his head, as this will only increase the abnormal extensor tone, as shown in this sketch.

(d) Both the neck and shoulder retraction can be inhibited by controlling the child as illustrated, which will facilitate head flexion and the bringing forward of the arms towards the mid-line

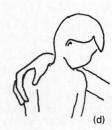

(d)

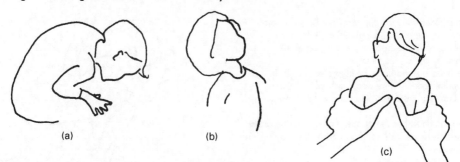

Figure 6.4 Children with low postural tone (hypotonia), because they lack stability at both shoulder and pelvic girdles, have poor head and trunk control.
(a) When placed in the sitting position they tend to 'flop' forwards at their hips.
(b) When their trunk is supported, their head either falls back or forwards onto their chest.
(c) Holding the child firmly around the top of his arms, and pulling his shoulders down and forwards, will stabilize his shoulder girdle and help the child keep his head up in mid-line with his chin tucked in

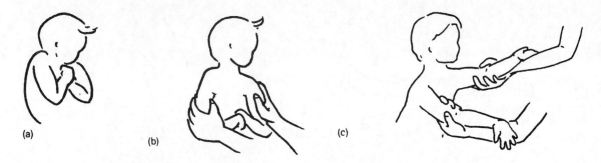

Figure 6.5 These sketches show how by careful control you can correct the position of the child's arms and at the same time **influence** the position of the rest of his body. The child in each of the sketches is sitting.
(a) A typical pattern of flexion seen in the *spastic* child. The arms are turned in at the shoulders: this is generally accompanied by straight hips.
(b) Hold the child over the outside of elbows and top of the arms.
(c) With one movement, lift and turn his arms out as you bring him towards you.
By handling him in this way, you can facilitate the lifting of his head, straightening of his spine and the bending of his hips

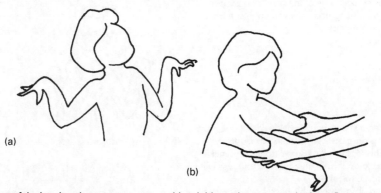

Figure 6.6 (a) A posture of the head and arms seen in some older children when sitting, who have fluctuating tone and intermittent spasms (athetoid type of cerebral palsy). The arms are flexed, shoulders hunched and turned out. The legs either flexed and turned out at the hips, or extended and turned in at the hips.
(b) With one movement, turn the shoulders in and down, extending the child's arms as you bring him forwards towards you. Handling in this way will facilitate the head coming forwards with an extended spine and flexed hips

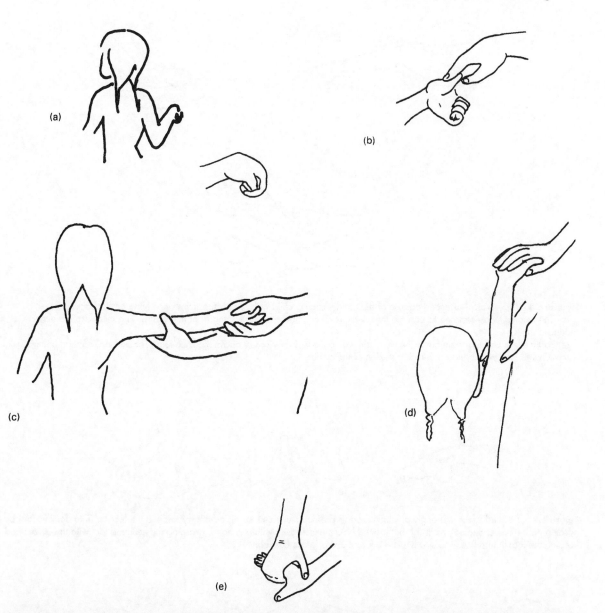

Figure 6.7   (a) An arm posture seen in some children with a spastic hemiplegia. The arm is flexed and turned in at the shoulder (which presses down). The forearm is turned in (pronated) so that the hand faces down, with wrist and fingers flexed and thumb across the palm (inset illustration).

(b) The **incorrect** way to extend the wrist and fingers. Pulling on the thumbs as illustrated increases the flexion of the wrist and fingers and there is also the danger that one might damage the thumb joints.

(c) The **correct** way to extend the arm, wrist and fingers. Turning the arm out at the shoulder, elbow straight with the forearm and palm facing up, facilitates the extension of the wrist and fingers, making it easier to keep the thumb away from the palm.

(d) The elevation of the arm in outward rotation inhibits the flexor spasticity and downward pressure of the arm and shoulder girdle. The abduction of the thumb with the arm in supination and outward rotation, and extension of the arm and waist, facilitate the opening of all the fingers.

(e) A good grasp to use when encouraging a child to support herself is an open hand with an extended arm

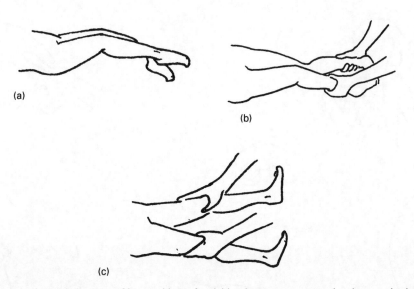

(a)

(b)

(c)

Figures 6.8 (a) A typical extended posture of hips and legs of a child with severe spasticity when lying on his back.

(b) The incorrect way of trying to part the legs, which will only increase the turning in of the legs, pulling them close together (adduction).

(c) Part the legs and turn them out at the hips, controlling the legs over or just above the knee joint. The outward rotation of the legs in extension will facilitate abduction and dorsiflexion of the ankles

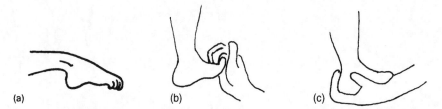

(a)　　　　　　　(b)　　　　　　　(c)

Figure 6.9 If a child's foot is strongly plantar flexed, a position illustrated in (a), do not try to bend the foot up (into dorsiflexion) by pushing on the ball of the foot, as in (b), but instead hold the knee bent with one hand, grasping the heel and foot with the other hand, keeping the foot in mid-line, and slowly bend the foot up as far as possible

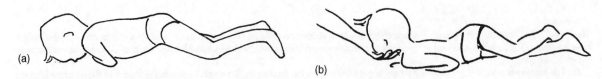

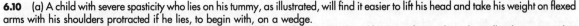

(a)

(b)

6.10 (a) A child with severe spasticity who lies on his tummy, as illustrated, will find it easier to lift his head and take his weight on flexed arms with his shoulders protracted if he lies, to begin with, on a wedge.

(b) When placing him on the wedge, do not lift his head first and then try to bring his arms forward, as this will only increase the pulling down and flexion of his arms and hips and the extension of his legs

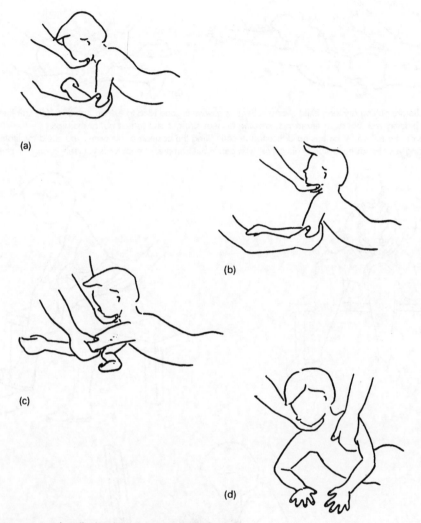

(a)

(b)

(c)

(d)

Figure 6.11   The correct way to handle the child illustrated in Figure 6.10.
(a) At the same time as you lift the head, start to bring the arm forward.
(b) Turn the shoulders out as you lift and straighten the arm – your point of control is over the elbow.
(c) Hold the head up, keeping the arm extended (off the support) until it no longer feels heavy and presses down at the shoulder. Place the arm on the support. Follow the same procedure with the other arm – do not let the head flex. Raising the child's head as you extend his arm will facilitate the extension of the spine, hips and legs.
(d) Lifting the shoulder up and over while at the same time rotating the trunk may be sufficient to facilitate bringing the arm forward with a child who has moderate spasticity.
Note: Other techniques of extending the more severely involved child before putting him in the prone position will be shown to you by your therapist

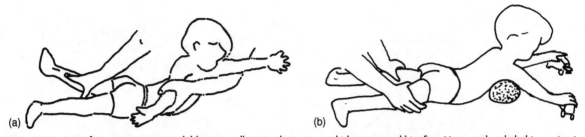

Figure 6.12 (a) Before putting a young child over a roller it is always a good idea to extend him first. You can then help him maintain this extension by placing your hands as illustrated, keeping his legs straight and turned out at the hips.

(b) When he is on the roll and if he has no difficulties in controlling the position of his arms, you could facilitate trunk and head extension by placing your hands each side of his pelvis, with gentle but firm pressure towards yourself, giving the child a point of fixation (stability)

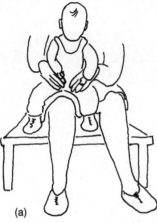

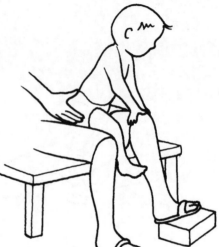

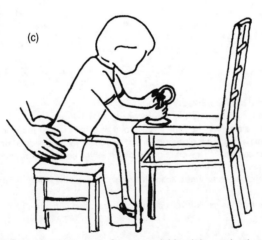

Figure 6.13 (a–c) These sketches illustrate various ways of giving a child stability so that he can keep his head in mid-line and trunk extended when learning to take his weight on open hands, or using his hands for play. When placing your hands on the child's pelvis, see that it is in a neutral slightly forward position, applying pressure downwards.

Note: Do not apply pressure with your thumb in the lower part of the child's back (lumbar region) to tilt the pelvis forward

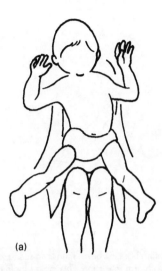
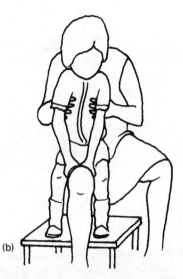

(a)

(b)

Figure 6.14   (a) Too wide a sitting base, as illustrated here, can increase the extension and inward rotation at the hips and legs of a child who pushes back when sitting – affecting his whole posture, although his arms are more affected than his legs.

(b) A narrower sitting base keeps the hips outwardly rotated, with hips and legs flexed. The arms and head are controlled at the shoulders which are lifted and turned in with slight pressure on the chest. The inward rotation at the shoulders with pronation of the elbows inhibits the retraction and outward rotation of the arms. Weight-bearing should be encouraged, with the arms extended

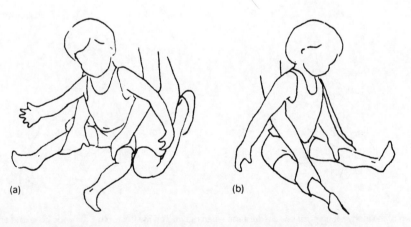

(a)

(b)

Figure 6.15   (a) When placing a child with moderate spasticity on the floor in long sitting, never sit him on the floor, and *then* try to bend his hips. Pull him towards you 'by the seat of his pants', so that the weight of his trunk is over his sitting base, keeping his legs turned out and apart as illustrated.

(b) Once a child learns to sit forward by himself, keeping his legs straight, encourage him to support himself first forwards, and then sideways.

Note: We would not recommend long sitting for a child who can only sit in this position by taking his weight on his sacrum, i.e. pelvis tilted backwards with a round back. These children are more secure sitting on a chair with their feet supported

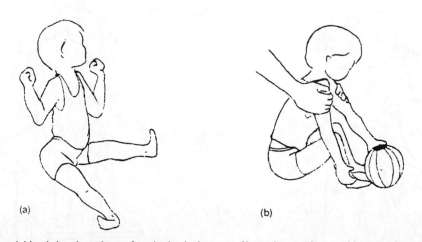

(a)

(b)

Figure 6.16 (a) A child with the athetoid type of cerebral palsy because of his wide sitting base is able to sit in long sitting, but often does so with excessive flexion at his hips, compensating by extending his head and trunk with arm retraction. This makes it difficult for him to move over his sitting base, to support himself or reach forward to use his hands.

(b) The child sits with his legs flexed and together, arms forward, with firm pressure over his shoulders which are protracted. He can then be encouraged to maintain a sustained grasp, in this instance using a ball. A good way to get a child to hold this position by himself is by getting him to hold his legs together by wrapping his arms around them

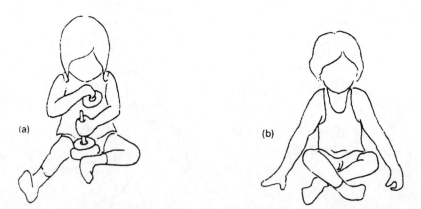

(a)

(b)

Figure 6.17 (a,b) Two of the many sitting positions children use when playing on the floor. Note the wide base and erect spine. Although cross-legged sitting is suggested for a number of young children with cerebral palsy, I think it is important to bear in mind that it is an asymmetrical position, i.e. more weight is taken on the under-leg, with weight on the outside of the feet – a position of the feet that a number of children have a tendency to develop later

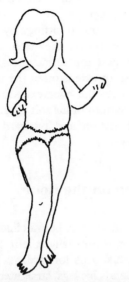

Figure 6.18 A typical standing posture of a child with moderate spasticity – hips and knees are flexed, with a flat lower back (lumbar spine) and the pelvis tilted back (posteriorly). Her standing base is small, with weight taken on the inner side of her feet making it impossible for her to take weight evenly on both feet, or to transfer her weight sideways onto one foot to take a step

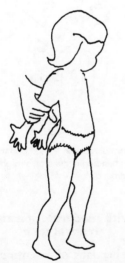

Figure 6.19 This shows one of the ways of facilitating in standing: hip and trunk extension, even weight distribution and weight shift from one foot to the other. The child's arms are extended diagonally backwards, i.e. outward rotation at the shoulders which are pushed up and forwards. Care must be taken to see that the child's weight is taken forward over the standing base

Ways of handling not recommended and the reasons why

It should be recognized that as we handle the child there is as much positive therapy in the avoidance of some movements as there is in the performance of others, provided that the reasons for avoiding them are clearly understood.

The following examples illustrate how by **our handling** of the child we can inadvertently increase postural tone, intermittent spasms and involuntary movements.

Pulling the baby up to sitting from lying on his back

The baby in Figure 6.20 is symmetrical: his head is in alignment with his trunk, his pelvis stable, hips and legs flexed and outwardly rotated. He has sufficient control of his flexor muscles to lift his head off the support and with help to assist in pulling himself up to a sitting position. A little later he will be able to come to sitting, keeping both legs extended on the support.

Pulled to sitting

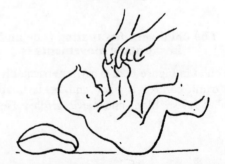

Figure 6.20 With sufficient control over his flexor muscles to overcome gravity the baby is able to assist with the movement

The child with moderate spasticity

The child in Figure 6.21, on the other hand, is slightly asymmetrical: her pelvis is unstable and the weight is taken over to one side. Although she has some head control, she does not have sufficient control of her flexor muscles to overcome

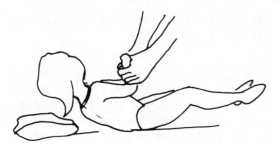

Figure 6.21   The child with moderate spasticity

the pull of gravity, and therefore, even with help, is limited in the amount of movement she can manage on her own.

Her mother, by encouraging her child to grasp her hands while her arms are flexed, has increased the flexor spasticity in her arms so that the child has to lift her shoulders to stabilize her head, at the same time rounding the upper part of her spine. By doing this, she reinforces the hyperextension in the baby's neck, making it impossible for her to flex her head forward with her chin tucked in.

This pattern of flexion of the upper part of the body also reinforces the pattern of extension, adduction and internal rotation at the hips and legs.

The child with fluctuating tone and involuntary movements

The child in Figure 6.22 is asymmetrical, his head and trunk control is poor and he is unable to stabilize his shoulder and pelvic girdles. He can-

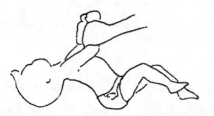

Figure 6.22   The child with fluctuating tone and involuntary movements. Pulling a child to sit who lacks shoulder and pelvic stability and has no sustained grasp increases head and trunk extension in the lumbar region and flexion of the hips and lower limbs

not reach forward with extended arms or maintain a sustained grasp.

Pulling him up to sitting, by holding him as illustrated, increases the extension of his neck and trunk, and the retraction of the shoulders. This pattern of extension of the upper part of his body reinforces the hyperextension of his lumbar spine (the bottom of his spine), and the pattern of flexion, abduction and outward rotation at the hips and legs.

Bouncing on the floor

Figure 6.23 illustrates how a child, when bounced on the floor, is normally able to keep his head in alignment, his arms forward. As he is lifted into the air he bends his legs, straightening them a little just before his feet touch the ground. Eventually, as he grows older, his legs will straighten in the air and his feet will be in a position to take weight.

Bouncing

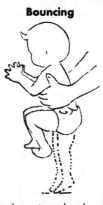

Figure 6.23   A normal reaction – head and trunk in alignment, arms forward. Legs bending in the arm, straightening just before the feet touch the ground

The child with moderate spasticity and low truncal tone

To overcome her lack of extension, the child in Figure 6.24 extends her head, chin poked forward, her arms flexed, shoulders protracted (forward), elbows back. She does this to compensate for her poor truncal tone and lack of shoulder and pelvic stability. In an attempt to get her feet on the ground, she has to flex her hips, legs extended,

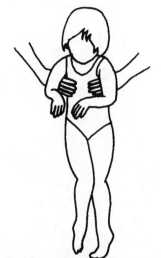

Figure 6.24 *The child with moderate spasticity* – Weight bearing on plantar flat feet (on the toes) increases the hypertension in the neck, flexion of the upper limbs and trunk, extension of the hips and legs

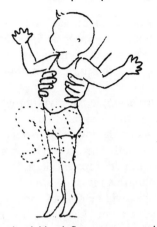

Figure 6.25 *The child with fluctuating tone and involuntary movements.* Either totally flexes in the air and collapses when the feet touch the ground, or totally extends

feet plantar flexed. She is consequently taking her weight on plantar flexed feet, i.e. on her toes.

The child with fluctuating tone and involuntary movements

These children, when lifted in the air, may either draw their legs up into flexion or extend them, and then when their feet touch the ground unable to support their weight, they collapse. If, in addition, they have strong intermittent spasms, when their feet touch the ground they may extend their head, arms and trunk, standing momentarily on their toes, then collapse or make continuous stepping movements (Figure 6.25)

Note: **Baby bouncer**. At around 7 months of age a baby, when he stands, often starts to 'bounce' by bending and straightening his legs. He does so when standing on his mother's lap, in his cot or on the floor, holding on to give himself extra support and stability. If he is put in a 'baby bouncer', because he has good head and trunk control and hip stability he is able to keep his head and body in alignment over mobile legs, putting his feet flat on the ground while he bounces. To a certain extent **he** is in control of the 'bouncer', and can stop and start bouncing at will.

The child with cerebral palsy, on the other hand, has no such control, and is therefore **controlled** by the movement of the **bouncer itself**, any asymmetry of posture and movement being accentuated.

The child with spasticity, as he takes weight on his toes, will increase his tendency to extend, internally rotate and adduct his legs, and the equinus position of his feet will be reinforced both in the air and when they come into contact with the ground. The child with intermittent spasms and involuntary movements, as his feet come into contact with the ground, will either draw them both up in a total pattern of flexion, or draw one leg up in flexion, with the other stiffly extending. He is also likely to push his body back into extension. We therefore **do not recommend** the use of baby bouncers for children with cerebral palsy, as the excitement and stimulation will only increase any abnormal patterns of postural tone and movement patterns present.

Kicking

When we talk and play with a baby who has cerebral palsy and he responds by kicking, we quite naturally want to encourage him to continue doing so. I would, however, advise you to **watch carefully** to see the **way** he 'kicks', as it is easy without realizing it to reinforce an abnormal kicking pattern.

Does he, for example, kick with only one leg, or pull one leg up into flexion while at the same time pushing the other leg down into extension? When 'kicking' with both legs, does he extend them, internally rotating his hips and legs, feet in plantar flexion (pointing his toes)?

Your therapist will be able to show you ways of handling that facilitate 'kicking' while taking into account your baby's particular problems.

Vigorous play

The majority of children love being thrown in the air and caught again, whirled round and round and joining in a rough and tumble. Unfortunately, the excitement and stimulation of playing in this way with the young child with cerebral palsy may increase tone in his muscles or result in an increase in involuntary and disorganized movements.

Figure 6.26(a–c) illustrates ways of enabling a child with cerebral palsy to enjoy this important aspect of 'father's play', by controlling the child's reactions so that he has time to make adjustments to being moved.

Handling during routine activities

Bathing, dressing and undressing a child is normally comparatively easy, as the child moves with you rather than against you. If, for example, you lift his arm or leg when bathing him, you will feel no resistance. When you put his tee-shirt over his head he will automatically push his head up through the opening. His natural self-protective reactions and his ability to balance when being handled enable him to adjust his position and, if he is uncomfortable, move or alternatively push his mother away.

The child with cerebral palsy, on the other hand, often feels insecure when he is bathed,

Vigorous play

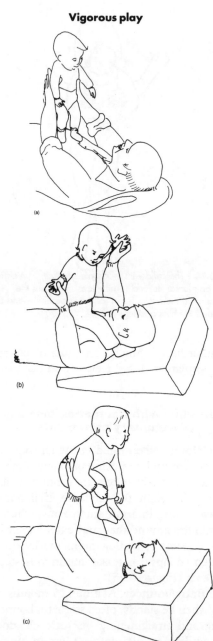

Figure 6.26 (a) While the baby bends and straightens his legs, his grandfather keeps his trunk in alignment, weight forward, by keeping his shoulders *up* and arms *forward*.

(b) To help his son keep his back straight and bend forward at the hips as he moves him in different directions, his father holds his hands, wrists extended, arms in extension and outward extension.

(c) To prevent his son pushing back as he swings him in the air, his father stabilizes his pelvis keeping his hips flexed, weight forward.

dressed and undressed. A child with increased tone (spasticity) is limited in his movements, reactions and responses and therefore is unable automatically to adjust his posture when being moved. A child with intermittent spasms and involuntary movements, although he is able to move, lacks stability and his balance reactions are exaggerated.

It is therefore important, **before** for example dressing, undressing and changing a baby's diaper (nappy), to make sure that he is in a **position** where he feels **secure** and is **symmetrical**, i.e. his head, trunk and pelvis are in alignment, and his **weight evenly distributed**. Suggestions on ways of doing this are discussed in the following chapters.

Once your child has achieved a new motor skill, be sure that you give him every opportunity to use and practise this skill while you handle him in **everyday situations** and during play times together, and later when you are teaching him self-help tasks.

Summary

In summary, when handling a child with cerebral palsy one should:

- understand the reasons for a child's difficulties in moving and how these vary
- how his abnormal patterns of posture and movement affect the whole body, and which handling techniques might minimize or change these reactions
- be sensitive to the changes in tone under one's hands, **taking away support as soon as it is no longer needed**
- give a child every opportunity to practise any new skill he achieves when being handled in everyday situations
- remember that physical, communication and intellectual skills cannot be taught in isolation.

Chapter 7

Early stages of hand function

- Visual/auditory awareness
- Problems affecting the development of hand skills
- Stages of early grasp and release
- Movement and play

Before a child can achieve independent function for daily living he needs first to use his hands for grasp, release, support and manipulation. As many children with cerebral palsy may need to rely on their hands for support, assist in mobility, push themselves to stand and later to walk, the **importance** of teaching the child **hand skills** at **each** stage of his development **cannot be** over-emphasized. In this chapter we will discuss the importance of visual/auditory awareness, the early development of eye–hand coordination, and ways in which we might help the baby with cerebral palsy acquire these basic skills, all of which are the prerequisites for skilled hand function.

Visual/auditory awareness

Choice of position

You should experiment to find a position that is comfortable for both yourself and your baby, one in which you can be face to face, and feel able to control his total posture if and when necessary.

Figure 7.1 illustrates a position that many mothers prefer, as their lap provides a slight incline and they can use their knees to keep their baby's head in mid-line, leaving their hands free. Alternatively, you may find handling easier if your baby lies on his side, using a wedge as a side-lier,

his back supported against the back of the couch, or have him lying beside you on your bed.

Encouraging visual fixation

How you encourage eye contact will of course be a matter of personal preference and vary according to your baby's responses. Your therapist will help you to understand the degree of eye contact you

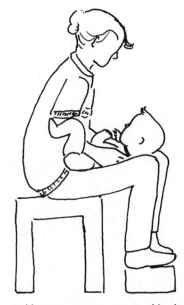

Figure 7.1 Stable support encourages visual/auditory awareness

can expect, and show you ways you might make eye contact with your baby.

Fortunately, during the early months your face is the most stimulating, versatile and interesting toy as far as your baby is concerned. At first to gaze at intently, then to focus on particular features. Later he will react to changes in expression, raised eyebrows, a frown, an expression of marked surprise and at around 8 months finds your face fun to poke at!

As long as your baby has no problems taking the breast or his bottle, an excellent time to encourage eye contact is during a feed or if he enjoys being bathed at bath time. Both are times when he will be relaxed, and occasions when you will be near enough for him to focus on your face.

As babies are attracted by the rhythm and various tones in an adult's voice and fortunately have no idea when one sings out of tune, a good way of stimulating a baby to listen, quieten and maintain eye contact is by singing or humming. Figure 7.2 illustrates a grandfather interacting in this way with his grandson. Hypnotic toys that are operated by an adult usually fascinate a baby and are an excellent way for stimulating visual fixation. Once visual fixation has been established, visual following starts to develop.

Ways of encouraging visual following

When you feel that you have made good eye contact with your baby, start to encourage him to follow you by moving your head from side to side, later up and down. To stimulate his interest, it is often worthwhile wearing a bright necklace or earrings.

A good way of encouraging a baby while he lies in his cot to listen and follow a moving object is by using a rattle. Shake the rattle gently until he looks at it, then move it slowly from side to side. If a baby has poor head control, he may find it easier to follow if a shawl or light blanket is wrapped around his shoulders, giving him a feeling of stability. Once he can manage to follow the rattle, moving his head as he does so, try to encourage him to follow while you hold his head steady in mid-line. You can play with a baby in a similar way when he lies on his tummy or sitting supported on your lap, and with a child who has sitting balance at a table (Figures 7.3 to 7.5)

Looking at familiar objects

As the first place your baby will start to develop head and trunk control against gravity is when he is being carried, make use of this opportunity of encouraging visual awareness. Draw his attention to rain on the window pane, look at shiny objects on a mantelpiece, stop in front of a ticking clock.

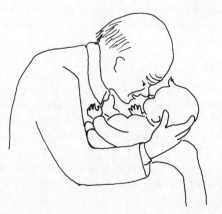

Figure 7.2 Stimulating a baby to quieten, listen and maintain eye contact

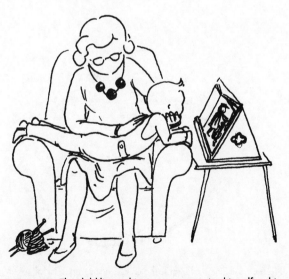

Figure 7.3 The child lies on his tummy, supporting himself on his elbows. His grandmother helps him keep his back extended and his head up, as they look together at the picture

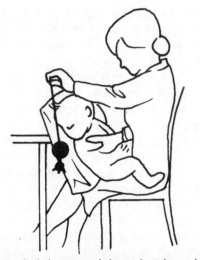

Figure 7.4   The baby sits astride his mother's lap and she prevents him pushing back by holding his arms forward across his chest. At other times she will hold his head in mid-line and get him to follow the ball without moving his head

If you have pets, such as fish in a tank, a cat or dog, as they will be familiar to your baby they will hold his interest and be fun for him to watch. As he grows older, draw his attention to sounds, such as the doorbell ringing, the telephone, water coming out of the tap, clicking on and off an electric

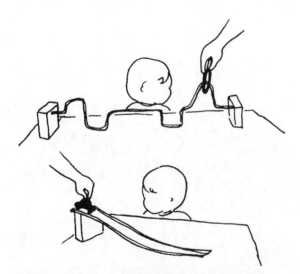

Figure 7.5   Sitting at a table the child is encouraged to follow an object as it is moved from left to right, right to left and later towards and away from him. Progressing to holding, looking and moving the object in his hand – moving it as directed

light switch and so forth – all objects you will later be helping him to use.

Stimulating visual awareness outside

If you should be fortunate enough to have a patio or garden and your baby spends time outside in his pram, nature will provide him with all the stimulation, movement and colour he needs: the sun reflecting light and shade; the wind providing spontaneous movements of flowers, branches and leaves on the trees; and even washing blowing on a line will attract your baby's attention. All you need to do is to see that he is placed in a good position to look at what is going on around him.

If a child has a visual defect, such as nystagmus, strabismus, poor visual acuity or other occulo-motor deficits, your therapist working with the ophthalmologist will give you specific advice regarding these problems.

Although the suggestions I have made are ways in which a mother and members of the family automatically play and interact with a baby, I have still mentioned them, as sometimes when a baby has cerebral palsy, either because he does not appear to respond or takes a long time doing so, we are apt to forget the **important role** eye focusing, visual fixation and visual following play **in the development of eye–hand coordination and hand skills**. They are an opportunity that should not be missed, rather than relying on cot toys and mobiles as the sole means of stimulating early visual awareness. The suggestions may also encourage the reader to invent and discover other ways of stimulating their baby to look and listen.

Mobiles

As soon as a baby spends less time sleeping during the day, he starts to learn more about the world around him through what he sees and hears. This is a time when mobiles have a special fascination for him. I would, however, strongly advise you **not** to buy a mobile that when wound up goes round and round, as this type can precipitate fits with some babies.

While a baby is at the stage of just 'looking and listening', I often think the home-made less sophisticated variety of mobile is best. That is to say, 'bits and pieces' you can find in the home, objects that move naturally and do not rely on an adult to activate them.

A mobile can for example be made from an old lampshade frame, wire coat-hanger or by making notches in a wooden coat-hanger. You can also attach various objects across a baby's cot using elastic cord, plastic-covered wire or even a fishing line.

When putting up a mobile or attaching anything to the sides or across a cot, always see that all the objects are **near enough** to be within the baby's line of vision. Remember that it will take a baby a time before he can focus from a distance. If in doubt, do get your therapist to advise you.

As a baby's concentration span is short, when lining up and suspending objects be sure to watch to see the ones that your baby finds the most interesting.

Objects you might suspend above the cot

Examples of things you could suspend over a cot are objects that:

- are **shiny** – milk bottle tops, a bracelet wrapped in coloured cellophane or tinfoil, strips of crepe paper, decorations left over from Christmas
- make a **noise** – small bells attached to coloured ribbons, string of coloured beads
- **reflect** – small plastic mirrors, painted lids, shiny coloured balls of the type used to decorate a Christmas tree.

Toys

Always see that toys are hung or placed at eye level and the correct distance away from the baby. At this stage, colour is an important factor in visual orientation, so choose toys in primary colours, avoiding pastel shades. The best toys are those that are simple to operate and can easily be adapted so that, as a child acquires the necessary skills, he can operate them by himself:

- toys that are visually stimulating and will encourage the baby to locate sounds are those

that reflect light, click, rattle or play a tune, such as musical mobiles, Mirror Chime About, Musical Fantasy, Play Sound Activity Cube and a Helter Skelter loop
- toys that encourage visual tracking include Touch 'n' Go Dump Truck by Torny, or one of the many 'Action' toys
- toys that provide the baby with visual and tactile experiences, i.e. those that can be given to him to hold, feel and look at, such as the Koosh and Koosh Krinks or a Sensaring
- toys that are good for getting the baby's attention are those with a surprise element, Teddy Bear-About, Bobbing Man Mobile or a Clown who, when a bead is pulled, moves its arms and legs up and down.

The early development of hand skills

The development of a baby's hand skills is closely linked and dependent on sensory input, postural control (stability) and gross motor patterns of movement, so that there are only a few variations in the order in which hand skills develop, with age serving just as a rough guide.

How does the lack of postural stability and the abnormal patterns of posture and movement affect the development of hand function in the baby/child with cerebral palsy?

- Because of inadequate trunk and pelvic stability he is unable to stabilize one part of his body while moving another.
- Abnormal patterns of posture and movement of the trunk, arm and hand affect his ability to reach, grasp, release and develop fine motor skills.
- His hands may be totally or partially closed in association with his total abnormal posture, or if there is minimal involvement with the posture of the arm itself. In addition, there may be sensory loss in the hand, found most frequently in the child with spastic hemiplegia.
- Because of poor or inadequate balance, a child may need to use one or both hands for support.
- Hand function may remain at an earlier developmental level. For example, a primitive hand

grasp (an object squeezed between the palm and two or more fingers) or mirror movements normally seen in babies and young children persisting beyond the time expected.

● Release may be immature or abnormally performed. For example, a child with increased tone (spasticity), releasing an object with a flexed wrist, fingers extended, or a child with intermittent spasms and involuntary movements (athetoid type of cerebral palsy), releasing an object by withdrawing his arm with an open hand and hyperextending his fingers.

There are a number of children who may have impaired hand function because of visual and perceptual problems, and others who find it difficult to **listen** and at the **same time** look at what they are doing. This not only affects their ability to use their hands, but also their speed of learning and concentration.

Not all the difficulties described will necessarily apply to every child, and many if present will, in a number of children, be modified in time.

It would obviously be a waste of time to try to teach or expect a baby/child with cerebral palsy who is **hypersensitive to touch** to become familiar with his hands, learn where his body parts are, how they move or the space they occupy, or, **if his hand is fisted**, to learn grasp and release. How can we help if either of these two problems are present?

Getting an open hand

As long as a baby/child has a primitive hand grasp, i.e. his hand closes immediately he touches anything, or his hand is fisted with the thumb lying across the palm, he will be unable to grasp or release in a purposeful manner.

It is therefore important, **before** encouraging hand activities, to try **first** to open his hand with the fingers straight, thumb out, the wrist extended. This can be done by turning the arm **out** at the shoulder with the elbow straight, forearm and palm facing up. Start by doing this with both arms out sideways (horizontally), then later with the arms forward – see Figure 6.7(c,d), earlier.

Another way you might try opening his hand is by stroking the outside of the hand towards the little finger or, with an older child, by pressing the heel of the hand on a firm surface, keeping the elbow straight, then pulling the fingers and thumb out from the **base**.

Once the baby/child's hand is open, get him to **take weight on an open hand**, applying gentle pressure through the shoulders.

A number of babies/children are able to use their hands despite the fact that their thumb lies across the palm. This applies particularly to those children where one side of the body is involved, i.e. spastic hemiplegia. If this persists, the transition of grasp from the outer fingers towards the thumb and index finger is blocked and the child's ability to abduct and adduct the thumb will not develop. Unable to use his thumb, the child has no alternative but to use a palmar grasp with an ulnar deviated wrist, i.e. the hand pulls outward and away from the thumb.

To minimize the chance of this abnormal pattern of the hand developing, I now, as **EARLY** as possible, use a thumb strap. Figure 7.6 illustrates a thumb strap that is simple and cheap to make. When used with a baby, as well as keeping the thumb extended and abducted it also holds the wrist in extension. With the hand held in this position, you will also find it easier to get the baby to **support** himself on an **open** hand.

Early tactile experiences

The baby who is hypersensitive to touch

When a baby is hypersensitive to tactile stimulation he will be abnormally responsive to being touched, withdraw his arms and hands when given a toy, and have problems with textures. Any tactile stimulation therefore needs to be added gradually, to begin with under the baby's own control so that he has time to adjust and respond.

The following are ways you might introduce early stimulation

● Hold the baby by his shoulders or upper arms and encourage him to look at his hands as you

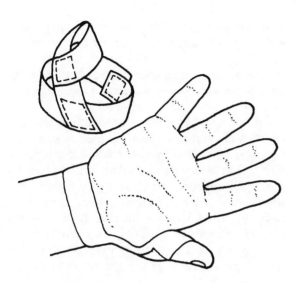

Figure 7.6 Thumb strap

rub, clap and press them together. Take one hand at a time over the front and back of his forearms. Hold his wrists and shake his hands, i.e. wave goodbye.

- Rub his hands over his face, top of his head and his tummy. Take both his hands and rub them over your face. Blow kisses, tickle and walk over the palms, back of his hands and up the back and front of his forearms.
- Place a toy between his palms that squeaks as you press his hands together. Place his hands around familiar objects such as his bottle.
- If you have a pet take his hands over its coat.
- Place familiar things in his hands that are rough, smooth, wet, dry, warm, cold and sticky. If he has reached the stage of putting everything in his mouth, remember that **size and safety is important**.
- Put your hand in a rubber, woolly or garden glove and get him to touch and hold your fingers.
- Draw your baby's attention to his hands and feet when you wash and soap them, swishing them in the water.
- Bend and stretch his arm, hands and fingers as you dry them. Do the same with his toes.

- Introduce turn-taking by placing two fingers in the palm of his hand and encourage him to relax his hand so that you can withdraw your finger. Place his hand in yours and open and close your hand around his hand.
- Finger and glove puppets are simple to make and stimulate a baby to look, touch and get hold of them. You can also add an element of anticipation and surprise by 'hiding' a finger and then suddenly getting it to reappear.

The following points may help you when encouraging hand activities

A child will only be able to bring his shoulders and arms forward, his hands towards mid-line if he is in a position in which he can maintain a symmetrical stable posture:

- his head must be in mid-line so that he can look at the toy in his hands
- check to see that the effect of grasping has not caused an abnormal posture or increased the tone in the rest of his body
- aim to get your child to grasp with his forearm in a mid position with an extended wrist. If he finds this difficult, get him to support himself on an open hand with the wrist and arm extended from time to time
- it is less stressful for a child to handle and play with toys and objects that are familiar to him
- a child should be encouraged to **repeat** anything he does well on his own, **even if** it was not what you had in mind.

If your child has difficulty in speaking when he uses his hands, encourage him to tell you what he is doing while he plays. This not only gives him an understanding of language so important for future speech, but also helps him start to **organize his thoughts so as to reinforce his actions**.

Early grasp

During the early months a baby's hands are only open when he is relaxed, asleep or after a feed. At around 3 months they are open most of the time, and if he should touch for example his vest or clothes he will automatically clutch at them in a crude and clumsy manner.

Although unable to reach out and grasp, if a rattle is put into his hand he holds it with his outside fingers, but just as he makes no attempt to handle what he sees, he makes no attempt to look at the rattle and is only aware of the tactile stimulus.

As he waves his arms about, he starts to get fleeting glimpses of the rattle in his hand, stopping at times with his arm still to look at it, then putting it into his mouth to explore its shape and texture, from time to time taking it out to look at it once again. This is an important **first step** in the development of eye–hand regard.

The baby with cerebral palsy

When some babies with cerebral palsy grasp, they often do so with excessive flexion of their arms, their shoulder turning in and coming forwards (protraction), and are apt to clench the rattle so tightly that it is difficult to get it out of their hand. If this should happen, keep his arm straight, turned out at the shoulder, forearm and hand facing up, before putting the rattle into his hand, or try giving him a rattle with a larger ring/handle.

If your baby finds it difficult to maintain his grasp when holding a rattle, hold your hand over his hand, keeping his arm straight, the wrist **extended**. When helping him take the rattle to his mouth, see that his arm is at shoulder level, his elbow **away** from his body. Once he is aware that he has something in his hand, move his arm smoothly in different directions, occasionally stopping and shaking his wrist so that he associates the movement of his arm with the sound of the rattle. Playing with your baby in this way, besides encouraging early eye–hand regard, also gets him to pay attention to what he is doing.

Some babies are hypersensitive in the oral area, and when the rattle touches their mouth the added stimulus may make them push the toy away, their head back. If this is a problem, your speech and language therapist will show you how to desensitize the child's mouth.

Toys

The best hand to mouth toys that encourage early grasp are rattles, teething rings or teethers which have large projections of different colours. They should be the correct size for your baby to hold, but not too small so that there is a danger of him swallowing them, and not too heavy.

Choose toys for holding and mouthing that can be safely chewed and when squeezed make a pleasant noise. For two-handed reach and grasp, the best type of rattles are those that have two handles that make different sounds and move in different ways when shaken. Mirrors always fascinate a baby and many have two handles. Avoid squeaky and soft spongy toys, and only later choose small, squeaky rubber animals. If in doubt which toys to choose, always ask your therapist for advice.

Visually directed grasp

A baby, when he first reaches out and discovers his feet and toes or when a toy comes into his visual field, grasps them first with flexed fingers, then later with the palm of his hand and two or more fingers. Although able to visually examine the toy in his hand and pass it from hand to hand, he still continues to learn more about it by taking it to his mouth.

The baby with cerebral palsy

The reasons a baby with cerebral palsy may be limited in his ability to establish visually directed reaching and discover where his body parts are have been discussed earlier in this chapter. The position in which you choose to work with your baby will depend on which, if any, of these difficulties apply. It can sometimes be difficult to help a baby with cerebral palsy maintain a stable symmetrical posture while at the same time bring his shoulders and arms forward to grasp, and you therefore may need to work with your baby first, **before** encouraging early grasp. The ways of doing this will be shown to you by your therapist.

Figures 7.7 to 7.9 illustrate ways, at different stages of a baby/child's development, that progress can be made from reaching out to know

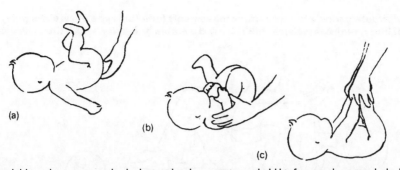

Figure 7.7   (a) If the child is to be encouraged to look at and at the same time to hold his feet, see that not only the hips but the lower part of his spine are off the support. Many children, when they try to reach out for their toes, push their head back and this immediately straightens their hips and legs.

(b) When the child takes his toes to his mouth, see that the legs are bent and turned out; help by keeping his arms forward and up at the shoulder. With the effort of taking his foot to his mouth, the bending of one leg may make the other leg straighten and the child will often lose his balance. To prevent this happening, have your other hand under the opposite hip. Work as quickly as possible to get him to hold both feet at once, taking one or both to his mouth.

(c) A child normally plays for many hours in this position, i.e. holding his toes while the legs remain straight and moving his legs up and down. Work for this pattern, which is a good preparation for long sitting later on, but do see that the legs are not stiff or turned in

his own boundaries to learning about others in relation to himself, and ways you might play with a baby or young child to encourage him to reach and grasp. Suggestions for drawing your baby's attention to his body parts are also discussed in Chapters 16 and 17 on bathing and dressing.

The young child with increased tone (spasticity)

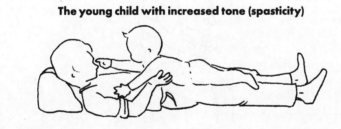

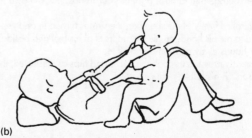

Figure 7.8   (a) The child lies on his father, who supports his son under his armpit so that he is able to take weight on an open hand as he reaches forward with the other hand to touch Daddy's face.

(b) The child sits astride his father, his feet flat on the floor. His father guides both his hands towards his face, naming his nose, eyes, mouth and ears as the child touches them. The amount of support he gives with his legs will depend on his son's ability to keep his trunk forward over his sitting base, which in this sketch he has failed to do!

The child with fluctuating tone and involuntary movements (athetoid type of cerebral palsy). To have an appreciation of body awareness these children need a stable base from which they can use their hands

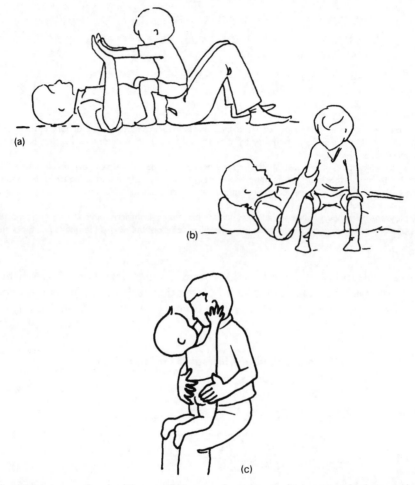

Figure 7.9   (a) The child grasps your hands while you pull him towards you keeping his arms straight, then quickly jerk him back a little. This will give him the feeling of grasping while at the same time you increase the tone in his trunk (making it firm) and improve his head control. Try also to encourage him to push against your hands; this will give him the very important pattern of reaching forward in a controlled way.

(b) The child is controlled firmly at the shoulder, the arm is turned in and kept straight by his side. He puts his hands on his knees and moves slowly forward to put his hands on his feet, in front of his feet and beside his feet, returning to the sitting position with his hands on his knees. Take your hands away as soon as possible.

(c) By giving firm steady pressure through the pelvis and hips as illustrated, the child is able to maintain the extension in his trunk while lifting his arms up to touch his father's ears

Reaching and swiping – a goal-orientated behaviour

Further coordination between hand and eye develops when a baby starts to pay sufficient visual attention to focus on an object that attracts him. Before the age of 6 months he will find it easier to monitor the position of his arm in relation to an object, if and when he makes contact it moves and makes a noise.

As he waves his arms about in a random fashion his early attempts to 'swipe' at a toy are poorly timed and coordinated, but with practice he hits his target and in time is able to get hold of the toys he wants and make them do what he wants.

It is interesting to note, that as he reaches out he opens and closes his fingers in anticipation of grasping, long before he is capable of doing so, reacting in a similar way when offered a toy to hold.

The baby with cerebral palsy

To help a baby with cerebral palsy master these skills we need, as previously mentioned, to see that he is in a position that gives him sufficient postural support and enables him to keep his head in mid-line and bring his shoulders and arms forward.

Toys

Toys should be chosen that respond to the lightest touch, rewarding the baby for his efforts. When playing on his own, Cot Toys, Cradle Gyms and Activity links Gyms, are all excellent at this stage. They all have simple activity toys that can be arranged in different combinations, such as mix and match links, toys that when touched spin, rattle and provide a variety of sounds and movement.

Toy manufacturers produce a wide range of these types of toys made in different designs, colours and materials. Their catalogues are well illustrated, with notes on safety, durability and play value, and are well worth looking through before making a final choice.

Encouraging voluntary grasp – the baby with cerebral palsy

As most children with cerebral palsy find it easier to reach, grasp and move their toys when supporting themselves on one arm, it is a good idea at least some of the time, to play with your baby sitting supported on your lap, with a table in front of him. A good game to play with a baby is to put a favourite toy on a soft piece of cloth just out of reach, and get him to grasp it with both hands and pull it towards him. At first he will just grab the toy, but in time will realize that his hands are pulling the toy towards him. In this way, he will learn to grasp and at the same time how to get something he wants.

Until around the age of 9 months a baby will look at a toy before grasping it, so when either handing the baby a toy or putting one down for him to play with, be sure that it is directly in front of him.

A way of teaching a child, while you hold his hands to maintain a sustained grasp with an extended wrist, is by using action songs. Here are a few examples, but of course all families have their own favourites: 'Ride a cock horse', 'Row, row, row your boat', 'See-saw', 'This is the way the pony trots'. I also find the 'Grand Old Duke of York' is a good way of getting a child to follow the actions while, for example, holding a favourite toy.

Ways of encouraging reach, grasp and manipulation at different stages in a child's development are illustrated in Figures 7.10 to 7.17.

Further development of hand function

As a baby's eye–hand coordination and fine motor skills develop, he begins to learn what he can and cannot do with things around him. He does this by patting, rattling, banging, clutching and pulling things apart. At this stage he still takes anything of interest to his mouth whether familiar or new, to suck, bite and chew. As soon as he has sufficient trunk balance and pelvic stability, and no longer relies on his arms for support, sitting becomes the most functional position for him to practise using his hands.

Preparation for reach and grasp

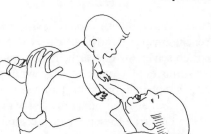

Figure 7.10   The gross motor skill of taking weight on extended arms with an open hand and extended wrist, in a variety of positions, precedes the development of voluntary reach and grasp. In this sketch the grandfather helps his grandson learn to support himself by stabilizing his pelvis

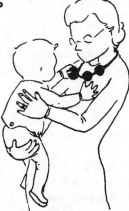

Figure 7.12   The baby's grandmother has a string of red wooden balls around her neck. She carries her grandson on her hip, supporting him so that he can bring both arms forward and they can be face to face as he plays with them. Little balls, small squares of foam or macaroni can also be used, gradually increasing the number on the string

Where previously he grasped towards the ulnar (outer) side of his hands with flexed fingers, he now begins to grasp using his whole hand in a squeeze-like grasp, his fingers against the palm. Between 7 and 9 months he begins to grasp an object towards the radial (inner) side of his hand using his thumb in opposition to two or more fingers. His ability to manipulate becomes more precise once he is able to oppose his thumb first to the **side**, then towards the base and middle part of his **index** finger.

Able to reach out unilaterally, using each hand separately, he transfers objects from hand to hand, and bangs them together.

At around 10 months he starts to **point**, by inhibiting the activity of the other three fingers. Pointing first at himself then at objects around him, he also becomes fascinated by spaces – poking and exploring them with his index finger. This **important achievement of pointing precedes**

Encouraging reach and grasp during routine activities

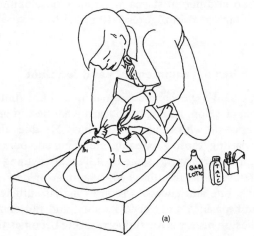

(a)

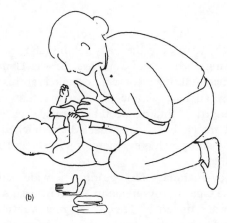

(b)

Figure 7.11   (a) When having a diaper (nappy) changed; (b) when being undressed

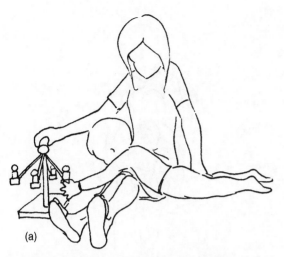

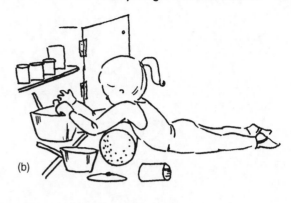

Figure 7.13 (a) A teenage sister takes a turn to play with the brother. Growing more accustomed to lying on his tummy and with fewer spasms, the child can lie on the hard surface of the floor.
(b) By using a roller in this way the immobile child can enjoy exploring the contents of a cupboard

his ability to oppose first his fingers with the tip of his thumbs and, in the following months, a precise opposition of the tips of his thumb with his index finger.

Having achieved a full range of grasp, a baby begins to use these skills in a more purposeful manner. Where previously he could only release, for example, a cube by pressing it against a hard surface, he can now release a large object in a crude manner by excessive extension of his fingers. By the time he can handle small objects, he begins to release in a mature manner.

From exploring objects, he finds out how things 'work' by putting them in and out of a container,

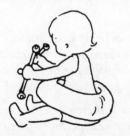

Figure 7.14 Sitting a child in an inflated rubber ring, as illustrated, or a similar shape in foam is a good way of helping a child who has just acquired sitting balance feel more secure when attempting to use both hands. The child in the sketch is grasping dowel rods with bells attached. Rods with flags or windmills, or with sleeves of different colours or textures over the rods, can be used.

building a tower of bricks, fitting things into one another, by understanding that some things can be pushed and pulled, others screwed and unscrewed.

As he becomes more proficient in using his hands, speech starts to develop which often helps him with the task in hand. It is about this time that we start to show him books, encouraging him to turn the pages, point to objects we describe and eventually to name them himself.

Movement and play

You have only to watch a baby while he plays: he is rarely still and seldom silent. When lying on his back playing with his toys he continuously kicks his legs and wriggles about. When on his tummy he is just as active. Interspersed with his play, he rocks on his tummy, lifting and waving his arms.

As soon as he develops sufficient stability and mobility at his shoulders and pelvis, still clutching his toys he will roll over onto his side and return to his back, later rolling onto his tummy, stopping to inspect his toy, then taking it to his mouth to explore it further.

In this way as he plays, besides practising new patterns of movement information – for example regarding distance, i.e. how far he has to reach to get a toy – the baby builds up a stable body image,

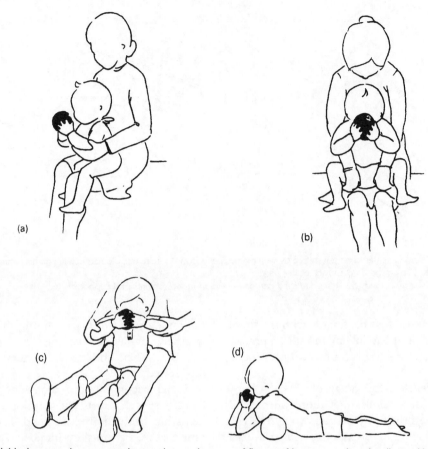

Figure 7.15   A child who can only grasp an object with a total pattern of flexion of his arms and trunk will most likely have difficulty holding a spoon and taking it to his mouth. The following four sketches illustrate positions that can be used to practise this movement using an apple, its round shape being easier for the child to hold than the handle of a spoon.

(a) Sitting astride his mother's knee the child first grasps the apple with extended arms. As he takes the apple to his mouth, his mother stops her child's arms from pressing down and turning in, by supporting him under his elbows keeping his arms away from his body.

(b) If a child with fairly good arms has a tendency to push back, extending his hips and legs as he lifts his arms, you might try controlling his legs as illustrated.

(c,d) Two positions you might use with an older child. Later, sitting at a table, getting him to support himself on his elbows as he takes the apple to his mouth

learns about himself in space and about relationships in the world around him.

The baby/young child with cerebral palsy

With so much emphasis on positions for play, please do not think that hand activities should only be encouraged in **a position only – this is not the case**.

In the baby/young child with cerebral palsy, because he has a problem in moving, his ability to build up a stable body image and to handle the environment will inevitably be reduced. It is therefore important that immediately he is able to reach and grasp, that when playing with him we encourage him to maintain his grasp while moving. For example:

● once he has sufficient stability and mobility at his shoulders and pelvis to grasp his toes with his legs in the air, roll him from side to side and return him to his back

● when handing him a toy or a rusk, get him to reach out for it

● when he starts to develop sitting balance, place his toys out of reach so that he has to support

Before a child can use *both hands* for skilled activities in sitting he must have good trunk control, pelvic stability and balance

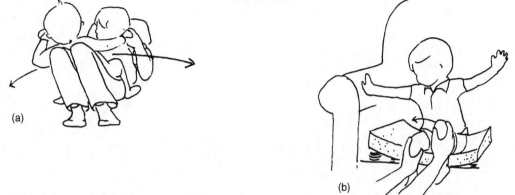

(a)

(b)

Figure 7.16 (a) A child with poor head and trunk control sits astride his father holding his hands. His father moves his legs sideways teaching his son to make the necessary adjustments, holding him by one hand as he becomes more competent. If his arms begin to feel heavy and start to push down he would then extend them above his head with the shoulders outwardly rotated (turned out)
(b) Balance reactions with a moderately affected child can be facilitated on a roll, ball or by placing a square of foam on the base of a chair, as illustrated. Always tip the child *slowly* to one side and wait a second *before* moving him back to the mid-line

himself on one hand while picking them up with the other hand

● when he is sitting on your knee, encourage balance reactions while he plays, by moving your knees so that he starts to make adjustments as his sitting base shifts while using his hands (see Figures 7.18 and 7.19).

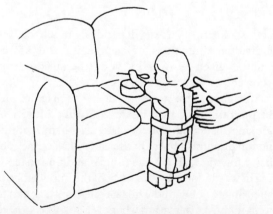

Figure 7.17 A young mildly affected child plays standing in front of a couch. The foam 'case' is used to give confidence rather than support. Strips of Velcro hold the foam together and the top of the case prevents the child from pressing his arms down

If your baby/child refuses to play, always **ask yourself why** – are the toys you have given him too difficult for him to handle, too easy and he is bored, or are the steps you have taken to break down the task inappropriate?

Playing with his toys is of course only one of the ways in which a child learns to use his hands. He also does so as he explores objects both inside and outside the home and, as mentioned throughout the various chapters, practising and using hand skills in all activities is the only way a child will eventually learn to be independent.

As the choice of toys for a baby will depend on the size of his hands, his ability to use them will depend on his powers of concentration and comprehension. The few toys we have mentioned should only act as a rough guide. It is always advisable to ask your therapist what she thinks would be the best toys to suit your baby's needs, so that you avoid buying toys he ignores because they are too difficult for him to handle or too simple and he soon tires of them.

Toy catalogues are well illustrated and offer a wide range of toys grouped into different categories, such as those suitable for various age groups, coordination of hands and eyes, sensory stimulation, two-handed play, grasp hold and

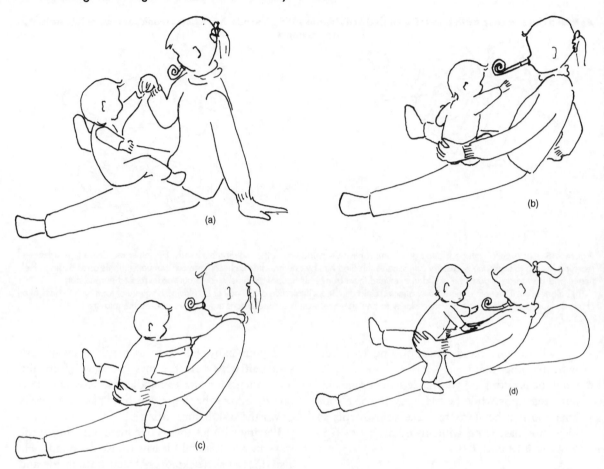

Figure 7.18 (a–d) These four sketches illustrate how one might encourage mobility, reach, grasp and release with a young child

manipulate, play touch talk, electrical reward toys and so forth. A number of toy manufacturers have also designed toys working closely with those in the caring professions for children with special needs. Useful addresses can be found in Appendix III.

Summary

In this chapter we have made no attempt to discuss ways in which you might teach a baby or young child with cerebral palsy how to transfer, put objects in and out of a container, to build

and so forth, as these depend so much on the individual difficulties of each child and advice will be given to you by your therapist during your child's treatment sessions.

What we have tried to do is to explain the **important** role that **basic building blocks** of looking, listening, touch, taste, eye–hand coordination and grasp have, in the early development of hand function, and as the sounds and understanding of words come before speech, the importance of speaking to your child while he plays, getting him to joint in the conversation whenever possible.

Even though a baby or young child with cerebral palsy may be restricted in his ability to move and use his hands, we can still help by teaching

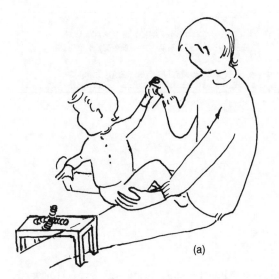

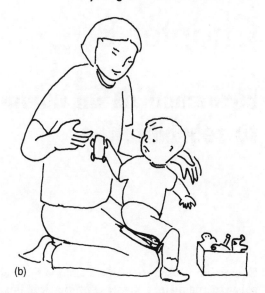

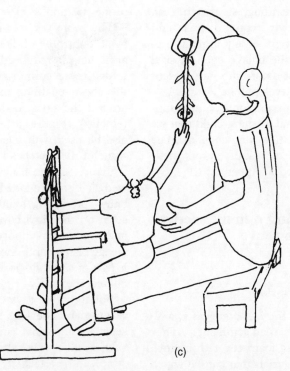

Figure 7.19 (a–c) Three sketches illustrating various ways of encouraging reach, grasp and release combined with trunk rotation

him the basic skills of visual, auditory and tactile awareness, so that he can make use of the abilities he has, using his hands in his own way, learning at his own pace.

Much of what we have said and many of the suggestions made, I am sure, are familiar to the reader, but I hope that within the framework suggested you will be encouraged to develop your own ideas.

Chapter 8

Equipment as an adjunct to rehabilitation

- Equipment providing (a) a firm base and postural support and (b) a movable surface
- Equipment for babies and young children

Equipment is used to enable a child with cerebral palsy to maintain a stable, symmetrical posture when lying, sitting or standing, so that he can practise and develop newly acquired gross and fine motor skills. The type of equipment prescribed will depend on the child's age, physical problems, whether or not deformities are present and the child's stage of development.

In this chapter we will discuss some of the equipment used with a baby and a young child that we will be referring to in the following chapters. The addresses of the equipment manufacturers mentioned in the text are listed in Appendix III.

Equipment providing a firm, secure base from which to move

Wedges

Description

A wedge is exactly what the name suggests, a V-shaped form which slopes at an acute angle. They are usually made of dense foam covered in vinyl, PVC or polyester, all materials that can be wiped clean which is clearly an advantage with young children. They are available in a variety of sizes, elevations and colours.

The elevation of the wedge shifts the child's centre of gravity towards his pelvis, making it easier for him to maintain his head and trunk in alignment, and stabilize his shoulder and pelvic

girdles so that he can bring his arms forward and hands into mid-line, particularly in the prone position.

The more severely involved child who has no head control and lies on his tummy with his arms flexed by his sides, may find a small chest wedge more comfortable, as it is narrower than the chest, enabling the child to bring his arms around the sides, taking weight on his forearms (elbows) (Figure 8.1a, b). A chest wedge can also be used with a large wedge, as illustrated in some of the sketches in this chapter.

Figure 8.2 illustrates a Tumble Forms Tadpole wedge, recommended for the mildly involved baby and young child. It has two Velcro strips sewn on the vinyl covering, with a small log roll and two lateral supports. A strap at the base of the wedge fastens onto the log roll. The wedge, which is part of a mobile positioning system, can be purchased separately.

For the more severely involved child we would recommend the Jenx wedge. It has Velcro strips sewn on the vinyl cover onto which accessories such as side walls, abduction block and webbing strap can be attached. The suppliers of the wedge also offer a customized service for making any size of wedge.

Note: With any equipment that has a foam filling, it is always advisable to check occasionally to see that no splits have appeared in the cover, in this way minimizing the risk of your child picking at the foam and putting pieces into his mouth.

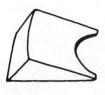

(a)

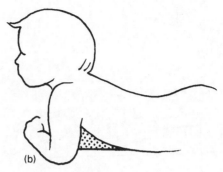

(b)

Figure 8.1   A small chest wedge, particularly useful for the more severely involved child

Suggested uses

A wedge, because of its elevation, makes it easier for some children when lying in the prone position to develop head control and trunk extension, shoulder and pelvic stability, visual awareness, mid-line play and eye–hand coordination. It can also be used to encourage gross motor activities such as rolling and crawling, and even as a means of facilitating weight shift when standing and walking (see Chapter 21, Figure 21.10).

However, it should be clearly understood that by putting a child on his tummy on a wedge **does not** mean of course that he will automatically be able to lift his head, extend his back and use his hands. While he may for example be able to lift his head and look around, he needs to support himself on his forearms (elbows) before he can handle toys placed in his hands, and later to transfer his weight onto one arm before he can reach out with the other.

Too often the value of a wedge is lost because the 'play area' is too low. The child just 'hangs' over the top of the wedge and in his attempt to reach his toys he lifts his head, his shoulders turning in and pushing down, his arms bending or stiffly extending with fisted hands. It is therefore important **always** to see that the play area is high enough for the child to be able to support himself on his forearms (elbows) or on an extended arm according to his stage of development (Figure 8.3 a–c).

Various other ways in which you might use a wedge are discussed in the following chapters, for example with a baby and young child, when changing a diaper (nappy), dressing, undressing, encouraging play activities, communication and social interaction.

Side-lying boards

Description

Side-lying boards are supplied by a number of different manufacturers in a wide range of sizes and with a variety of accessories. The majority have adjustable padded slanting backboards and slightly angled lying surfaces, hinged for storage and easy carriage.

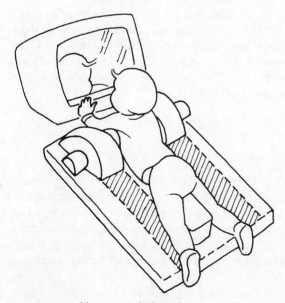

Figure 8.2   Tumble Forms Tadpole wedge

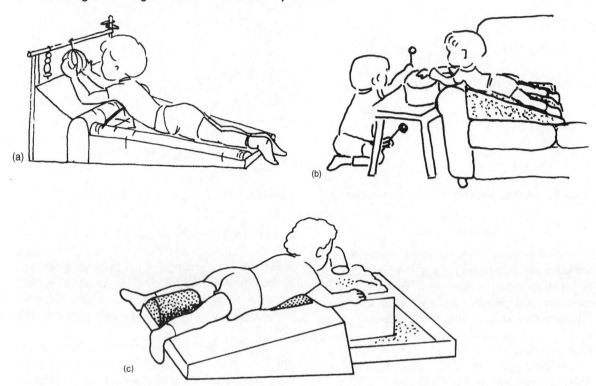

Figure 8.3   Three ways that you might use a wedge to encourage symmetrical weight bearing and reaching forward while playing

Figure 8.4 illustrates the Jenx side-lying board that we have used for young children. The board has Velcro strips over the length of the lying surface, which facilitates easier positioning of the wide restraining straps. Accessories for the side-lying board include a set of foam blocks for head and trunk support, a third bridged block for the legs, and a stand that raises the board 500 mm (20 in.) above the floor level. The James Leckey side-lying boards are also recommended.

In the UK, when your therapist decides that it would be helpful for your child to have a side-lying board for use at home, she will contact your Community Occupational Therapist or local district social services to see if one is available on a temporary loan.

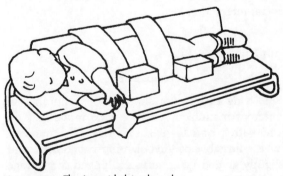

Figure 8.4   The Jenx side-lying board

Suggested uses

A side-lying board provides the more severely involved child who is excessively extended, and will most probably spend part of his day in a supportive seating system, with an alternative position that will enable him to keep his head, shoulders and arms forward and bring his hands together in mid-line.

When a child is placed in a side-lier, the following should always be carefully checked:

- that his head is flexed and positioned in midline, his shoulders and arms forward, his under-leg extended as much as possible, the upper leg semi-flexed
- that the knee and lower part of the upper leg are **supported** so that they are prevented from turning in at the hip and pressing against the lower leg
- that suspended toys and play activities are placed within reach and at the correct height so that they are within the child's line of vision.

Prone standers and upright standing frames

Undoubtedly there is a place for the use of equipment to promote standing and for use during the pre-standing phase. In keeping with the general philosophy of this book, that every opportunity should be exploited to its fullest therapeutic potential, so I believe should the use of this type of equipment. It is, of course, of paramount importance to have clear criteria for its use and sound objectives.

Implicit in a prescription for prone standers and upright standing frames are that they must be adjustable and accommodate for growth and meet the changing needs of the child as he becomes more competent, thus needing less control.

It is not my role to recommend any particular prone stander or upright standing frame, as they can only be prescribed after a full assessment and as with all such equipment monitored to ensure that it is fulfilling the child's needs. I will therefore just mention a few that are most generally prescribed.

When a baby first stands he takes weight through slightly bent legs and therefore his pelvic/hip stability is maintained by active flexion at his hips, and there is little activity in the muscles that straighten his hips (the hip extensors). This means that the baby has to rely on his arms for stability so that he can remain upright, which he does by supporting himself on his forearms or elbows, then later on extended arms (see Figure 5.15, earlier). At first his pelvis is in a fairly neutral position, but as he develops the ability to extend the muscles in his lower back (the lumbar region), his pelvis assumes a forward (anterior) tilt and he starts to bend and straighten his legs simultaneously.

Although the child with cerebral palsy will not have developed the physical abilities and stability throughout his body that a child normally has before pulling himself to stand, it is important that he experiences being in an upright position for his physical, emotional and social development, and to prevent or minimize the development of contractures. Prone standers and upright standing frames have been developed to enable a child to stand and maintain an acceptable posture while at the same time allowing movement in a limited range.

Prone standers

Prone standers are normally prescribed for children with low tone (hypotonia) who have poor upper trunk control, the child having difficulty in stabilizing one part of his body so that another part can move. They can be tilted from various degrees to the upright, with postural support provided by padded chest and lateral supports, pelvis and knee supports, pommels and foot plates. Trays or a working surface can be purchased as an optional extra. The prone standers most frequently prescribed are the Thalia Prone Board Z1708/2 (Figure 8.5) and the James Leckey Prone Stander (Figure 8.6).

Upright standing frames

Upright standing frames are prescribed for children who have good hand and trunk control, but are unable to stand unsupported or need to use their hands for support. Postural support is provided by wide bands of vinyl for the chest and buttocks attached to the vertical poles of the frame and held in place by Velcro fastenings. The knees are supported with foam knee blocks. Adjustable sandals or heel blocks are also supplied, with adjustable trays and postural asymmetry straps as an optional extra.

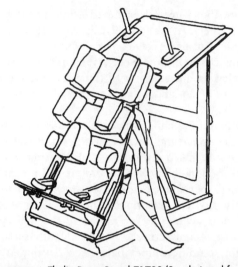

Figure 8.5   Thalia Prone Board Z1708/2 – designed for small children

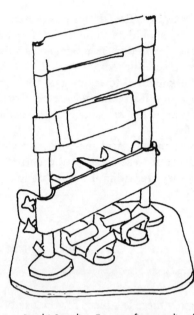

Figure 8.7   Bambi Standing Frame – first standing frame for small children (approximately 0.75–0.85 m tall)

The upright standing frames most frequently prescribed for young children are the Bambi Standing Frame (Figure 8.7) and the Flexistand (Figure 8.8). I personally find the Flexistand for

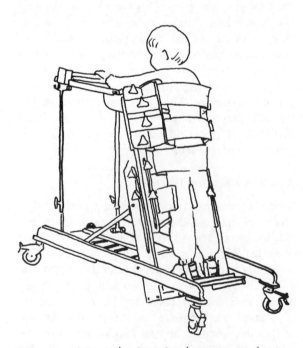

Figure 8.6   James Leckey Prone Stander – nursery and junior size

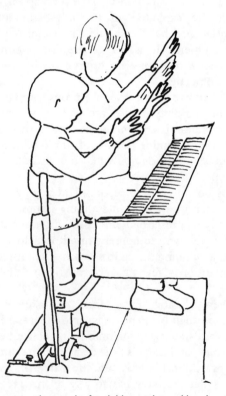

Figure 8.8   Flexistand – for children with good head and trunk control

children who need **only minimal** support, i.e. are at the stage of learning to get from sitting to standing, excellent for enabling the child to enjoy a variety of activities both on his own and with the family (see Chapter 13).

Note: An extension to the base of the frame may be necessary with an older child to give the frame extra stability.

Following a detailed analysis of the early standing posture and the problems of available postural supports in standing, Green *et al.*, 1993 identified the therapeutic requirements in standing needed to provide a normal standing posture, allowing the child to move within his base of support before moving out of it. The Chailey Standing Support, (Figure 8.9) was then developed by these researchers to meet those requirements.

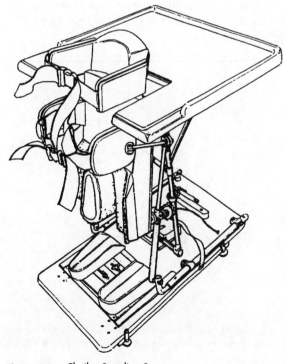

Figure 8.9 Chailey Standing Support

Equipment for play, coordination and balance

Rolls

Description

Rolls come in a variety of colours, lengths and diameters. They are made of combustion-modified foam with flame-retardant covers made of tough reinforced polyester, or vinyl. Rollers with a flat bottom are also available.

Note: When a child straddles a roll, if he does so with his legs flexed and adducted, hips internally rotated with his feet plantar flexed, this indicates that the **diameter** of the roll is too large.

Suggested uses

A roll can be used with a child lying on his tummy or straddling it to facilitate postural alignment, trunk rotation and balance reactions. As a roll only moves in one plane, unlike a therapy ball that moves in a frontal and lateral plane, some children find it easier to work first on a roll (Figure 8.10). Other ways in which a roll can be used for play activities are illustrated in the following chapters.

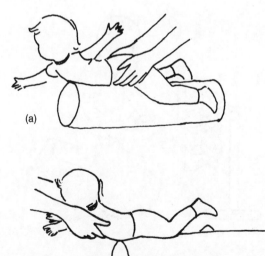

(a)

(b)

Figure 8.10 (a, b) Starting to facilitate balance reactions in the prone position

Inflatable therapy balls

Description

These balls can be purchased in a wide range of colours and sizes, and in varying diameters. All are covered in wipe-clean materials. Included in the Ayres Collection (Mike Ayres and Co.) is a Sensoball, which has a bobbly textured surface giving a child additional tactile experience.

Suggested uses

Therapy balls are used to increase movement experiences, facilitate weight shift and balance reactions in prone lying, sitting, standing and walking. A good way of introducing young children to being moved is to sit on a small ball one-self with the child on your lap. Figure 8.11 (a, b) illustrates ideas for using a SMALL ball for balance and play, with a young child with moderate spasticity, and Figure 8.12 (a–d) with an older child.

Note: Only use a small ball with young children and **never** allow a child to lie or sit on a ball unless you are present to supervise.

When using a ball that needs to be inflated, **always see that it is firm**. If it is allowed to become soft, the child will just sink into it, and the purpose for which they were intended, i.e. to facilitate balance reactions, will be lost.

Simple equipment for babies and young children

Hammocks/cut-out foam wedge

Description

When buying a hammock, get one made of sail-cloth, reinforced cotton or a similar material, as a baby's hands can so easily become entangled in those made of open mesh.

Figure 8.13 illustrates a design for making a hammock. If needed, extra pockets can be made for a firm pillow to put behind the head and under the knees to prevent the baby from slipping down. The hammock can be made firmer by insetting small wooden rods into pleats at the top and the bottom.

A hammock can be suspended between the uprights of a cot, or at about a metre from the ground, between the lintel of the door posts or two trees in the garden. Great care should always be taken to see that it is fixed securely and safely (Figure 8.14a, b).

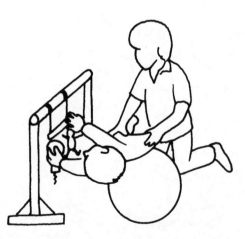 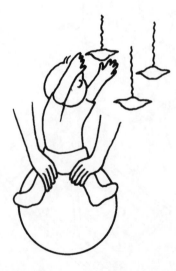

Figure 8.11   (a) A mother uses the movement of the ball to encourage her son to lift his head and rotate his trunk as he reaches towards his toys – helping him by stabilizing his trunk and keeping his legs apart. This is a pattern of movement he will use later when he starts to roll over.
   (b) Here, the ball is used to facilitate weight shift and balance as the child plays

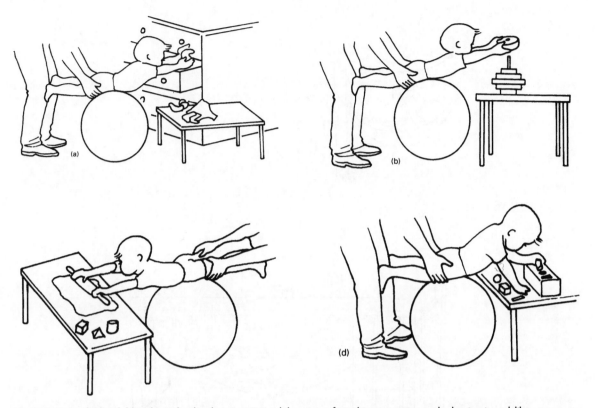

Figure 8.12   (a–d) The child in these sketches has just attained the stage of reaching, grasping and releasing in a deliberate manner when lying on his tummy. His mother stabilizes his pelvis, his feet flat against her legs, helping her son keep his head up and back extended while he plays

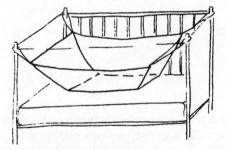

Figure 8.13   Design for a hammock

- minimizes any tendency to extend
- brings the head into mid-line
- brings the shoulder and pelvic girdles into alignment
- brings the shoulders and arms forward, hands in mid-line
- brings the baby's hands and later his feet into his visual field.

Figure 8.15 illustrates a cut-out foam section in the shape of a hammock, which we have found gives a young child similar support.

The support given by both a hammock and cut-out foam:

Suggested uses

Both hammocks and cut-out foam wedges can be used to facilitate the development of visual awareness, mid-line play, eye–hand coordination, and early reach and grasp. All theses aspects are discussed in greater detail in the following chapters.

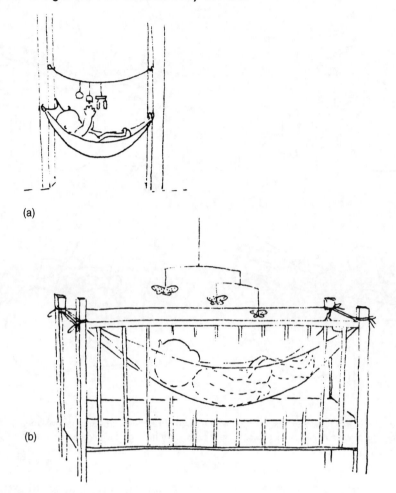

(a)

(b)

Figure 8.14 (a) Slung between the door posts when you are working near by. (b) When a baby is resting during the daytime

Note: A baby should not be put in a hammock during the day unless an adult is nearby, or to sleep in at night time.

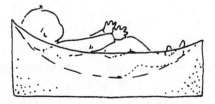

Figure 8.15   Foam section cut out to provide a hammock shape

Since all 'therapeutic' equipment is prescribed for a specific purpose, as your child becomes more competent your therapist will check to see if he is as able out of the equipment as he is with the support it provides, or perhaps whether any modifications need to be made.

When speaking of equipment for a baby we should not of course forget **ourselves**: our laps make a soft but firm stable base, we can use our hands for additional postural support, our legs make excellent rolls, we can act as a wedge and provide a movable surface.

Part III
Integration of treatment and handling

Chapter 9

The parents' contribution to early learning

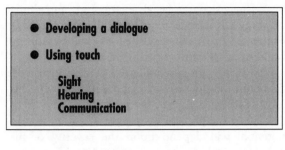

- Developing a dialogue
- Using touch

  Sight
  Hearing
  Communication

It is universally recognized that parents have an important role as educators of their child, especially during the early formative years. In this chapter we will look at the ways in which a baby learns during the early months, with particular reference to the part that his mother plays in this early learning process while she tends to his needs throughout the day. This is a time during which a partnership develops between mother and baby, providing both with an opportunity to share and learn together, each guiding and modifying the growth of the other.

A dialogue develops very early on between a mother and her baby while she feeds, baths, changes diapers, dresses, undresses and carries him. As she handles him she automatically gives him visual, tactile and auditory clues. Later, in everyday routine situations, she will encourage her child to develop functional and communication skills, all of which will be based on this fabric of early learning, part of one skill being integrated with another until a more complex task is achieved.

Naturally she is not alone in this task for although a father's interaction is different from a mother's, and that of siblings and other family members, each in their own way provide opportunities and encouragement for learning. It is through continuous and progressive interaction with his parents and various other members of the family, in secure and familiar surroundings, that a child learns and grows, experimenting and

practising new abilities and skills while at the same time maturing both emotionally and socially.

Clearly the baby or child with cerebral palsy is just as dependent on this early learning/interaction, but his movement disorder and abnormal responses may interfere with the natural process, creating barriers to learning basic skills. It is also possible that sometimes the apparent emphasis on the movement aspects of his development may mask or detract from the importance of other aspects of early learning.

In the following paragraphs I have outlined how a mother normally interacts with her baby and in later chapters discuss how this is integrated with handling techniques in the total management of the child with cerebral palsy.

It is generally accepted that all babies at birth share common characteristics on which future personality and attainment will be based, that is to say, while every baby is born with the capacity to learn, his rate of development is influenced to a certain extent by his personality. Some babies are vigorous and active, others placid and slow, each progressing at his own pace, with considerable variation in motivation and drive.

The baby with cerebral palsy, although he shares these same common characteristics, will most probably lack the spontaneous behaviour and ability necessary to interact as positively with his mother and the environment. His mother therefore will need to be aware of how much handling her baby can tolerate, and guided by his visual signals, facial expression and body movements balance more carefully the intensity of her input. In this way she, too, will be able to build up a social ritual with her baby.

The baby with cerebral palsy is also born with the same ability to learn and interact with his mother during routine situations as any other child, but the pace of his progress and his future potential will depend upon the severity of his handicap, including any associated problems that may be present. He will need help for a longer period of time in organizing his movements, and any sensory input will have to be timed and graded more carefully, while his reactions are carefully monitored.

After a few weeks of repeating the same procedure day after day, every mother develops a routine and a method of handling her baby. This will be one that she feels most comfortable with and meets the needs of her baby.

As so much of a baby's learning is dependent upon the early interaction and dialogue that exists between himself and his mother as she sees to his daily needs, it follows logically that **any treatment/management programme for the baby with cerebral palsy should be incorporated into this daily routine**. Working in this way has advantages for both mother and baby, giving her the opportunity to **combine** specific techniques of handling with her own mothering skills. The baby, as he is handled and moved, becomes aware of his body parts, as he feels pressure through his skin, muscles and joints in different positions, and later learns to orientate himself in space. As this sensory input is vital if the baby is to progress smoothly from gross activities to fine motor skills, I thought that it might be helpful to the reader if we looked briefly at a mother's role in providing sensory input during the early months. For the sake of clarity I have separated discussion of the different sensory inputs from the development of the motor system. It should be emphasized, however, that in function **the sensory motor systems are inseparably linked**. That is to say, interacting one with the other they enable the baby to become mobile against gravity and finally to attain an upright position and use his hands for functional activities.

How does a baby learn?

A baby learns by:

- touching
- looking
- listening and communicating.

Touching

The tactile system is one of the most mature systems the baby has at birth, providing him with a means of early communication with his mother, as he experiences the feeling of his body weight against her as she supports him. To begin with, most of a baby's reactions to sensory stimulation will be reflex in nature, some elicited automatically by his mother as she handles and moves him. If, for example, she touches the side or middle of his lips the baby moves towards the part that is stimulated; in this way he roots to find the nipple (rooting reflex). If a finger is placed in his mouth he sucks automatically (sucking reflex). If one strokes, or puts a finger in the palm of his hand, the feeling of touch and pressure will cause the baby to immediately close his fingers around it (hand grasp). See Chapter 5 for further information regarding these primitive reactions.

All babies vary in the type of tactile stimulation they enjoy. For example, some like the pressures and warmth of being cuddled and rocked, whereas others prefer the sensation of being gently stroked, a preference a mother recognizes early on, and so we see the beginnings of early social interaction emerging. When a baby has sufficient voluntary control to actively put his thumb or fingers into his mouth, he has for the first time a means of comforting himself as and when he pleases. He can suck his thumb or fingers to console himself when he is tired, unhappy or bored or, when happy and contented, to enjoy the sensory experience it gives him.

As soon as a baby is able to maintain his head in alignment with his body and has developed sufficient trunk and shoulder girdle stability, he is able to bring his arms forward off the support, and through tactile stimulation explore and become familiar with various parts of his body.

At first, he enjoys the tactile experience of clasping and unclasping his hands, pressing the palms together, moving his fingers and wrists, then putting his fingers back into his mouth to suck, although at this stage with hardly any visual attention. Gradually, as he becomes more competent visually, he starts to look at his hands as he moves them, initially holding them immediately in front of his face, then moving them away from himself, watching the movement of his fingers before sucking them once again. Although unable to reach and grasp a rattle, if one is put into his hand he is able to hold it, taking it immediately to his mouth to explore with his lips and tongue. The tactile stimulation of mouthing the rattle provides him with information regarding its texture and taste and at the same time gives him an opportunity to exercise the musculature of the oral area, developing patterns of movement that he will use later for eating and speech.

A baby also enjoys the sensation of rubbing one foot against the other and against various surfaces, and crossing and uncrossing his ankles, often rubbing one foot against the shin of the other leg, which serves a useful purpose, that of desensitizing the soles of his feet.

So we can see that although a baby's control over his voluntary movements is minimal, he is still able to build up an awareness of his body parts through the sensory experiences of touch and visual clues. As he gains more voluntary control and becomes more proficient at using his hands, further exploration will be possible. He becomes aware of how parts of his body relate to one another, and the relationship of himself in space and to objects around him. This eventually helps him to understand 'what is me' and 'what is not me'.

Looking

From his birth a mother gradually enters her baby's visual world, providing them both with an ideal opportunity to interact one with the other. Visual contact occurs at a distance of around 18–21 cm (7–8 in.) during these early weeks. The baby's most frequent visual contact with his mother at this time takes place during feeds, when from time to time he will pause between bursts of sucking and gaze at her intently, attracted by the variations of light and shade, her hair and facial outline, and in time being able to focus on other distinguishing features.

It takes a long time for a baby's eyes to develop physically; his first eye movements occur in response to changes in his position, as his mother sees to his daily needs. At first his eye movements lag behind those of his head, but in quite a short time they will adjust to both head and body movements, following the direction of the movement. The combination of touch, change in position and the visual cues he receives provide him with sensory information about any changes in his position that takes place.

During the early weeks, when placed on his back a baby often lies with his head turned to the side, his arms in a 'fencing' position, which is a position imposed on him by one of the primitive reactions (asymmetrical tonic neck reaction), a posture that from time to time brings the baby's hand into his field of vision (see primitive reactions in Chapter 5).

As his head becomes steadier, the baby begins to fixate on a stationary object and research has shown that at this time he responds more readily to black and white, and shades of dark and light, rather than colours, and to simple designs rather than complex ones. When he first starts to scan he does so by moving his head and his eyes together, his eyes moving in rather a jerky manner, at first horizontally then vertically, as he selects what holds his attention. Finally his visual organization is such that he is able to track a moving object. As his eye sensitivity increases and he starts to accommodate to distance, he becomes competent at picking out details of people and objects at a distance.

It is well known that babies reach out with their eyes long before they have the ability to reach out with their hands to grasp, so the choice of cot toys are important, and is discussed in the early stages of hand function, Chapter 7.

When a baby first starts to smile, a new and exciting dialogue develops between mother and baby, through turn-taking. Fascinated by his mother's face, the baby at this stage rather than looking at one feature as he did previously, will look up and down repeatedly from her hairline to her smiling mouth, her eyes and chin.

As she speaks to him, he responds by smiling, cooing, shouting and wriggling, at first moving his hands and fingers, later with 'signalling' movements of his arms which take on a repetitive pattern in a rhythm of bursts and pauses. Studies have shown that during this time of pre-speech and vocalization, not only are there movements of the head and whole body but more complex movements of the fingers which include pointing of the index finger. This type of behaviour is in contrast to the stillness of his posture and the seriousness of his expression when looking at a stationary object. With the development of head control the baby now has the ability to avert his gaze at will, and so becomes an active partner in this social play. **This non-verbal communication forms the basis of an important two-way relationship between mother and baby.**

As the link between auditory and visual stimuli develops he will begin to recognize that voices and faces go together, that father and mother look and sound different and that both differ from strangers. His dialogue with adults will rapidly grow and change in character, as we will see when discussing the beginnings of communication in the next section.

Listening and communicating

Following studies of the various of ways in which a baby reacts to sound from an early age, it has been established that he is able to distinguish between the sounds he hears. While he will remain calm and still when spoken to softly in short repetitive sentences, changes in levels of sound and very high or low sounds will startle him or make him cry. Continuous gentle sounds or singing, on the other hand, he will find comforting.

At first, the baby enjoys repeating the sounds he makes and begins to imitate the sounds of his mother and other adults. He then learns how to both start and end a 'conversation' at will, by remaining still and silent or, as we mentioned ear-

lier, by just looking away, perhaps reminding us that the art of communication is to be a good listener! These early 'conversations' normally start as a result of the baby's spontaneous behaviour, with his mother's coming in to support and elaborate his responses and then waiting for him to resume. In this way a rhythm of turn-taking takes place, the baby now having a means of being an active participant in the dialogue, and by his response it is clear that at this stage **his preference** is for his mother to imitate the sounds **he** makes. A favourite pastime at this stage is copying and 'blowing raspberries' which he soon becomes adept at using as a ploy to attract attention.

Although joining in and interacting well with his mother at this time, he will not necessarily be looking at her while she is speaking, and will be around 2 years of age before visual and vocal activities are well coordinated.

As the baby develops sufficient inhibition to remain still and pay attention, and has an understanding of what comes next, anticipatory games such as 'Round and round the garden', 'This little piggy goes to market' and 'Pop goes the weasel' becomes his favourites. The baby enjoys the sound and rhythm of these songs, responding by smiling and gurgling and shouting, and later clapping his hands, encouraging us to repeat the game.

In the beginning the dialogue between a mother and her baby will obviously be one-sided, her conversation directed 'at him', often interpreting how he feels in different situations. For example, expecting him to anticipate what is going to happen as she prepares his bottle: 'You know what is going to happen next'. Wanting his bath to be a happy experience, she will say, 'This is fun, now is the time to kick and splash'. Well aware that he is going to scream when she cleans his ears, she says, 'You don't like this bit'. A few months later her response to the same situation has changed to 'It was not so awful was it?'. As soon as she is free of the responsibility of moving her baby from one position to another and no longer has to support him when he sits, she directs his behaviour using verbal control, urging him to cooperate, at first by gesture and speech and then by speech alone. For example, 'Lift up your arms so I can take your sweater off', 'Push your foot into your shoe', 'Hold on tight and you won't fall', 'Let go of the flannel so I can wash your face', 'Sit still while I zip up your jacket'.

I have emphasized the importance of early communication, as not only does it play an important role in the baby's social development, but **speech is also an important tool for organizing and reinforcing movement**, often used by a child later when learning new skills. When a child has cerebral palsy, this is an area that can so easily be ignored during his early years, either because we feel that he does not understand and we become frustrated because progress is so slow, or we feel that we must concentrate all our efforts on helping him to move. However, as stated above, speech is a very useful tool in learning motor tasks.

But if a child with cerebral palsy does not have the opportunity to listen to speech and be spoken to throughout the day, how is he ever going to learn to imitate speech and expand his language experiences? Different facets of language and communication skills **should not be in addition to, but part of** any child's treatment/management programme introduced throughout the day and in various situations. Your speech and language therapist will of course advise you on the basic skills necessary at the different stages in your child's development, and in the event that your child has a particular problem with speech, feeding, or language development she will provide specific advice and treatment.

Summary

In this chapter I have tried to illustrate how the naturally occurring sensory inputs of touching, looking and listening are used by the baby as building blocks in the development of gross and fine motor skills, each of these interlocking with the other and with the development of the motor system so that the child continually expands his sphere of competence. I have also tried to show the new parent how to make the most of each opportunity as it is presented throughout each and every day.

In later chapters on dressing, bathing and all the other routine repetitive activities of daily life, this theme is repeated and the specific ways of modifying normal handling to help the child with cerebral palsy make the most of this learning experience are described.

Chapter 10

Speech

Helen A. Mueller

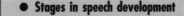

- Stages in speech development
- Problems
- Handling
- Early cooperation

Some major stages in speech development

The newborn expresses his needs through body movements, facial expression and crying. These first sounds are totally nasal and monotonous at the beginning. Soon incidental sounds can be heard when the baby is moving, e.g. kicking, feeding or even falling asleep; he can hear the vowels and intonation of our speech, although in a very limited way.

During the third month when making 'happy' sounds, his voice becomes less nasal and is produced more through his mouth, whereas crying or whining will remain nasal. Throaty sounds begin while the baby is lying mainly on his back.

At about four months the baby will start repetitive babbling, especially when he is left alone. This means that the sounds he is making are no longer purely accidental; it will be noticed that lip sounds occur more frequently when he turns onto his tummy. He will now start to turn to the source of the noise or sound and try to watch the mouth of the adult who is speaking.

At about 6 months, when the baby progresses to sitting and begins to chew (see Chapter 18 on feeding), lip and tongue sounds start to develop and rhythmical repetitions are more frequent, and in this way chains of syllables are formed. Hearing is more differentiated and includes high frequencies, for example consonants.

At about 8 months these syllable chains start to become more organized, i.e. broken up into single and double syllables such as 'ba-ba' and reversed – 'a-ba'. The variations in pitch and volume increase and a lot of self-imitation can be heard. In effect, the first little dialogue takes place.

From 9 months onwards, the first meaningful words are being used, even double syllabled words such as 'Mama', and imitation of rhythmical sounds combined with movement starts.

At about 1 year old the baby begins to understand such constantly used expressions as 'give it to Mummy', particularly if the sounds are accompanied by gestures; he will begin to imitate adult speech by its intonation and thus starts his baby language.

Approaching the end of the second year, he will start to drop this baby language and will try to express himself by combining two words and eventually three-word phrases, but we must remember that at this time his understanding of language is far greater than his ability to express himself verbally. This accounts for the stuttering so often experienced between the age of 2 and 3 years and which will be overcome with increasing use of the speech apparatus; it is most important that parents should recognize this and carefully avoid paying any real attention to it, as it is merely an interim stage in progress towards speech.

At 3 years of age the child begins to start putting together simple sentences and is able to dissociate speech from gestures although, to a limited extent, facial expressions and physical gestures generally accompany speech.

When we consider these developmental stages certain conclusions can be reached:

- that speech develops out of movement and human contact.
- that body movements and sound production are linked in early infancy – later of course the child has sufficient control to hide his feelings and keep a straight face when speaking.
- that the foundations of speech are laid in infancy.
- that speech development does not start when the child says his first words, but is dependent upon contact and the stimulations arising from his surroundings from birth onwards.

These facts must guide us when we are dealing with the speech problems of the child with cerebral palsy.

When a child has a motor handicap, his tools of speech, breathing, voice and articulation, facial expression and gestures will also frequently be involved and sensory input is more or less limited, which then reflects in language development.

Speech and the child with cerebral palsy

When a parent speaks to a child who is spastic or ataxic the child will be slow in making any sound or assuming any facial expression; the athetoid child, however, will have almost an excess of facial expression – grimacing and often an extreme of pitch and loudness in his voice. Each of these reactions is unusual and therefore strange to us and we are inclined to interpret them as indicating a lack of understanding or of intelligence; very likely we then give up trying to communicate with him or confine our talking to a minimum, probably thinking 'he does not seem to understand anyway'. By our reactions we are depriving the child of some of the most important stimulations, without which he cannot develop his language ability, involving thought patterns, speech and language.

If, on the other hand, the child shows no signs of any reaction to sounds and noises and you begin to be doubtful about his hearing ability, do not hesitate to take him to your doctor. In those rare cases where there is the possibility of hearing defect, early detection and training are of the utmost importance for language and speech development.

Preparation for speech

If you handle your child as advised in the preceding chapters you will be helping him to improve his head and trunk control and at the same time helping him towards better feeding, thus giving him largely what he needs for the development of speech, i.e. an almost normal breathing pattern, coordination of the movements of his mouth and tongue and the possibility of making sounds without extra effort, leading to reasonably effortless articulation.

As in most other activities, the child with cerebral palsy should be in a stable position and one which will not allow any grossly abnormal patterns to occur. Figure 10.1 shows a suitable position for a young child. Since we all make use of other senses in communication, such as lip-reading when we are listening to someone, your position when you are talking to the child is most important, for example, handling him in such a way that he has good head control. Always try to be in front of him at his eye-level, or slightly lower, so that he does not have to look up to you as this will probably throw him into a pattern of hyperextension;

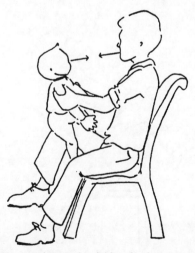

Figure 10.1 Speaking to the child so that he can watch your mouth without having to look up and controlling him from his upper arms or shoulders for a good head position

breathing and the effort to speak tend to cause this movement anyway, so guard against it by sitting or squatting down at the child's level (Figure 10.2b). You can also help your child before he gets ready to make sounds by controlling him from a suitable 'key-point' (see Chapter 6 on basic principles of handling), thus facilitating babbling or speech.

For speech and babbling the baby needs to have delicate, coordinated movements of his lips, mouth and tongue; if these continue to function abnormally, oral control (see Figure 18.5, later) might be found helpful – with a baby this might consist of lip and tongue play to induce babbling in positions, such as those shown in Figures 18.1 and 18.2, in the chapter on feeding. Demonstrate with your own mouth and voice while you stroke lightly his upper or lower lip or move his tongue sideways or, with light control of his jaws, open and close his mouth to obtain chains of sounds such as 'ababa, bababa', etc. Never try to practise single sounds or certain mouth positions, as that would be unnatural and would tend to increase the child's tendency to block and get 'stuck'; these little babbling plays should be pleasant and short; at the same time we must remember that while results should be anticipated, we must not expect the child to succeed on the first occasion in imitating perfectly the sounds that you are making.

Some common problems

When your child reaches the age when specific sounds need to be made or, having been made, need to be corrected, do not tell or show him what or how to do it, nor expect him to learn from trying in front of a mirror, as his brain damage prevents him from translating auditory or visual commands (especially when they are 'mirror-like') into the correct movements.

It is important to remember that we should never practise isolated sounds with a child with cerebral palsy. We must not forget that it is not lack of intelligence or effort which prevents the child from speaking correctly but that his difficulties are due to his **sensorimotor involvement**. Undue persistence in our efforts will only increase the child's frustration by reinforcing his already frequent experiences of failure; you are performing a much more useful service by helping him to facilitate the necessary movements. This is admittedly a difficult undertaking when we consider the precision, fluency and speed of the movements necessary to produce articulate speech. In some

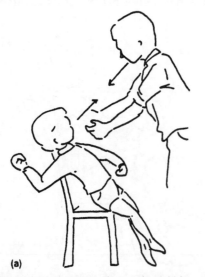

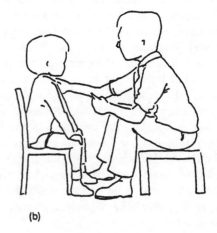

(a)

(b)

Figure 10.2 (a) *Wrong*. Speaking to the child from above throws him into an extensor pattern, making phonation difficult.

(b) *Right*. Speaking to the child at the same eye-level, helping him with head control from his shoulder or upper arm or by pressure on his lower chest with your flat hand

cases of course it may be essential to seek the assistance of a speech therapist.

Speech problems caused by abnormal breathing cannot be corrected through 'blowing' exercises, as these would only increase spasticity and in such cases it is advisable to consult your physiotherapist or your speech therapist.

If the child's voice is weak it is not a good idea to tell him to speak louder, as he can only do so with great effort and this will merely mean an increase in spasticity. Aim rather for better trunk and head control, as this may help his breathing and in turn should improve the volume of his voice. An open mouth is always a passive mouth, whether it is due to hyperextension or lack of muscle tone, and you will need the help of your physiotherapist or speech therapist to deal with this problem. You can practise mouth closure at home, during mealtimes and sleeping times while watching for good head control. Pressure above the upper lip, back, not down (see Chapter 18 on feeding), can be applied in between times, or you can stroke his lower lip two or three times; there is no need to say anything when you are doing this. Remember that mouth closure is essential for breathing through the nose, and for swallowing, articulation, dental health and dental occlusion.

Mouth closing will not improve by continually telling the child to keep his mouth closed and must be treated as part of his overall disability. Thumb-sucking will certainly counteract your efforts and, if it is essential, should be replaced by a 'dummy' as this, of course, can be discarded so much more easily in the very early stages of its use. A helpful method is to try to direct the child's interest towards a toy, or some absorbing activity which might be going on around him. Mouthing (experimenting with hands and objects at and in the mouth) is an entirely different thing and most certainly has its place in the development of speech; it represents an important sensorimotor experience and should be encouraged in the young handicapped baby (see Chapter 18).

Remember that all these preparations for speaking must be integrated into the daily life of a child in early infancy, in the hopes that when he is ready to talk, what we have described as his 'speech tools' will be available and under reasonable control.

Sensory input

It has already been pointed out that the baby receives and takes in speech, including facial expressions and gestures, with all his senses, not merely that of hearing. Because of his motor problems your baby may be deprived of part of these sensory experiences, and therefore you will have to try to bring them to him; do not, however, bombard him with sensory stimuli as a young child's perception is not yet organized, i.e. is not yet able to distinguish the important from the unimportant, or to put things into proper sequence. The brain-damaged child might be slow in maturation of perception anyway, and if, in your natural anxiety, the rate of progress you wish him to make is too fast, he will merely become frustrated, retire into himself, or lose interest altogether.

A baby learns and forms concepts by mouthing, handling, manipulating, playing and listening to your talking about the objects you are showing him. Use the parts of his body, simple elementary toys, the things that you use when feeding, bathing, dressing him and so on. Do not expect the young child to maintain his interest and to want to take part in such play for more than a short time, nor expect any immediate verbal reaction from him, let alone imitation of your talking – stop while he still has fun and he will be eager to go on the next time.

It is normal for a young child just to listen, watch, manipulate and even laugh, but not 'say' anything until possibly many days later. As play is the form in which he will absorb and learn during the first few years of his life, make the occasion one of play rather than a teaching situation, use objects of different colours, shapes, textures and sounds, even tastes and temperatures; name each of them and talk a little about them and what they are used for; **all this will help to develop the sensory avenues which are necessary for the formation of language**.

Rhythm plays an important part in the early stages of development; therefore, for the child with cerebral palsy, reinforce rhythmical verbal play with rhythmical body movements, e.g. clapping hands. This is an essential activity if the child is to learn to use his hands independently of each other. Later on, of course, nursery rhymes with suitable actions and words should be introduced.

Attempting speech

When the child attempts babbling or speech but without very much success, all the joy will be taken out of it for him if you try immediately to correct his attempts; **remember that it normally takes a child about 5 years to reach a reasonable level of speech**. The pleasure of playing with speech is a very important factor in speech development and must be taken into account. Let the child play with speech, let him experiment before trying to help him, but be careful, however, not to become too excited at his first successful attempts and not to start urging him to repeat; too much fuss makes a child withdraw just as easily as neglect or constant correction.

Look upon his efforts to speak as being normal and let him see by experience that speech in day-to-day living is necessary and of course interesting.

Gestures

During the first year of life, gestures are essential. When you go about your daily activities speak to your child mainly about those activities that directly concern him; name objects first, then the verbs for the activities and so on and eventually construct little sentences. We must not, however, run the risk of overemphasizing the importance of gestures as otherwise the child might not develop beyond them either on the receptive or the expressive side; the danger would then be that he would never learn to dissociate language from gesture.

We must give the handicapped child plenty of opportunity to express himself, no matter how fragmentary or unsuccessful his first attempts may prove to be. If we keep reading every need or wish from the expression in his eyes or from his gestures; if we answer every question for him; if we always speak for him – he will have no need or incentive whatsoever to talk and the valuable and sensitive phase for the development of speech will pass unused. Ask him simple questions, letting him feel by your intonation and facial expressions that you expect a reply and one that lies within his mental and verbal capacity. Ignore his gesturing or nodding of the head more and more and, this is most important, do not forget to be patient in waiting for his answers, as they will often be slow and delayed in coming.

Personal interaction

We hope that what we have said will leave you in no doubt as to the importance of close contact between yourself and your child, as you help him to build up 'inner language' which is so essential for his future speech development. Television, radio, discs, tapes and so on, however excellent their presentation, have only a very limited value and place in the child's speech development and can never replace personal contact as you help your child build up his vocabulary. For example, while reading a book do so by speaking slowly, explaining any new words, stopping frequently to repeat and explain their meaning – personal touches that are so important but impossible when technical devices are used.

In our efforts to help the child to form concepts, we should start by teaching him about his own body, the objects around him in his cot, his playpen and so on, by these means gradually widening his horizon by talking about familiar objects he knows and uses in his room. Later take him to the window and talk about the familiar scene outside, let him see the postman coming in to deliver the letters, the milkman with the milk and so forth. He should then be ready to look at the first simple picture books representing objects with which he is familiar, and from these he can go on to pictures that represent everyday simple situations.

When choosing books be sure to take the child's limited experience into account. A child who is fairly immobile or has, for example, never been to the country cannot be expected to recognize the farm animals in the pictures he is shown.

Choose books carefully, finding ways and means to enlarge the child's world despite his physical handicap. When you show him things in the picture books, name them, talk about their use, their special characteristics, their colours and so on, gradually introducing nouns, adjectives and verbs. Remember, however, that this cannot be done all at once. Later, as he progresses, a children's picture dictionary may be found useful. Have short pleasant sessions and you will find that the child himself will keep asking to look at the pictures over and over again; 'feed' him little at one time so that he can absorb and stay interested.

The age at which articulation of a specific consonant, or the use of the first word emerges, must never be of primary concern to us, as it is known that it differs greatly among children. Remember that what will really count in the future of the child with cerebral palsy is not merely perfect articulation, but the ability to use language and thus be able to speak and express himself without undue physical effort and tenseness and in this way being easily and clearly understood.

I have tried in this chapter to stress the importance of **early sensorimotor preparation** and the part the parent can play in helping the child towards effective speech. 'Augmentative communication' might become necessary or helpful for your child. For advice on the best possible choice, right time, careful introduction and practice, as well as individual adjustments on technical devices, consult your specialized speech therapist (see Chapter 11 on communication and technology).

Chapter 11

Communication and technology

Marian Browne

- Communication skills
- Augmentative communication systems
- Technology in communication
- Practising augmentative communication

Developing communication skills

Communication is fundamental to every aspect of human life. The need for easy communication is basic to healthy social, emotional and cognitive development. Every child should be able to express himself quickly and clearly with as little effort as possible. The young child with cerebral palsy frequently grows up understanding more than he is able to express through speech or actions as a result of impairment of motor skills. This discrepancy often increases as the child grows and develops skills of understanding, while the ability to talk lags far behind.

Speech development often begins late and develops relatively slowly in children with cerebral palsy. All those who are at risk of speech problems therefore benefit from the introduction of alternatives, or strategies which can be used in combination with speech, to help them express themselves. Development of general communication skills can also be encouraged at a very early stage – often this is before we know the extent to which articulation may be impaired. If a child does not attain intelligible speech, then no time has been lost in providing alternative or supplementary means of expression.

The contribution of technology

Developments in technology have made it increasingly possible to reduce the disparity between understanding and expression. Computers can now be controlled through use of the slightest movement – even, for example, movements of the eyes, or a light touch of a finger. As computers have become more compact, so a wide range of aids have become available for use as a means of communication. These developments have added to the now well-established use of computers in the classroom and at home as a means of writing and learning.

Augmentative communication systems

Speech and non-verbal aspects of communication

Communication is a complex process and involves many skills. Speech is just one component that we use in combination with many others to convey our 'message'. The use of eye contact, eye movements, facial expressions, gesture and body posture all play a vital role in relaying information. Developing these 'non-verbal' skills with the combined help of a physiotherapist and speech and language therapist can bring tremendous gains in expression.

Signs and symbols

For many children with cerebral palsy, an additional specialized means of expression is required.

This is called an 'augmentative communication system'. It may be a 'manual' system, entailing the use of gestures or signs, or it may be 'graphic', involving pictures or symbols to which a child can point. Manual systems (sign languages) are commonly taught by a speech and language therapist and have the advantage of being free of equipment. They do nevertheless require a 'listener' to know the system and this may present a problem to children who have many friends and relations who may not be able or willing to learn sign language.

Children with cerebral palsy more frequently benefit from the use of graphic communication systems because impaired control of hand movements makes the use of signs very difficult. There are a number of graphic systems, ranging from simple line drawings or photographs, to complex symbols (such as Blissymbols) which give the user the potential to say anything with only a limited symbolic 'alphabet'. A combination of signs and symbols is used by many to make communication as easy as possible in any given situation. It may, for example, be quicker to use signs at home, but in the classroom a picture or symbol system may be needed to 'talk' to other children (Figure 11.1)

Supplementing speech

The use of speech can be very frustrating indeed for some children with cerebral palsy. The harder the child with spasticity tries to say something, the stiffer he becomes and the more his voice may elude him. Repeated attempts at the same word may become less and less clear. For the child who has involuntary movements (athetosis), the effort to speak may unbalance him and give rise to even more movements which he cannot control and which make talking even more difficult. Many children therefore benefit from an augmentative system for use in situations where they know talking will be difficult. The very presence of such an 'augmentative' strategy may so relieve the pressure on speech that less effort is used and speech production thereby becomes more successful.

Encouraging speech to develop

Experience has taught us that any means to enable us to communicate more effectively is 'self-reinforcing'. A child who finds that by pointing to a symbol he can choose a game will naturally want to use this strategy to indicate preferences in other situations. Research has demonstrated that children who use augmentative communication systems are less frustrated and more successful in education than those who have no effective means of expression. Far from discouraging the use of speech as many parents fear, augmentative systems have been found to have the opposite effect.

Early intervention

Poor communication skills interfere with social and emotional aspects of development. Many children become passive as a result of communication impairment. Children should be able to express themselves as young as possible, so that during early formative years they can participate more fully in social interaction. Even before their first birthday, and before reliable assessment of understanding is possible, children may be encouraged to point with their hand or eyes to the toy they would like to play with for example. Through the experience of being offered choices, children quickly learn how their preferences may be expressed.

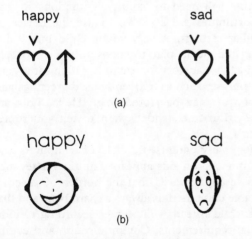

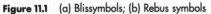

Figure 11.1 (a) Blissymbols; (b) Rebus symbols

Communication through technology – who can benefit?

The field of technology is expanding constantly. Computers can be operated by increasingly ingenious means, making their use accessible to the majority of children with cerebral palsy. For those whose hand function is too restricted to use a conventional keyboard, access to communication aids and computers may be achieved through the use of switches or adapted keyboards.

For many young children with severe levels of disability, the use of a switch provides a means through which movements can be used to control the environment. This idea of 'cause and effect' is the basis of early communication. A child may learn, for example, that 'when I move my arm, the music always comes on'. Once this basic idea has been grasped, then the activity can be developed. A child may turn his head one way to turn some music on, for example, and the other way to touch a switch that activates another toy.

Electronic communication aids

The use of electronic communication aids provides the opportunity of 'talking' through the recorded (digitized) speech of another person, or through electronically synthesized speech. This may open up many new possibilities such as talking on the telephone, interrupting others or speaking to a whole group of people at once. It does not matter if a child is unable to read, for messages may be stored and recalled through pictures or symbols. Electronic aids can therefore be introduced to children of pre-school age, and of a whole range of learning abilities (Figure 11.2). They will, however, never totally replace the use of 'low tech.' communication systems. The need for battery recharging and the occurrence of temporary technical faults all mean that a back-up will always be necessary.

Writing and talking

It is common for parents to assume that a child who can learn to read and spell will have no need for an augmentative communication system. Writing and talking are very different, however, and everybody has a need for both. Written language is highly structured and follows precisely the rules of grammar to ensure that the intended meaning is conveyed without ambiguity. Speech, however, is much less rigidly structured, for the speaker has at his disposal the use of gesture, facial expression and intonation to help convey his message efficiently. The child with cerebral palsy needs to be able to write, but he also needs a sign or symbol system to enable him to communicate more quickly and easily in conversation.

Choosing a communication aid

The decision to select a communication aid is usually made with the help of a specialized team. The choice is always to some extent a personal one. It will also depend on whether the aid will be used as a main means of 'talking', or as a supplement to another means. There are a number of Communication Aid Centres where children may be assessed by a team of professionals and where they may try different means of accessing a computer, a selection of software, and communication aids. Children may be referred to such a centre by a teacher or a therapist, or by parents.

Extensive practice and advice from a speech and language therapist is needed to become confident in using a communication aid socially. Initially, parents will need to 'contrive' situations so that opportunities are available to use the device in familiar settings. A very young child may enjoy using the aid in play to choose a toy or to help read a familiar story for example. Often some general phrases such as frequently used greetings and responses may be stored (e.g. 'Hello, how are you?', 'I'm fine', and 'I want to tell you something').

For many parents, the field of computers and communication aids appears daunting. They may be assured, however, that the burden of selecting suitable equipment is always a shared one and that each child's needs will be met according to individual requirements. Communication and equipment needs will gradually change with time as

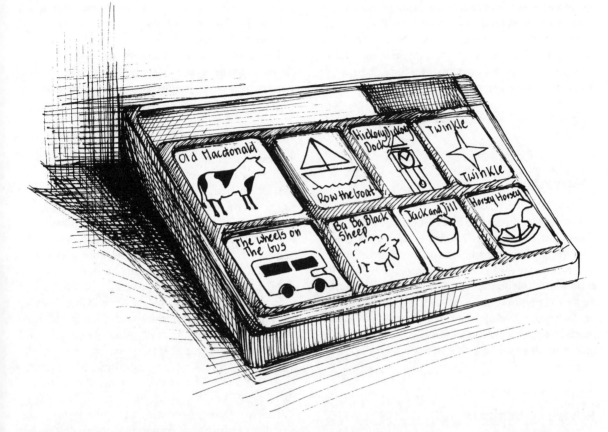

Figure 11.2 Alphatalker communication device. The child may press the appropriate picture to select a nursery rhyme to sing. Any song or message can be recorded into the device and appropriate pictures or symbols inserted for each child's individual use. Available from Liberator Ltd.

children encounter new challenges and as the picture of physical capabilities unfolds.

Other uses of technology

Early learning with a computer

Technological equipment has many applications for the child with cerebral palsy reaching beyond the areas of communication and literacy. The simple skill of controlling a switch can open the avenue to using a computer to assist in the learning of many concepts. There is now a range of software which can be of great value in learning early concepts such as shape, number, colour, positions

and spatial relationships, to name but a small selection.

More advanced uses of technology

The use of a switch can also be applied to controlling the movement of electric wheelchairs. 'Environmental control mechanisms' have also been available for some time. These are devices which may be linked to a computer, and which give a disabled person the possibility of turning on lights, the television or the video for instance.

The touch screen

A recent addition to our resources is the 'touch screen'. This is a frame that can be fitted around a computer and that enables a simple touch on the surface of the screen to activate a program. It has been found to provide an excellent means for helping children learn to look at their own hand movements (i.e. to develop eye–hand coordination) and to develop skills of visual perception through play. Touch screens are now in widespread use, and are often available in local clinics or schools.

Motivation

Communication should not be considered 'work'. Care should be taken to make 'talking' fun and rewarding. The use of electronic equipment is as much for play and entertainment as it is for education and independence. Its use must not be limited to supervised sessions with a parent, teacher or therapist. A child's own motivation to use a piece of equipment is perhaps the most important factor in determining the success of its application.

Where to begin

The starting point for every child is to make choices in everyday situations. At home, this may be done by showing him a choice of two things to play with. Present one toy at a time, and place them in front of him, one to each side. Ask your child to show you which one he wants to play with. He may do this by looking at one more than the other, by moving a hand towards it, or by smiling at it. Whichever toy you think he prefers, play with it immediately. Do not waste time by asking him to show you again because the message seemed unclear – this is frustrating for everyone. If your child has difficulty in controlling the movements of his eyes, he will be helped by providing support for his head in the mid-line.

Repeat this procedure in as many situations as possible, and your child will soon learn how to make you select the right toy. It is not important initially if he does not know the names of the toys

– by choosing and then playing, he will learn about the objects, and also become more confident in expressing himself.

There are many situations in which simple choices can be made: you can show your child a choice of two books to read, two tee-shirts to wear, different foods at teatime, and so on.

Introducing pictures

The next step may be to ask your child to make a choice by looking at photographs of two toys. In this way he can refer to things that may be out of sight. A simple book of photographs may be made up so that your child can have his 'communication pictures' with him at all times (Figure 11.3). To begin with he may only be able to choose between two pictures on each page, but he may soon progress to four pictures as control of hand or eye movements improves. He will probably love to have pictures of his family and friends to show other people. Parents and other caretakers will then need to create situations to provide the opportunity for using the communication pictures (e.g. 'Who would you like to read you a story?', 'Which toy would you like to bring to Nana's?').

The use of hand-pointing or 'eye-pointing' can also be reinforced in other games. In 'hide and seek', for example, a child may point (with a hand or by 'looking') to show somebody where a toy has been hidden, or to find an object in a very simple 'I spy' game ('I spy a teddy bear – can you find it?').

Using a switch

The first step in using a switch is to control a simple toy in play. This may be done even before a child is a year old. Several companies supply battery-operated toys specifically for use with a switch. A 'battery toy adapter' (a small disc attached to a socket which can be squeezed into the battery compartment) provides an inexpensive way of adapting any toy for use with a switch. Switches themselves can be reasonably purchased by mail order and have standard plugs (Figure 11.4).

Children can experiment with a switch and toy in play. By placing the switch in different posi-

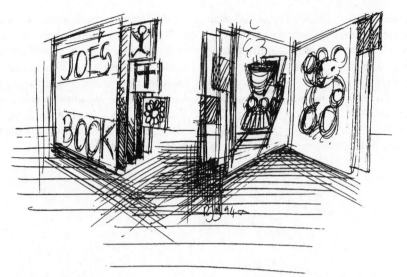

Figure 11.3 A simple picture communication book. The pictures are grouped in topics marked with tabs at the side of the pages. A child can choose a toy by pointing to the relevant picture

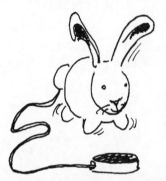

Figure 11.4 A toy rabbit operated by a Tash 'cap' switch (Technical Aids and Systems for the Handicapped Inc., Ontario, Canada)

tions, it is usually possible to work out where to secure it for easiest access and control. If a child is sitting, it is often helpful to place the switch on its side so it can be activated by a simple outward movement of a hand to the side – the switch may be stabilized against a flat surface by use of Velcro. For some children, supported side-lying (against the back of a sofa with a wedge, for example, or in a side-lying board) is the position in which they can most easily see and control the switch in front of them.

It is important not to reinforce movements which cause an increase in tone (make a child very stiff) or make him asymmetrical. With the excitement of controlling a toy, it is common for children with spasticity to become stiffer, but this must be minimized. A physiotherapist will be able to suggest ways in which this can be done. For many children the optimum position to use their arms or hands is when supported in a prone standing frame. In this position, try to ensure that the child's head stays in the mid-line so that he can see his hands and the toy without turning away. It may be helpful to support the head using 'oral control'.

The child with athetosis often experiences an increase in involuntary movements with effort and excitement. In this case the child can be assisted by holding his head and trunk stable so that he can see clearly, and begin to isolate the movement which controls the switch. Our aim is to find a movement that we are sure the child is controlling, and that is not happening 'by accident'.

Priorities for parents

Beyond the basic use of a switch in play, and of simple pictures for communication, the advice of an expert is very important. Our goal for every child is to enable him to attain the highest possible quality of life. Communication is fundamental in this; our physical, psychological, social and emotional wellbeing all depend on it. Therefore, it may perhaps be considered our most important goal for the child with cerebral palsy.

In working towards this end, there is no need to be deterred by our inability to predict exactly how well speech or motor skills will develop. We know that communication is self-reinforcing and that those children who communicate well via one means can readily adapt to changes that further broaden their communicative potential. 'Talking' should be fun for every child, and technology provides us with a variety of ways which can help us to reach our goal.

Chapter 12

Music and music therapy

Diana Thornton

- Sharing the language of music
- Music therapy
- Developing a music dialogue

Music

All of us are musical beings whether or not we consider ourselves to be gifted in this way. Imagine a baby's experience in the womb. For nine months he heard the rhythmical beating of his mother's heart; her breathing; her voice rising and falling in phrases and patterns and he felt the rhythmical movements of her body. He will also have heard the more chaotic sounds of digestion (and indigestion!) and of blood rushing, all syncopated against the strong heartbeat. The child is born well versed in the patterns of human rhythms, speeds, timings and phrases. He was already 'dancing' in the womb in time to music from outside his mother and it could be said that the basis of human artistic endeavour in the fields of dance and music is this common experience of life in the womb.

The relevance of this to you and your child is that you have a common language in music which you can share together. Many people are anxious about music, feeling that they are tone-deaf or that they simply do not know what to do. It may be that you have not thought of music on such a basic level before – I hope you are reassured of your capabilities.

Music may be used to amuse your child – allowing him to listen to tapes or the radio. It is far more beneficial, however, if it is used 'live' by you to add to your repertoire of games together and to enrich your interactions. If you know songs

and rhymes, use these (there are many available on cassettes which you could learn if you feel you do not know any suitable ones). Otherwise why not make up your own special songs? They need only be a few words long with a very simple tune, or you could put your own words to a tune you know. These could be used at special times; for example, you could have a bath song and a dressing song.

Such songs help you when you feel you are running out of original things to say. They may also help your child by exaggerating your words, phrases and patterns of speech. Songs may also give him a familiar landmark so that he knows what to expect. Humming to yourself is a way for a child with a visual defect to keep tabs on you if you are not directly involved with him.

Responding to the sounds your child makes is important in his development of communication skills and speech, as outlined elsewhere in this book. It may be that you will feel freer in imitating his vocal sounds, whatever they may be, and responding to him if you think of your responses as music rather than speech. Listen to the rhythms of his noises or watch his body rhythms. You can use both these as the basis for a game, tapping his rhythms back to him. You could clap or could tap the rhythm on the child's body or on his chair so that he feels the vibrations. Even a child with a hearing impairment will be aware of these vibrations and will enjoy rhythmic play. If your child is able to, you could set him up over a wedge with instruments or with an upturned plastic bowl to bang with a spoon – you do not need special equipment.

Different sounds can be explored by putting sand, lentils or beans into empty plastic bottles or balloons before you inflate them. Tie up bottle tops or scrunchy paper in a silk scarf for him to play with. Make sounds back to him with your voice or another 'instrument' so that you get a dialogue going. He may be slow and his rhythms uncontrolled, but it can be a most rewarding way of playing together.

Music therapy

Music therapy is a specialized way of interacting undertaken by a trained therapist using proper musical equipment. It is used with both adults and children who may have a wide variety of problems. The essence of the therapy lies in making music together. Using the child's sounds, rhythms and any sounds with instruments which he may be able to make, the therapist will build up an interaction and relationship with him. Because she will be a skilled musician, the therapist can use all of the child's tiniest signals as a musical cue. She will respond to these by singing or playing an instrument (e.g. the piano, clarinet or violin), or by playing some of the instruments set out for the child.

By responding to all of his actions as if they were intended and meaningful (e.g. stereotyped sounds or movements), the therapist may change the meaning of these actions for him. For instance, he may begin to use them to gain a response. This may increase his repertoire of communicative skills and change an unproductive action into a productive one. This is paralleled in normal child development. The child's use of the sound 'dadada' does not at first refer to 'Daddy' until it is given that meaning by those around him, who respond to it in that way. Similarly, a stereotyped action may become meaningful if responded to as having a musical meaning.

The musical dialogue which grows up between child and therapist may be the most prolonged and subtle interaction the child has taken part in. His experience of being physically disabled and having language difficulties may leave him excluded from many everyday interactions taking place around him. The music therapy may provide a bridge into any sense of isolation which this may cause.

The child can influence the music-making immediately, because the therapist responds to him at all times and changes her music accordingly. He will usually be well aware that the sounds the therapist makes are directly related to him. This can give him a great sense of potency and can be a most stimulating and exciting experience for him. Coupled with the sheer enjoyment which is usually part of music-making, music therapy is an activity in which children are often highly motivated. This is true whether their experience is primarily one of listening or of taking part more actively.

The music may help the child to organize his movements and the therapist may work particularly on helping his physical coordination (e.g. in beating a drum). She may also work on an emotional level. This may involve expressing feelings for the child in the music which he is not able to fully express for himself, or she may support him in expressing frustration, sadness or glee. This may give him a sense of being understood and of being able to share his feelings rather than being burdened with them, unable to share them successfully. The therapist may also listen to the child's sounds, observing their unique patterns and use them to help her understand his state of mind. She may talk to him about his feelings and put them into words as well as into music if this is appropriate.

If you are interested in music therapy for your child, it may be available at school or from a clinic. Otherwise contact the Association of Professional Music Therapists (see Appendix IV). Equivalent organizations exist in most countries.

Chapter 13

Play

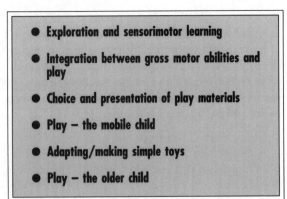

- ● Exploration and sensorimotor learning
- ● Integration between gross motor abilities and play
- ● Choice and presentation of play materials
- ● Play – the mobile child
- ● Adapting/making simple toys
- ● Play – the older child

It is mainly through play that a child learns during his early years. As previously discussed, a baby begins to learn about the world around him from what he hears, sees, touches and tastes, with his mother interacting with him and providing help only when needed. Once aware of himself, he learns about others in relation to himself. As eye–hand coordination develops he begins to explore objects around him: grasping and putting them into his mouth, he starts to become aware of their shape and texture, that some taste pleasant while others are unpleasant.

As his physical abilities and hand skills develop, his fingers become his main source of information and he starts to concentrate on what he is doing with his hands, learning first by chance and later by repetition and practice.

He learns what he can and cannot do with his toys and familiar objects

Familiar objects and toys are now the tools a child uses for further exploration and development. He finds that they have a top, bottom, inside and outside. That if an object is hard it cannot be squeezed, but if it is soft it can. He learns that he can put objects in and out of a container, at first emptying them all out at once and, at around 18 months, in an orderly and systematic manner. He discover that he can build by putting one thing on top of another with a tower of two small bricks, or can hold an object steady with one hand while using another. He also discovers how to assess the amount of effort needed to get the desired result; for example, that some toys move more easily and go faster when pushed, others when pulled. Able to make choices, he now only plays with those toys that interest him, discarding others.

He learns about the qualities of objects in relation to one another – which fits, goes on top, in front or behind; the width and height of objects in relation to one another; to match and discriminate between basic shapes with and without colour, and to match like objects.

The child with cerebral palsy

Play also provides a child with cerebral palsy with a medium through which he can develop intellectual, emotional, communication, gross and fine motor skills. But because of his physical difficulties, and depending on the severity and type of cerebral palsy, including any impairment of vision and/or learning, his progress may be slow. Poor perceptual ability, a short attention span and difficulty with recall or short-term memory, if present, will all mean that to gain the most enjoyment and benefit as he plays the child with cerebral palsy will need considerable help, guidance and support.

However, although a child with cerebral palsy may lack many of the normal gross motor patterns of movement that are necessary for him to use his hands in a skilled coordinated manner, **if we help him make use of the skills he has, however limited they may be, he will be able to learn as he plays**. We can do this by:

- seeing that the position he is in provides him with a secure base, and the necessary stabilization, so that arm and wrist fixation are possible
- choosing toys that are at the child's developmental level and ability and are the correct size for him to handle
- paying attention to his preferences by allowing him to choose those toys that **he** enjoys and that interest **him**
- being aware of his tolerance level and his ability to concentrate
- allowing him to explore at **his** own speed and initiative, giving him help only where necessary
- giving simple directions using short sentences.

When playing with your child, always remember that it is his interest and curiosity in the toys he plays with as he tackles the problems they present that is important, **not** that he necessarily completes what he set out to do.

The importance of concentration

Children are often easily distracted and it is difficult to hold their attention even for a short time. They soon tire of their toys or games and want to move on to something else, and with a child with cerebral palsy this stage is often prolonged.

It is most important that we should know and appreciate the maximum amount of concentration a child is capable of giving, for if we ask too much of him he will lose interest, become frustrated and cease to try. Lack of achievement will soon lead to boredom. He will return to the toys and games he knows and understands, and so be deprived of learning and gaining new experiences. The frustration tolerance of a child with cerebral palsy is also often low, and if he does not succeed at the second or third attempt, he gives up. This applies especially to the child of higher intelligence who

knows what he wants to do, but cannot control his movements sufficiently to allow him to do it.

Here are two suggestions that may help your child to concentrate. When giving him toys, offer only two from which to choose, then put away the one he does not want. See that he is not surrounded by things that will distract him – an open toy cupboard, for instance, a pet or other activities going on in the room, playing by the window and so on. He will eventually, of course, have to get used to things going on around him without interruption of his play. One has to remember that although normally a child can pick up a new toy and play with it, he often needs quite a lot of help to understand how it works. So when you give your child a new toy, show and explain to him exactly how it works, not once but many times. Stay with him, see if he can manage and that he understands what you have told him. You may find that he would play and use his hands more easily in another position or if he had more support giving him better balance and stability.

Play that involves sensory motor learning

The following are some ideas that you might try with your child once he is able to open and close his hands but **still has an immature grasp**.

Fill a jar, cardboard box or plastic container with dried beans, macaroni or marbles, and let him play and move them around as he wishes. He will have fun and enjoy feeling them and the sound they make.

Put a handful of the same objects in the middle of a tray. With straight arms using both hands at the same time, help him to sweep them up to the top, bottom and to the sides of the tray, repeating with you if possible the direction in which he is moving his hands. When he gets the idea, you can get him to use one hand only, which will involve crossing the mid-line of this body. Later you could play with him in the same way using finger paints.

A child needs to become aware of objects as a whole before he can appreciate their parts and their relationship to one another. A good way of starting to help him to do this is to explore the everyday objects he would normally get hold of and play with by himself. For example, you could use unpeeled fruit such as an apple, orange or a banana, helping him hold, feel its shape and texture, naming the fruit and the way it feels as he handles it.

The more severely handicapped child

As play only **starts** when a child **succeeds** in making something happen, if he seems to have no interest in his toys, we need to think of ways and activities that with little effort will get a reaction. Examples are simple commercial toys such as a 'Jack in the Box' or a favourite toy of mine, 'Pop-up-Men', that only need the slightest pressure for the men to pop-up, and later can be used for colour matching and imaginative games. For a baby, you could try a Deluxe Discovery mat, with its surprising sounds and soft textures, or encourage him to splash his hands in the bath, resulting in floating toys moving about in the water.

A way I often use is either to put a collection of toys on a child's lap, or have him sitting in a confined space and crowd his toys around him, even sitting on some of them! This often stimulates the child to look and start to push them away. Seeing something happen as a result of his own actions, he is stimulated to try again. Watching and touching and later trying to get hold of a balloon or bubbles blown into the air are other simple ways of getting the severely involved child's interest.

If a child frequently just throws his toys on the floor, you can try either tying them to his chair, a belt or thick piece of string around his waist, or attaching smaller toys to an old cushion.

Even if a child cannot use his hands or speak, he is sure to have some way of indicating what he wants. For example, if you are building a house with bricks, have a book with different pictures of houses and get him to act as 'foreman' and 'direct proceedings', choosing the type of house he wants you to build, the type of roof, the number of windows, and where he wants the door to be, and so on. In this way, when the house has been built he will know that he has taken an active part in its construction.

The moderately affected child

It is up to us to see that play activities are presented in such a way that the child is able to succeed, to make his own choices and to vary the way he wishes to play, experimenting on his own, **not** directed by us. We should only help when he gets into difficulties or asks for our help.

The following are some ideas you might try

Water play

Use a large basin of water or, in the summer, if you have a child's paddling pool let him play in the pool. See that the objects he has to play with are as varied as possible: ones that sink or float, and those that make a noise when banged together. Later a plastic bottle funnel, sieve or colander, all giving a different effect as he takes them in and out of the water, can be used. Playing in this way he learns about how liquids behave and how they behave in a container. Making the water cloudy with some bath foam is a good way of getting a child to use both hands automatically as he plays with the bubbles and searches for objects that have sunk to the bottom. A squeezy bottle cut in half makes a good home-made chute to send things down into the water.

Sand play

Again you need a variety of objects for the child to play with. Different size spoons make good spades, a wooden spoon for stirring, a soup ladle to pour sand from one container to another, a perspex or plastic box is fun for the child to fill as he can see how much is in it. James Galt play buckets (N41444H) are ideal for water and sand play – one sprinkles, one pours and one empties through a spout through its side (but you may need to pad the handle if he has insufficient grasp), and also the Galt Flotilla (N6954G), a collection of 10 brightly coloured small boats in a variety of types and sizes.

Simple items

Newspaper or tinfoil can be made into a light safe ball. One can hide a favourite toy in a loose paper parcel and play pass the parcel. Make a mask or a simple spyhole in the paper. You can also make simple finger puppets by either drawing faces on them or using transfer stickers.

Play foam can be used for making patterns on a mirror. Finger paints for making hand, finger and foot prints.

Books

Looking at a book together is a very special **quiet time** for parents whose child has cerebral palsy. To begin with, look at the pictures in his own scrapbook or photograph album, then later have one picture to a page with objects he is familiar with such as a cup, spoon, shoe, ball or car. Avoid those that have pictures of animals or things he may never have seen.

Show him and name only two pictures at any one time, until he becomes familiar with them. If there is a picture of a dog or cat, tell him the noise they make and get him to copy you.

Encourage him to hold the book with you, but as learning to turn the pages is difficult for a child, start with a book with a hard back or let him practise with an old magazine, as inevitably he will tear the paper to begin with.

Play throughout the day

All children are curious and learn not only by playing with their toys but by exploring familiar objects in the environment, both inside and outside the home.

There are a number of children with cerebral palsy who, although able to use their hands while sitting, are not sufficiently mobile to explore their environment on their own. This, I think, highlights the importance of encouraging play **throughout the day in everyday situations,** rather than putting aside a special time for a 'play session'.

Make use of things around you

When in the **bedroom** let him look at himself in the mirror, play with his brush, bounce and roll about on your bed. While he is being **dressed**, allow him to play with a sock, or his shoes. In the **bath**, give him his flannel or sponge to play with, and let him help you put his towel back on the rail when he has been dried. When you are both in the **kitchen**, give him a saucepan and wooden spoon, empty cereal box, or yoghurt container, empty squeezy bottle. Let him taste hot and cold food while you cook. Many children with cerebral palsy dislike getting dirty. If you are making pastry, give him his own bowl, moisten the flour and get him to copy you as you knead the flour. Encourage him to take his finger around a bowl that has held custard or a mixture that he likes. In the **garden**, if you are for example potting a plant, encourage him to help you put the soil in the pot, brush the leaves, and later have his own garden plot.

Integration between gross motor abilities and play

As a child becomes more mobile, his play extends to learning about moving through space, by climbing in and out, up and down, under and over objects. He learns to judge the size of a space he can squeeze through, which heights are dangerous to jump from and which are safe.

If his ball rolls under a chair, he works out the best way to get it out. If he climbs onto a chair to get a toy, he decides how he can get down without dropping it. He bumps into furniture until he realizes that it is solid and he must find a way round it.

The young child with cerebral palsy who has the ability to balance and is mobile

A young child who has the ability to balance and is mobile should **not** only play when sitting. If he does, he will miss the chance of gaining many new experiences. By moving around while he plays, he will use new patterns of movement and acquire new experiences and skills. For example, if he has learned to move from sitting to kneeling upright, play games and place his toys in such a way that he can practise this sequence of movement.

Organization of self

It is very important at this stage for a child to become aware of the space that surrounds him as he plays. This should include the space behind him. Encourage him to move in different ways, backwards, forwards and sideways, crawling, upright kneeling and walking. Games that include throwing a bean bag over his shoulder or passing a ball over his head, and guessing from a sound behind him what object you are holding are all ways of encouraging this awareness. Miming to nursery rhymes, conducting or moving to music, and playing on see-saws, slides and swings, are ways of playing that will help a child to understand the relationship between space and his own constantly changing position.

Games such as 'London Bridge is Falling Down', 'Ring-a-ring o'Roses', 'Oranges and Lemons' and 'Statues' will assist in teaching him the concept of 'up and down, round and round' and so on. Obstacle courses are a good way of teaching a child to climb over and under, through, sideways and around objects. 'Hide and seek', and getting him to roll over and crawl on verbal command, are all good active games.

The transition from play to function

In time, a child uses the basic skills that he has learned and practised when playing with his toys to manipulate simple functional objects in the home. For example, he may like to open and close cupboards, drawers and doors, but will not be able to manage objects that screw and unscrew until much later.

He starts to enjoy feeding himself, if in a somewhat messy manner, and begins to cooperate more when washed, bathed, dressed and undressed. Later, he likes to imitate his mother while she polishes, picking up things when they fall over, be with her when she gardens, pass her the shopping when she puts it away in the cupboard and so forth. He begins to follow short verbal commands, 'Put your mug on the table', 'Bring me your shoes so I can polish them', 'Sit on the chair so that I can put your socks on', etc.

Choice of Toys

The following are ideas for **simple** toys found mostly in the home. No attempt has been made to state any particular age group, as so much depends on the ability of the individual child to use his hands, as well as on his level of intelligence, and powers of concentration and comprehension. Your therapist will advise you on the most suitable toys and games to play with your child.

A **heavy ball**, for example, is easier for children with involuntary movements and intermittent spasms to play with, as their movements are so disorganized and clumsy that the ball is apt to roll away. A child with spasticity, on the other hand, can play best with a smaller solid ball, as his grip is apt to be firm and he will have difficulty in lifting and letting go of a heavy ball. A child with a spastic hemiplegia should play with a large beach ball to encourage him to use both hands together. When a child can only grasp a bat or stick, a ball attached by elastic enables him to play with the ball. For the child who may want to throw and catch a ball but is unable to hold it, a bean bag can be used instead of a ball. They are easy to make and can be made of bright washable material, in many shapes, weights and sizes. Velcro mitts and contrasting ball are also good for encouraging the use of both hands and make catching easier and more fun.

A **medium size** ball can be used for a young child to push when he first starts to walk, and as a movable base for an adult to sit on with a child sitting on her lap, when encouraging balance reactions.

Velcro or a magnetic strip attached to building bricks will make it easier for the child to build. Large lightweight wooden bricks can be used for games as well as building. It is as well to remember that children get as much fun knocking down as they do building! Many early learning games designed to help the child with activities, such as grouping and matching, involve the use of cards

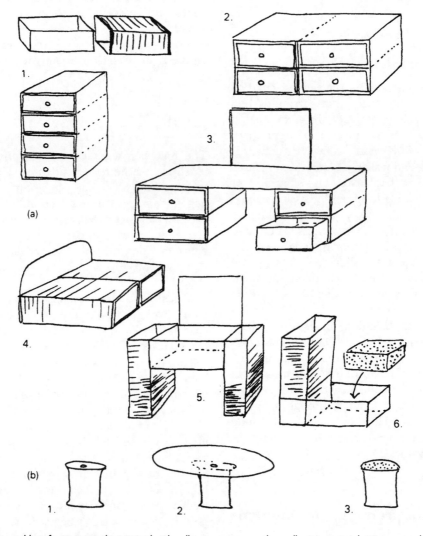

Figure 13.1   All matchbox furniture can be covered with adhesive paper or other adhesive material. Mirrors can be made of plain cardboard covered with aluminium foil.

   (a) 1. Chest of drawers (upright) – 4 whole matchboxes covered.
       2. Chest of drawers (side by side) – 4 whole matchboxes covered.
       3. Dressing table – 4 whole boxes with cardboard top and mirror.
       4. Double bed – 2 matchbox covers, headboard, covered with material.
       5. Washbasin stand – 1 inner box, 2 matchbox covers, with mirrors.
       6. Chair – 1 whole matchbox, a piece of foam in the base for padding covered with material or cotton wool.
   (b) 1. Cotton reel as a base for 'furniture'.
       2. Circle of cardboard glued to top of reel forming a table.
       3. Small circle of foam attached to reel forming a 'stool'

with pictures of for example different fruits, or all the articles associated with bathing. The child is required to pick out and place the appropriate card with its picture in the correct place or group. For the child with cerebral palsy, this may be more difficult because he is unable to manipulate the thin card. However, by gluing the cards to bricks he is then able to play the game.

Poor or clumsy coordination of the child's arms, hands and fingers often makes it difficult for him to hold his toys and at the same time to move them around. If, for example, your child enjoys playing with cars, either give him a friction car or place a magnetic strip on the car, and on the end of a short stick. Felt stuck on the bottom of a toy will make it easier to move over a polished surface.

A doll's house made from large wooden or cardboard boxes is best for the child with cerebral palsy, as the 'rooms' will be big enough for him to put his hands inside, and by using larger 'furniture' he will find it easier to move the objects about (Figure 13.1a,b). In a similar way, a simple garage can be made at home (Figure 13.3).

Coloured wooden or plastic cotton reels make excellent counters and can easily be fitted over a board of wooden pegs. Small empty plastic bottles (make sure that they have **not** previously contained anything **toxic**) can be used for guessing games and are a useful size for the child to hold. Fill them with different things to smell and of varying weights and sounds. 'Squeezy' bottles can also be used as a home-made set of skittles.

Something that is found in most kitchens – a kitchen plunger with a suction cap – can be used to give a child a lot of amusement while at the same time he learns. By fixing it either perpendicularly or horizontally and using different size rings, the child can be encouraged to stack them on the stick plunger. We have found varying sizes of curtain rings useful.

A popular toy with most children is an Activity Centre. For the child with cerebral palsy, a home-made Activity Centre can be made on a larger scale and designed specifically to meet his needs (Figure 13.2).

Discovering shapes

Once a child begins to discover that objects have a shape (i.e. round, square, triangular, oblong), collect objects of different shapes with him, and then

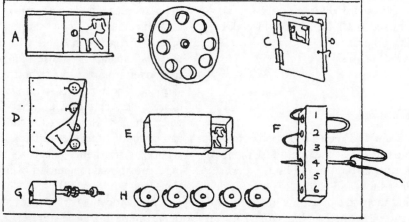

Figure 13.2   Home-made Activity Centre
A. Sliding door – or small runners with a picture behind the door.
B. Telephone dial.
C. Hinged door – with hook fastenings, photograph or child's own drawing pasted inside.
D. Material with buttons – inside is a felt head of a flower or butterfly attached by a popper to the material.
E. Matchbox – filled with a series of small cards or small buttons, etc.
F. A threading block – very popular with most children.
G. Large bolt mounted horizontally on block with crewing nuts.
H. Removable cotton reels fitted on pegs with corresponding colours or corresponding numbers

find pictures of them to cut out. Get him to draw round them with a pencil, then later copying and drawing the various objects for himself. In this way he will not only learn the names of objects around him, but also what they are used for, why they are made in a certain shape, the different colours in which they are made and what you can do with them.

When he gets to the stage of recognizing shapes, start by getting him to master one shape at a time. You can do this by having a series of cardboard boxes that will only take one shape, starting with a round; when he has mastered this, a box that will only take a square, and so forth. Then a box that takes a round and a square so that he has to make a choice. (See also 'Shape recognition' below.)

An excellent 'posting box' can be made from any square transparent type container so that the child can enjoy the pleasure of watching the pieces as they fall through. The container can be divided into three or four section with firm pieces of cardboard, so that apart from posting different shapes the child can be encouraged to fill each section with, for example, dried peas, beans, macaroni pieces or different size buttons. See whether he can name, or even point to, the section you name, then let him see what happens when you take away the cardboard divisions and the contents become mixed – ask him to try to pick out pieces of similar objects.

Keeping a scrapbook

Encourage your child to keep a scrapbook of common objects around the house, including the food he eats. Begin with a room in the house, perhaps the kitchen. First show and name the objects, then see if he can find them in a magazine or paper, and cut them out and paste them in his book. You can enlarge on this idea when you go out for a walk together, collecting leaves, flowers and so on, and press them in his scrapbook. If you should have a Polaroid camera, take photographs and make a special album of family, friends, pets and familiar places, all of which will **encourage recollection** and **speech**.

Making his own collection

In addition to the toys brought for him, a child usually gets great pleasure in playing with the odds and ends he finds around the house, or collects in the garden or on walks. All children are great collectors and hoarders, and if they cannot walk or move around the house they are not only denied the pleasure of exploring and finding out things for themselves, but also of acquiring a private collection of their own. It is up to us, if a child is severely handicapped, to take him out to explore his surroundings or bring things to him so that he can find out all about them and keep those he particularly likes. A large magnifying glass is an excellent way of helping him look at and explore his collection in greater detail, especially interesting if you have visited a pond or river and have a jar of water to put the objects in. An outsized magnifying glass with small 'legs' at each corner can also be of great interest if placed over a patch of earth.

Making music

All children love music. Listening to the radio or CD player is fine, but it is far better to encourage them to make their own music. Severely handicapped children, who cannot hold a stick to bang a drum or bang it with their hands, can make a satisfactory noise if a piece of elastic is tied over the top and bottom of the drum. 'Squeezy' bottles filled with sand, buttons, dried beans, etc., can give a variety of sound effects when shaken. Bracelets for the wrists and ankles can be made of leather or felt and small bells sewn securely onto them. This is a good way to encourage music-making and movement at the same time (see Chapter 12).

When choosing toys, do not always go to the toy department in a large store. The kitchen and general sundries department will often have things that can be fun for your child and easily adapted as toys. Shops that sell products from India and Asia have a variety of door-chimes, mobiles, handbells and so forth. Craft shops with products from Europe and Russia also have an excellent selection of simple games and toys.

Toy libraries

Toy libraries have been set up in most countries throughout the world. Some are run by volunteers, others by parents themselves or by professionals with a special interest in play, such as nursery and school teachers, health visitors, therapists and psychologists. They can be found in a variety of locations: in nursery and primary schools, health centres, hospitals, public libraries, mobile vans and play buses.

Toy libraries provide a selection of good-quality toys for children with physical, speech and language difficulties, visual impairment and learning problems. Many also have a reference library of books, booklets and catalogues which specialize in various aspects of play activities and toys.

The advantages of using a toy library are twofold. First, it enables a child to have a variety of toys of particular value for developing special skills at different stages in his development; secondly, it enables parents to discuss the various learning situations possible with each toy and gives an opportunity for an exchange of ideas between parents and members of the library and parents with one another.

Parents can apply to become a member of the National Association of Toy and Leisure Libraries (NATLL) which will enable them to receive mailings including the quarterly membership magazine *Play Matters*, discounts on the NATLL's publications, advice, support and information. International links are maintained by the NATLL through the International Toy Library Association, and they can provide the addresses of toy libraries throughout Europe and the rest of the world.

Simple games using everyday objects

Many of the everyday objects in the home can, with the application of a little thought and sometimes adaptation, be used in an interesting and amusing way to encourage learning, and at no cost to you.

For matching

Use food or soft drink tins or cans, making sure of course that there are no sharp edges, and preferably brightly patterned and coloured ones. As a moving object often presents a problem for a young child to follow, roll the tin towards him from different angles in the hope that he will follow it with his eyes, then later see if he can push the tin back using both his hands. If an added stimulus is needed, put some dried beans, peas, etc., into the tin – the sound will help attract his attention. Take a number of tins and fill two of each of them with similar objects; by shaking them the child may be able to match similar sounds.

A useful way to teach the child to learn how to match is by sticking sets of transfers, drawings, cut-out pictures, etc., on the lids and bottoms of margarine or yoghurt cartons, then getting the child to match the picture on the lid with the same picture on the base.

Strips of materials such as carpet, emery paper, silk, woollen or fluffy materials stuck on a tin can be used to help a child identify the texture of the material by feeling. See that the strips are broad and do not put more than three different materials on one tin. Sew or bind together 5 inch (12 centimetre) squares of knitted material, carpet, curtains, etc., then take loose pieces of similar materials to encourage the child to match them.

The shoes and socks of the family can also be used for sorting and pair matching or helping you sorting out the washing. For the older child, folding up dusters, dish cloths and sorting them into appropriate piles is a useful exercise.

Manipulation

Many food packs of the same product can be bought in different types and sizes, some with screw-on lids and others with lift-off lids, and so on. These can all be used to encourage fine movements of hands and fingers.

Bowls and containers, such as those made by Tupperware, or, if you have one, an old shoebox, are also useful in helping to get fine coordination of the fingers, by tying pieces of wool, ribbon, string or plastic twine together in a length and putting it in the container. Then cut a small slit in the lid, pull one end of the wool or whatever through the slit as a 'starter', and get the child to pull the length through the slit. As it comes through, the child should wind it over a stick or something similar – a little competition could be devised to see which of two children completes the winding over the stick first.

Children are always fascinated with objects that seem to disappear and appear. One way to do this is to take a large empty matchbox, either square or oblong with divisions in it; place different objects in each compartment, then let the child open the box by pushing. Another way is to make a hole in the lid of a small cardboard box and another one at the side of the box near the bottom. The child then puts a marble or something similar into the box and then has to shake it to try to get the marble out of one of the holes.

It is hoped that what I have said in the foregoing will be sufficient to prove that everyday objects in one's home can provide many sources of ideas to combine simple play with learning. My experience with children, whether they have or have not got a handicap, satisfies me that young children get as much enjoyment playing with simple things found in their homes as with expensive toys. This is probably one of the reasons why when a child borrows a toy from a toy library, the toy is returned but the box is missing!

Some dos and don'ts when playing

Keeping advice and help to a minimum

In our efforts to improve the physical function of children with cerebral palsy we may tend to interfere with and direct their play too much. We all tend to make the mistake, when a child is playing, say, with his bricks, of 'advising' him to 'Try the small one on top of the large one', or when he tries to take the lid off a jar, 'Don't pull, turn the lid round and unscrew it'. Then again, as he attempts to push his large model car through a narrow tunnel, 'You will never manage that, try the little car'. The point stressed here is that the child will learn

far more if he sees the large brick fall off, fails to get the lid off the jar by pulling or fails to push his big car through the tunnel.

As a child with cerebral palsy does not learn as spontaneously and easily as a child normally would, it is important that we balance this help by allowing him to make his own mistakes, asking for help when he feels he needs it. All this calls for patience. Some children can only manage to play for 5 minutes at a time, whereas others may play the same game quite happily for 20 minutes. Try always to understand what new things your child is attempting to do and give him the appropriate materials and opportunities, helping him only when he is in real difficulty.

Far too often, children with cerebral palsy, lacking in experience and in imagination, never get past the stage, when playing with their cars, for example, of lining them up and then returning them straight to their box, or pushing their trains around and around in the same direction. A good way of helping a child use his imagination is by building a garage for his cars, so that he can pretend to fill them up with petrol and oil, to wash them and so on, as he may have seen the garage man do (Figure 13.3). No child learns unless he is interested, and it is therefore up to us to stimulate his interest by helping him think of new ideas and situations as he plays. Make sure that it is possible for him to participate actively in the various games, for this is the only way by which he will benefit and learn.

Imitative play

Between 2 and 3 years of age, children begin to be interested in activities going on around them as well as playing with their toys. Anything that Mummy uses or does is fascinating and must be examined and tried. They continually watch and imitate their mother as they play; they want to polish with a duster, to stir with a spoon; to try to wash, dress and undress and take care of their dolls in the same way as their mother looks after them.

Play now becomes more varied, and symbolic play develops – dolls have tea parties, are put to

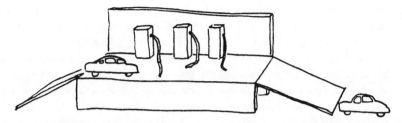

Figure 13.3 Petrol pumps made from wooden blocks, with feed hoses made from piece of cord nailed to side

bed, scolded and praised. If there is a new baby, they are only too anxious to have a live 'doll' to play with, if given the chance. When there are older children in the family, they watch and copy them, listen to stories about school and enact the various episodes with their toys.

The child with cerebral palsy

The child with cerebral palsy often has the same desire to join in the activities of his mother, brothers and sisters, but his handicap prevents him from doing so. If he is to have a chance of enjoying these new experiences, he must be helped.

If you are polishing and dusting, give him a duster; even the more severely handicapped child can polish for you while he sits in his chair. For example, a child who drags the toes of his shoes when he walks can be put in charge of cleaning and polishing them. It may even encourage him to try harder to lift his feet! A child who can walk, but does so in a rather disorganized manner, can help polish the floor if you wrap dusters over his shoes. This should help to improve his coordination, and consequently his balance, as well as giving him pleasure in helping you.

The kitchen is another place where your child can help and learn at the same time: let him help to cut out some pastry cases, give him something to stir, put the salt in the potatoes for you, let him make his own buns. Show and explain to him what you are doing, for example, when you make a cake or sweet, give him some of the ingredients to pour into the bowl or let him help you to weigh them. He will be learning all the time as he watches and helps you.

Remember that there will be many questions he would like to ask, but, either because his speech is poor or it takes him time to put his ideas into words, he loses the opportunity. The head of a school for handicapped children told me that often when children are asked at school for example how pastry is made, they reply 'You get it from a frozen packet and roll it out', or when asked where milk comes from, 'From a milk bottle'. This is what they have seen and, if the first answer is accepted without question, the full extent of their knowledge.

Shape recognition

A child at around 4 years of age begins to group together similar shapes and objects, and later to identify them when asked, for example, which is the circle, the square. He does this by matching shapes, picking one out from a group of shapes, seeing the shape in three dimensions, imitating, copying and finally reproducing the shape when asked.

The child with cerebral palsy

Difficulty in recognizing and differentiating between various shapes and forms is one of the many factors which may prevent the child with cerebral palsy from learning to read and to write. It is therefore worth while spending time helping the child to feel, to recognize and match different shapes as he plays. This can be done by teaching him about **one shape at a time**, mastering and recognizing that one shape before introducing another. The following example illustrates how you might do this with a circle. Give your child a ball and describe its shape, then take his fingers and place them round the ball, letting him feel it in his hands. Let him see, because of its shape, how it rolls, then take a square and show him why, because it has corners, it cannot roll. Find objects of the same shape, i.e. different sized balls, an orange. Later, get him to make the shape in play dough or flour dough. You can then show him the round shape in a quoit or other ring and how this circle is a space through which he can see, pass things through, or place over objects. Then point out to him the same round shape in cups, lids, saucers, saucepans.

When out for a walk, collect some round stones, point out the round of the wheels of the cars and buses, the round flower beds in the park and so on. In this way he will learn to associate a particular shape with many objects, thus extending his awareness of the things around him. Place a round sweet among some square ones and invite him to find the round one. Later, collect together a mixture of round and square objects and ask him to place them into two different groups. He should then be encouraged to make the same shapes with his fingers in sand, flour, with finger paints, with a pencil or crayons. A supermarket is also an excellent place for a child to learn colour, size, shape and texture or when unloading your shopping basket at home.

Some children find it difficult to grasp and lift an object but are ready nevertheless to learn abut the concept of shape and form. A magnetic board is useful for such children. It can be placed flat on a table or propped up at any angle from the perpendicular to the horizontal, or even attached to a pegboard on the wall. The makers of magnetic boards also supply figures, letters, shapes and a variety of designs which are easy for the child to handle as little effort is required to move them around the board. You can buy magnetic strips for use on a flat magnetic board that can be attached to any toy.

When a child is learning to place shapes in a simple form board, he will sometimes find handling them easier if you start by giving him shapes that have a knob on the top. These should not be too large or they may distort the outline of the shape for the child. Begin by taking one shape at a time out of the board and letting him put it back; then take two, and when he has mastered the three

shapes take them all out at once and let him replace them. Later, turn the board around and ask him to replace the shapes.

When a child has difficulty in using his hands this will take time and patience, but continue to persevere, as the learning and understanding of shape is a very important step for many skills, including as mentioned when he starts to read and write. Your occupational therapist will analyse the particular difficulties your child presents with and show you exactly how you can help him.

Simple puzzles

A child's first puzzles should have clear simple pictures with a well-defined background and foreground, as a picture with too much detail will only be confusing for the child. Before he tries to do the puzzle let him really get to know the picture, then take one piece out and let him replace it immediately so that he becomes familiar with each shape. In this way it will be much easier for him to understand how each piece fits the whole.

The field of perception is a most specialized one and your child's occupational therapist, and later his teachers, will give you expert advice on how to follow up his training. This will include, for example, learning how to distinguish between tall and short objects, a comparison difficult for the child with cerebral palsy who spends so much of his time on the floor or sitting in a chair, and therefore builds up his concept of the size and height of things around him in a limited way. This point has been demonstrated to us even by a child of 11 years who, when she stood up for the first time, was amazed to find that the refrigerator, tables and chairs were so much smaller than she had thought.

Colour awareness

A child also learns about colour in a definite sequence, first by learning a primary colour, which he will soon recognize, although when shown another colour in comparison he will often be unable to identify the second. Once he has learned to identify the primary colours he should begin to match similar colours, describing them by name and, finally, naming the colour of things around him.

We hope that, in the foregoing, it has been made clear how **learning through play** is essential for all children, and that in the process they are being prepared for the basic learning experiences which they gain when they go to nursery school. The following sketches illustrate some of the ideas which will help to utilize the child's 'play activities' as the basis for future learning and as a means of progress towards independence. Also illustrated are some of the problems and suggestions for play specifically for the child with a spastic hemiplegia.

Choosing the correct position to play

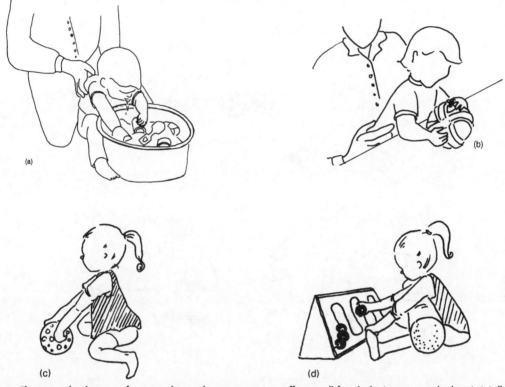

Figure 13.4 These two sketches are of a young boy with severe spasticity affecting all four limbs (spastic quadriplegia): (a) illustrates what happens when we choose the wrong position for him to use his hands, and play materials that are at his chronological age rather than his developmental age; (b) shows the correct position and toy

(a) As the child's weight is back on his sacrum in order to come forward, he rounds his back with his knees semi-flexed. To stabilize his head, he lifts his shoulders, chin 'jutting' forward with a hyperextended neck and open mouth. Because the bowl is too high, the only way he can get his arms up and forward is by turning them in at his shoulders with fisted hands, making it impossible for him to get any sensory feedback from playing in the sand

(b) Sitting securely on his mother's lap he is able to cone forward and support himself on his forearms (elbows). If he is then given a simple toy to play with, like a ball, even though he can only move it around in his hands he has made something happen and he has started to learn

(c) Many children with moderate spasticity and poor balance i.e. spastic diplegia, prefer to sit as illustrated when playing as it provides them with a wide base. This should be **discouraged** as there is always the possibility in this position of flexor contractures of the hips, knees and ankles developing with abnormalities of their feet

(d) Illustrates an alternative position you might try. Placing a small, light roll over a child's legs above the knees often makes it easier for them to keep their arms forward and to bend forward from the hip joints rather than the trunk – see also Figure 13.9

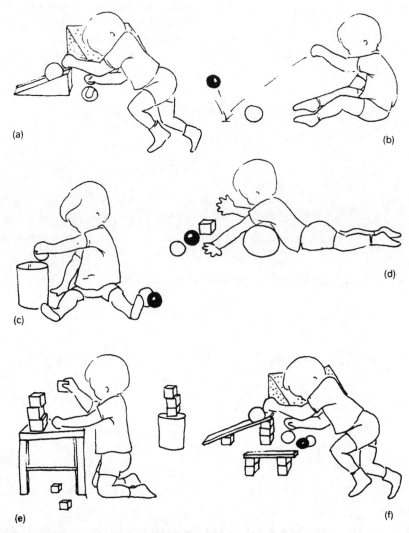

Figure 13.5   Learning basic perception from balls and blocks for children with **limited ability**
  (a) Provide a ball to coll, feel, etc.
  (b) Introduce more balls – soft, and of hardwood, rubber, etc.
  (c) Drops in container for sounds
  (d) Introduce a block with the balls, to discover difference in feeling, purpose – block cannot roll
  (e) Remove balls – introduce more blocks – child learns about building towers, bridges, etc.
  (f) Replace balls with blocks and experiment with the possibility of complementing each other, e.g. make ramps with blocks to roll balls down, build towers for balls to knock down, etc.

Figures 13.6 – 13.10   These sketches illustrate ways parents, when playing with their child, can help him practise newly acquired gross and fine motor skills

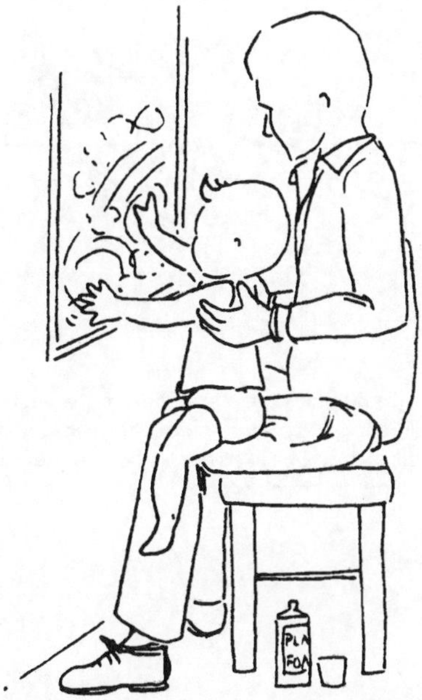

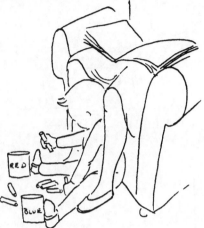

Figure 13.8   The child plays on the floor. His mother controls him at the shoulders with her legs and at the same time provides stability at the hips with her feet

Figure 13.6   Child sitting astride his father's knee makes shapes out of play-foam on a mirror. His shoulders are lifted up and pressed forward to help him give pressure with his hands

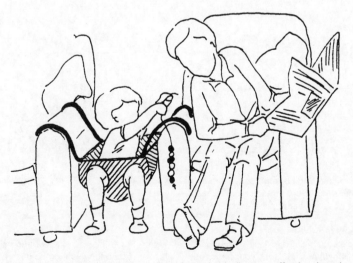

Figure 13.7   Sitting on a 'Safa' bath seat the child learns to thread wooden balls onto stiff nylon thread

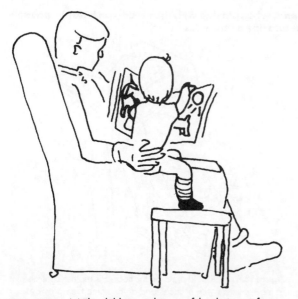

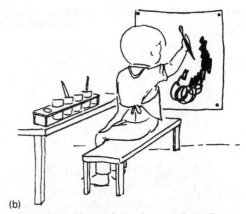

(b)

Figure 13.9   (b) By placing the stool next to the wall, as illustrated, and attaching a large piece of paper to hardboard or a blackboard, the child has to rotate his body as he paints; this is good for his head and trunk control

Figure 13.9   (a) The child sits on the arm of the chair, one foot on a stool and the other on the seat or chair, his father stabilizing his pelvis. He helps to hold the book, pointing to the pictures as his father names them

Figures 13.10 – 13.13   Practising and developing the skill of upright kneeling for children who are beginning to pull themselves up to standing

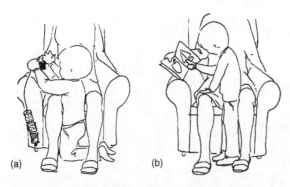

(a)   (b)

Figure 13.10   (a) The child maintains an upright position, being controlled between his mother's legs. He is threading cotton reels covered with different materials, e.g. sandpaper, fluffy material, paint, etc.

(b) The child stands supported by his mother's legs. He is looking at a book with simple bold pictures – tracing around the picture with his finger – while mother says: 'Take your finger up, around, down, under, across, the middle' and so on

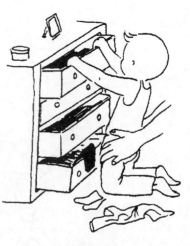

Figure 13.11   Playing in kneel-standing position – keeping the hips straight and weight on both knees. If the child is rather 'wobby' at the hips give pressure down as illustrated

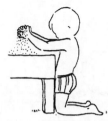

Figure 13.12 Playing with sand helps to teach the child the movements necessary for washing his hands

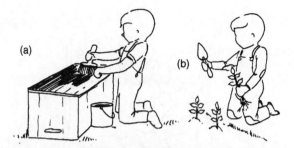

Figure 13.13 (a) Washing and painting a large wooden or cardboard box using a painter's brush. The brush is easy for the child to hold and encourages him to make large sweeping movements.

(b) Making use of upright kneeling while putting plants in the garden

Ways of encouraging a child at different ages and stages of development to move from sitting to standing while he plays

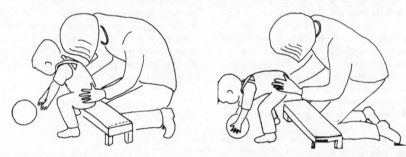

Figure 13.14 Stabilizing the child or his hips helps him to keep his weight forward with flexed hips as he reaches for the ball with extended arms

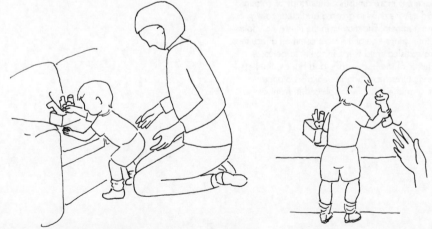

Figure 13.15a,b A sofa provides a good secure base when encouraging early independence – add an extra cushion if necessary.
(a) learning to stand up and support himself with minimal help
(b) weight bearing on an extended arm plus rotation

Standing

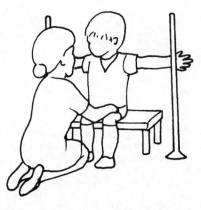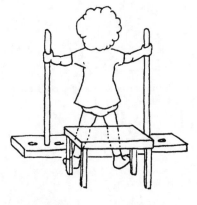

Figure 13.16　Playing with two sticks, as illustrated, is a simple way of teaching the child to grasp, regardless of the position of his head, a difficulty that often arises when he starts to dress and undress himself. Start with his arms out at the sides, straight and turned out at the shoulders, this will help him keep his back straight. He should gradually learn to do the following movements with the sticks at first out at his sides, as illustrated, and then in front of him, keeping his head in the middle and looking at you – as in (1) and (2) below. In (3) and (4), however, he looks at his hands as he grasps and lets go of the sticks

(1) Grasp both sticks, arms remaining straight and steady.

(2) Letting go a stick with one hand and grasping again, without any movement in the other arm

(3) Turning his head to look at his hand, as he grasps and lets go of one stick. He may need help in keeping the other arm straight while he does this

(4) Grasping and letting go of one stick with his head turned away from it. To make this more amusing, stick strips of coloured tape on the sticks and ask the child to grasp a particular colour, or for the older child use numbers. The mother in the illustration holds the child's legs together. Since one of the most common difficulties found in the cerebral palsied child is the inability to perform independent movements of the head, arms and hands, the legs often part or the pelvis turns, upsetting the child's balance

(5) The two sticks should eventually be placed in front of the child

Figure 13.17　A way of combining grasp with movement; the poles are placed in the holes at the extremities of the board. This calls for the widest extension of the child's arms and eventually the two poles are placed in the holes directly in front of him. The child is encouraged to get up from sitting and vice versa. The variety of hand movements suggested in Figure 13.17 can also be used; to begin with the plank (with holes) is used to provide stability and it can gradually be discarded as the child reaches the stage of being able to walk with sticks

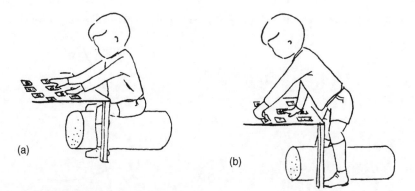

Figure 13.18 (a) The child in the illustration is matching up cards
(b) A roller with a low table in front encourages the child to move from sitting to standing while he plays

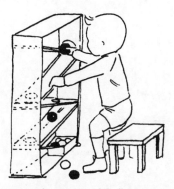

Figure 13.19 A simply constructed 'ball run' to encourage play at different height levels, or use a cabinet with drawers at different levels. As the child explores, you can get him to stop at the height he finds most difficult, or slowly get him to move up and down as he plays with the different levels of drawers

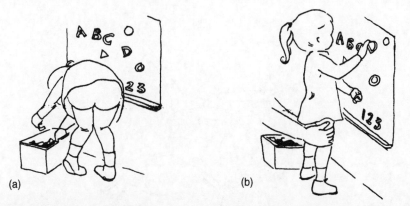

Figure 13.20 To prevent the child becoming stiff when she plays in standing, place the things she is playing with on the floor.
(a) Note that the effort of bending down causes the legs to turn in and the child to go up onto her toes.
(b) To stop this abnormal pattern, hold at the knees or high up on the thighs, turning them out and see that the weight is well forward. Tell the child to straighten her legs. Maintain this control as she bends down to get another letter from the box

Figures 13.21 – 13.23   A variety of ways of learning to practise balancing when standing

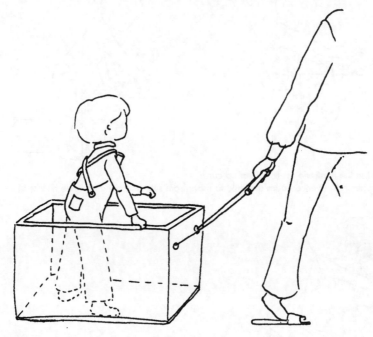

Figure 13.21   An enjoyable way of learning to balance while automatically developing arm-support and grasp. Later the child can learn to push and pull the box himself

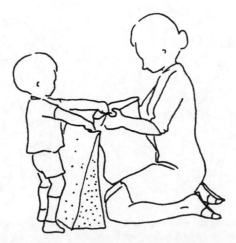

Figure 13.22   The child supports himself by holding onto a foam wedge. Mother holds a bag with objects such as comb, brush, spoon, cup, apple, pencil and sock in it. The child guesses *without* seeing what is in the bag – the purpose is tactile perception

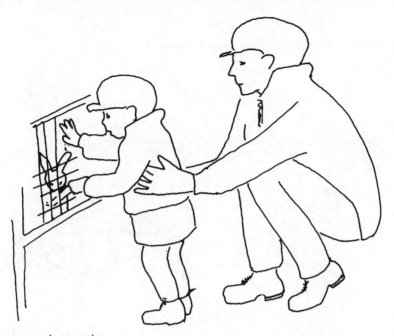

Figure 13.23 Practising standing outside

Figures 13.24 – 13.28   Games and toys that will help a child establish good eye–hand coordination

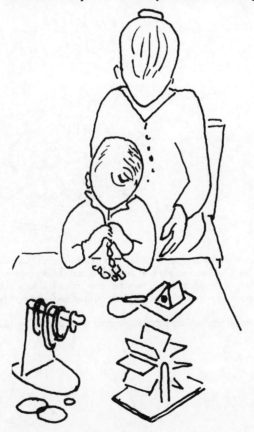

Figure 13.24   A child will usually find it easier when learning a precise motor skill when he needs to hold with one hand while using the other, if he sits at a table supporting himself on his elbows as illustrated

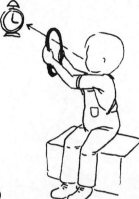
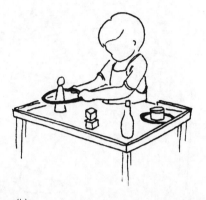

(a)

(b)

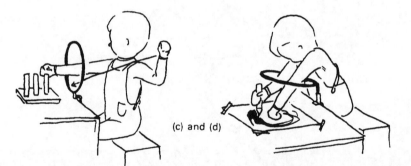

(c) and (d)

Figure 13.25 These sketches illustrate various games using a quoit ring that will help a child with fluctuating tone and involuntary movements to stabilize his shoulder girdle, keep his head steady and in mid-line and develop eye–hand coordination

(a) Using the ring as a camera and focusing it on different objects in the room. For the older child you can play 'I Spy' in this way.

(b) Placing a ring over an object without touching it. A number of rings can be used and care must be taken to see that no ring touches the other.

(c,d) A ring clamped on the table as illustrated can be used if the child cannot use his hands because his arms keep 'flying' outwards

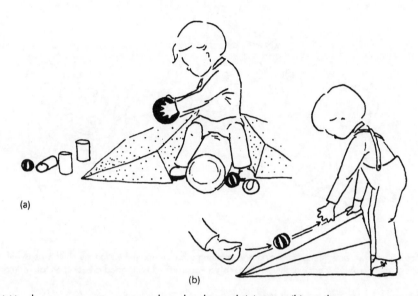

Figure 13.26   Activities that encourage movement and eye–hand control: (a) sitting; (b) standing

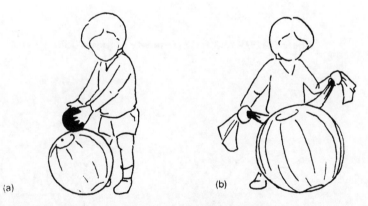

Figure 13.27   Play that needs good coordination between eye and hand when standing
    (a) Balancing one ball on another, using only the fingertips, then slowly moving the ball forward with the legs, while the small ball remains on the top
    (b) Moving a ball in all directions as the child walks about guiding it with a towel held in both hands

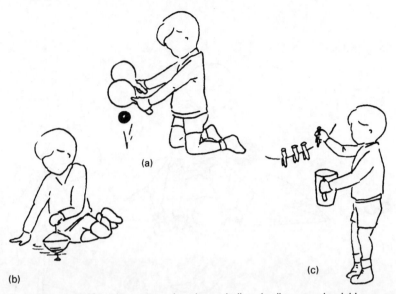

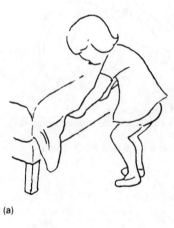

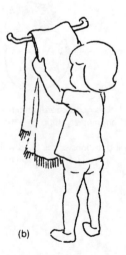

Figure 13.28   (a) Playing with two bats; lifting, bouncing and catching a ball. In the illustration the child grasps with the whole hand; if the index finger is held straight along the back of the bat, the movement used will be a good preparation for writing and eating with a knife and fork

(b) Working mechanical toys such as a humming top

(c) Movements that involve holding with one hand while we move the other come into all our functional activities – leading to the hardest of all, i.e. doing different movements with each hand

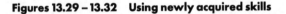

Figures 13.29 – 13.32   Using newly acquired skills

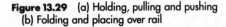

Figure 13.29   (a) Holding, pulling and pushing
(b) Folding and placing over rail

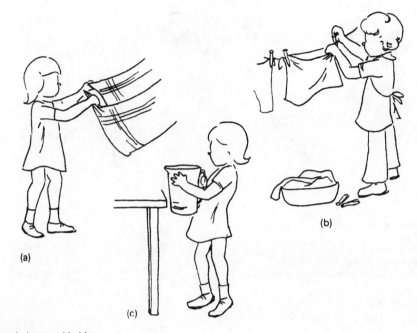

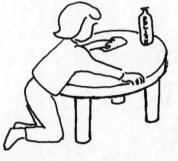

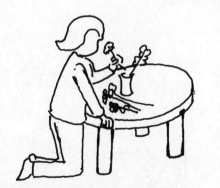

Figure 13.30 (a) Shaking and holding
(b) Finger–thumb opposition, placing pegs on a line
(c) Holding weight, lifting and pouring

Figure 13.31 Activities that involve using only one hand

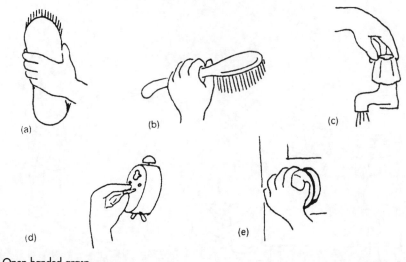

Figure 13.32   (a) Open-handed grasp
  (b) More refined grasp
  (c) Finger–thumb opposition
  (d) Finger–thumb opposition – finer coordination
  (e) Grasp combined with wrist movement against resistance

Figures 13.33 – 13.37   Ways a child with cerebral palsy can learn from the stimulation of playing with a brother, sister and friends

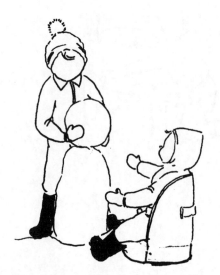

Figure 13.33   Making use of a triangle chair outside

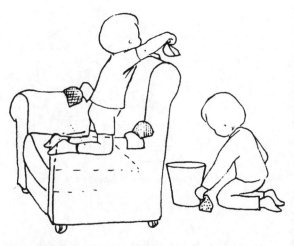

Figure 13.34   Using the back of the chair for upright-kneeling – throwing bean bags into a bucket combines movement and eye–hand control and grasp in exercise

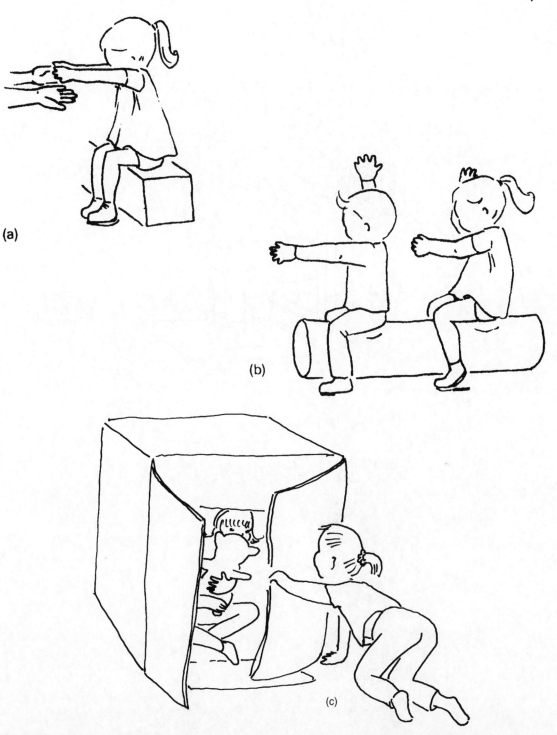

Figure 13.35 (a) Imitation by following a verbal command: 'Place your hands on top of my hands' – 'underneath my hands', and so on
(b) Imitation by copying. Sitting first behind her brother and later in front of him, she copies the movements he makes
(c) Using a large cardboard box as a 'house'

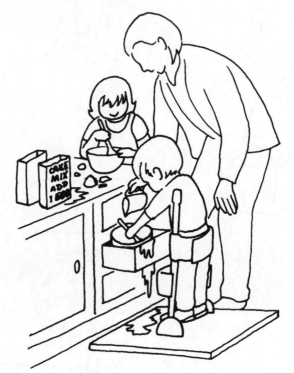

Figure 13.36 Brother and sister learning to cook together

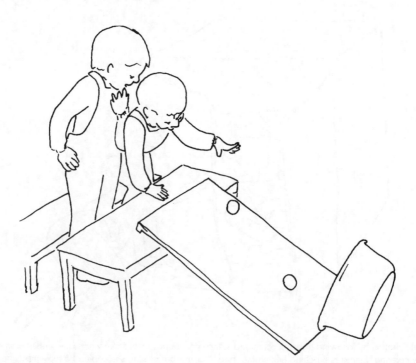

Figure 13.37 Twins compete with each other

Figures 13.38 – 13.39   Coordination and balance

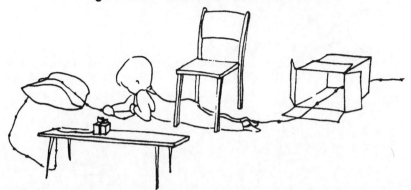

Figure 13.38   An 'obstacle course' made by leading a piece of rope under and over various objects teaches a child more about himself in relation to objects and to use his hands for support and grasp as he makes his way to the end of the rope. As an incentive for effort, drop a small 'prize' in a box attached to the end of the rope so that he has to unwrap the parcel to get his prize

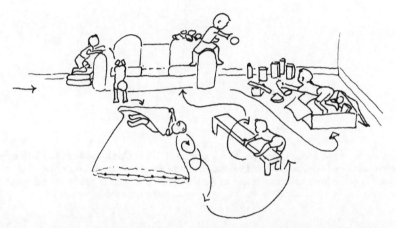

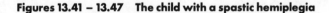

Figure 13.39   Some ideas you might use when making an obstacle course for the older more mobile child

Figures 13.41 – 13.47   The child with a spastic hemiplegia

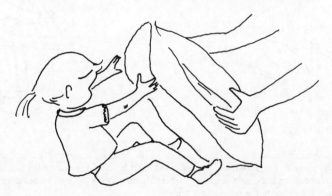

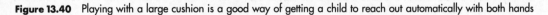

Figure 13.40   Playing with a large cushion is a good way of getting a child to reach out automatically with both hands

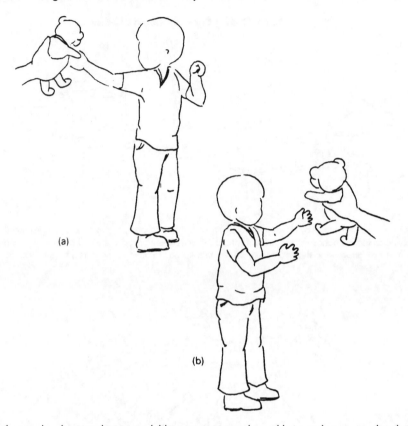

Figure 13.41   (a) When you hand toys or objects to a child it is important to take trouble to see that you are directly in front of him. If you stand, for example, on his unaffected side, as illustrated, you can see how the abnormal patterns of the whole of the affected side are reinforced – even the head is pulled more towards this side as the child looks and reaches out for his teddy bear

(b) If handed to him in the mid-line and slightly to the left, he becomes more symmetrical

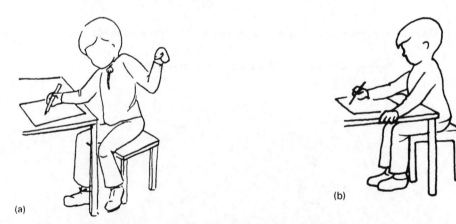

Figure 14.42   (a) When you look at this sketch you can see clearly how the child's asymmetrical posture affects his whole body. This setting base is unstable: as he turns his head towards his unaffected hand to write, the associated reactions, i.e. increased tone in the affected side, pulls his hip and shoulders back, arm flexed with a fisted hand. Unable to move his hand across the paper from left to right, i.e. cross the mid-line, he pulls the paper to the edge of the table

(b) Sitting on a symmetrical stable base he is able to bend at the hips and bring his trunk over his sitting base. Although associated reactions will still be present, he is able to minimize their effect by holding the edge of the table

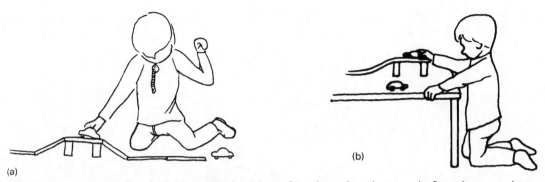

(a)

(b)

Figure 13.43   (a) A position which a child with a spastic hemiplegia often adopts when playing on the floor. This is a similar asymmetrical posture to that seen in Figure 13.43(a) and should be discouraged

(b) Kneel-standing is a good position for play. This position helps the child to take weight equally on both legs, with straight hips. As he uses his hands he has to balance, making adjustments in his whole body. Playing in this way will help to improve his standing balancing and therefore his walking

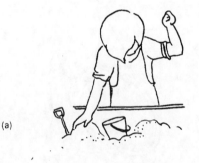

(a)

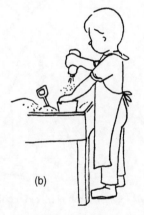

(b)

Figure 13.44   (a) Associated reactions in standing

(b) The associated reactions are minimized by getting the child to support himself on an open hand. *Note*: the sandpit is at waist height, enabling the child to bend forward from his hips with a straight back

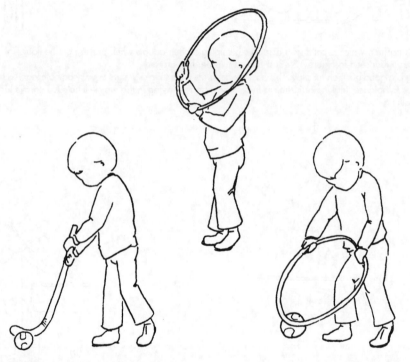

Figure 13.45 If the child can only hold a ball as illustrated, it is better to give him a stick, bat and ball, or hoop and ball to play with

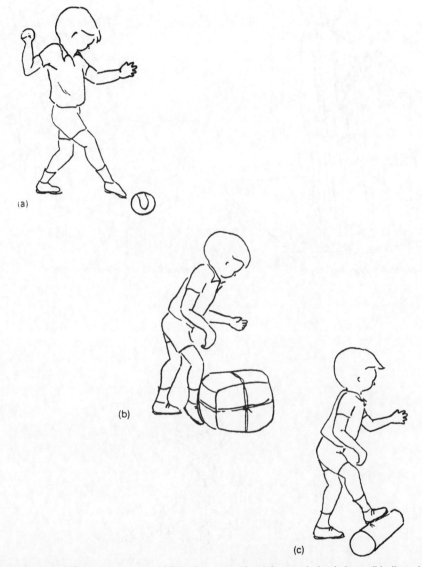

Figure 13.46   (a) It is not a good idea to encourage a child with a spastic hemiplegia to kick a light small ball; unable to stand on his affected leg, he will kick the ball as illustrated, leaning his body backwards, increasing the stiffness in his leg and the bending of his arm

(b) Kicking a parcel or medicine ball which gives resistance is good exercise for the child. He moves the parcel or ball while his leg is bent, his body-weight coming forward

(c) The child moves the roller by pushing it along with his heel

Figure 13.47 – 13.49   Helping in the home and the garden

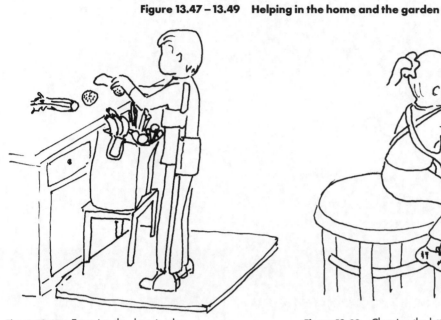

Figure 13.47   Emptying the shopping bag

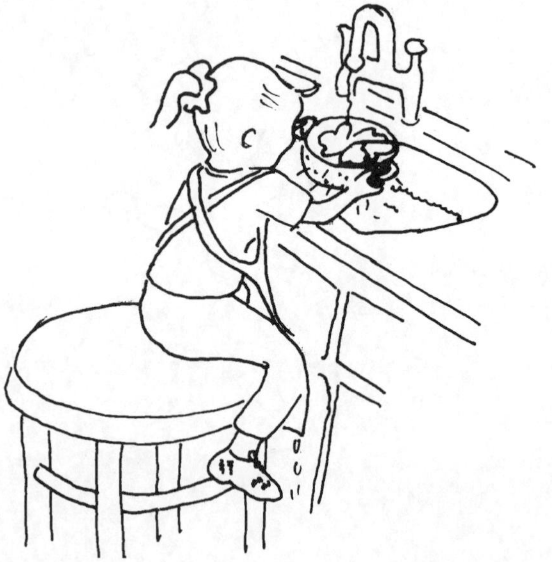

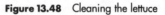

Figure 13.48   Cleaning the lettuce

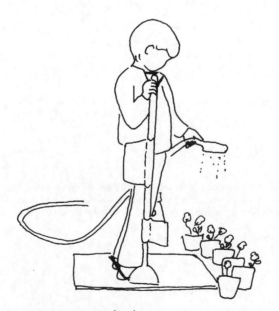

Figure 13.49   Watering the plants

Part IV
Handling during routine activities

Chapter 14

Sleeping

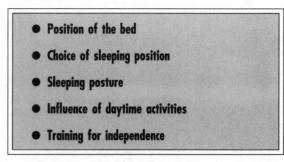

- Position of the bed
- Choice of sleeping position
- Sleeping posture
- Influence of daytime activities
- Training for independence

Night time presents parents whose child has cerebral palsy with some of their hardest trials. Many of these children are poor sleepers, which is understandable as they use very little energy during the day, and for various reasons may need frequent attention during the night.

In this chapter we will discuss the importance of the position of the bed, mattress and bedclothes and how these influence a child's sleeping position. Various daytime activities that can be used to help the child acquire the possibility of attaining good/comfortable sleeping positions are described.

The cot or bed

The importance of the position of the cot or bed in the room

The majority of children with cerebral palsy have a tendency, when lying on their back, to turn their head more to one side than the other, at the same time pushing back against the pillows. This could, in time, predispose to deformity of the spine and the development of asymmetry of limb posture. It is therefore important to take into account your child's particular problems before deciding on the best place in the room for his cot or bed. We will illustrate the importance of this by assuming that the child always turns his head to the right.

Look first at Figure 14.1, which shows the **incorrect** position. You will see that all the stimulation comes from the right; the windows, electric light and the child's toys are all on the right side. Only the wall is on his left, so that there is no incentive for him to turn in this direction.

Now look at Figure 14.2(a,b) which shows the **correct** position. All the stimulation now comes from the left, encouraging the child to look in this direction.

The bed

Preferably, a child with cerebral palsy should progress from sleeping in a cot to a bed at the same age as any other child. You may feel that you want to delay doing this, either because you are concerned that he will be unaware of the degree of danger in getting too near the edge of the bed, or you may have noticed that be becomes frightened that he might roll off when you put him on your bed. If this should be the case, it is worth while considering getting either a low, box-framed bed, using portable rails or placing a solid chair against the side of the bed.

The mattress

We all move when we sleep, repeatedly adjusting our positions during the night. If you have ever had the misfortune to sleep on a soft mattress, you will have experienced how difficult it was to roll over, and how very stiff you felt the next morning. This may give you some idea of the difficulties and discomfort a child with cerebral palsy faces if he does not have a firm mattress, particularly as he is already limited in his ability to move.

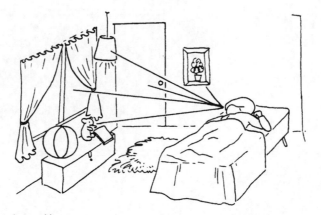

Figure 14.1   Incorrect sleeping position

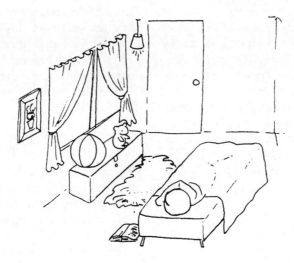

(a)

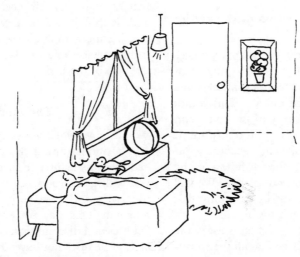

(b)

Figure 14.2   (a,b) Correct sleeping position

If you do not have a firm mattress, you could try putting a hard board under the length of the mattress or a very firm pillow under the top, so that the mattress is at a slight slope, making it easier for him to move and adjust his position.

Blankets, duvets, sleeping bags

Use light, warm blankets or duvets, as heavy ones add to the child's difficulties in moving.

Note: A high-tog duvet is not advisable until a baby is over 1 year old, as it can be too warm for the baby.

Young babies who are restricted in their movements and dislike having blankets tucked in are often more comfortable and it is easier to move if they sleep in a sleeping bag.

The majority of children with intermittent spasms and involuntary movements are relaxed when they are asleep, although there are children who move so frequently in bed that it is difficult to keep them covered. A number of parents have tackled this problem by sewing tapes to the four corners of the blankets and tying them under the mattress.

Pillows – neck cushions

Do not give your child a pillow unless it is absolutely necessary and, if he should have one, see that it is firm.

A neck cushion is sometimes the answer for children who frequently extend and keep their head turned to one side. The neck cushion designed by the staff at the Bobath Centre for the older child or the Cervipillow designed to fit the contours of the neck are recommended (Figure 14.3).

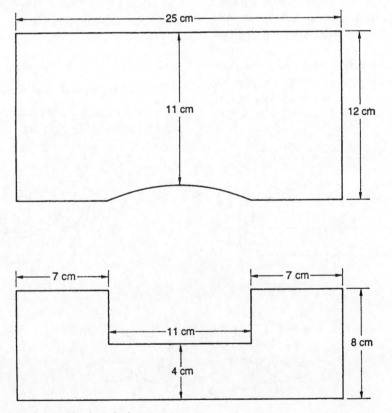

Figure 14.3 Neck cushion designed by the Bobath Centre

The problem of persistent head-banging is discussed in Chapter 3. Baby Bumper Pads are helpful for those children who persist in doing this.

Common problems and practical suggestions

Sleeping positions

Unless for any special medical reason your baby needs to be put down to sleep in a certain way, it is always best to have him on his side when asleep, until he can roll over by himself and choose his most comfortable position. This, of course, may not be possible to begin with, either because it is too difficult to flex him sufficiently to place him on his side and once there he immediately extends pushing himself onto his back, or because, lacking any stability, he just 'flops' onto his back.

We are not, of course, suggesting that you put your child to sleep in a position which although good for him is uncomfortable but rather that, having observed his preferred sleeping position, you may then use pillows or other aids in order to reinforce the good aspects of the position and to control or inhibit the negative effects, in this way minimizing his problems. Meanwhile you can use daytime activities to get him accustomed to lying on his side.

The baby with increased postural tone (spasticity)

When sleeping on his back, the baby with increased tone is inclined to push back and adopt an asymmetrical position of his head, trunk and limbs.

Parents have found that they can prevent or certainly reduce this problem by placing a firm support under the sides, top and bottom of the mattress, thus forming a shape similar to that of a hammock. Another method used is to raise the top of the mattress and then using a small rolled-up blanket, which is placed around the baby's bottom and tucked under the mattress. In this way his hips are flexed and his pelvis is in a neutral position. A neck cushion may also be helpful if he predominantly turns his head to one side. Figure 14.4(a,b) illustrates an alternative way of man-aging the baby's posture using a C&S Seating T positioning roll which can be purchased from Mary Marlborough Disability Centre in conjunction with a Taylor Therapy head support which has side blocks that are adjustable to fit the child.

The baby with low postural tone

Here the picture is completely different, with the baby 'falling' or 'flopping' into the mattress rather

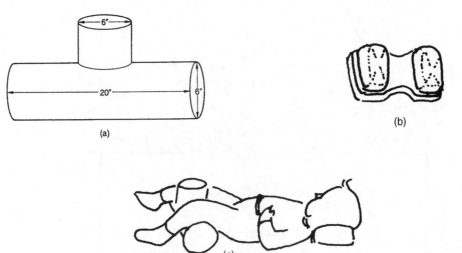

(a)

(b)

(c)

Figure 14.4   (a) Positioning roll; (b,c) Taylor Therapy head support

than pushing back. His posture will probably be asymmetrical, head turned to one side, his arms flexed (or one flexed, the other extended in outward rotation at the shoulders), hips outwardly rotated, legs abducted and knees on the support (Figure 14.5a).

To enable the baby to maintain a symmetrical position, any postural support should give him sufficient stability at his shoulders and pelvis to enable him to bring his shoulders and arms forward, and hips and pelvis to a neutral position. for

a small baby this can be done by rolling up a blanket which is placed around the baby's bottom and along each side as far up to the armpits, as illustrated in Figure 14.5(b).

An alternative way of providing stability at the shoulders is by using a shawl or soft scarf to form a figure-of-eight over the shoulders, maintaining firm pressure as you take each end over the shoulders and diagonally across the trunk (Figure 14.5c). If the baby is inclined to lie with a 'short neck', i.e. with his chin poked forward,

Sleeping

Sleeping

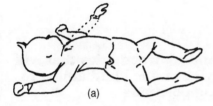

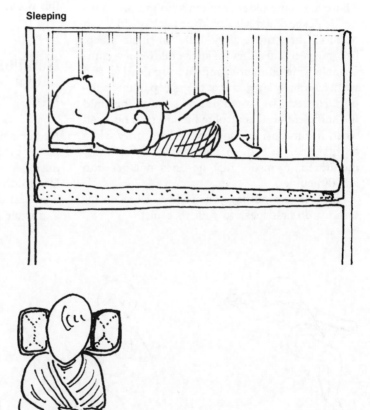

Figure 14.5 (a) Postures adopted by babies with low posture tone when on their backs
(b) A rolled up towel around the baby's bottom and up to the armpits, providing symmetry and posture support
(c) Alternative support using a shawl or soft scarf and Taylor Therapy head support

you could also try using a Taylor Therapy head support.

It must be remembered, however, that wrapping a baby in this way is a form of outside aid and, as such, is opposed to our objective of getting the baby to learn to adjust his position and move by himself at night. Therefore, while it may be useful as a temporary measure, it should not be used permanently. The support given by the shawl or scarf should gradually be reduced in the hope that it can finally be discarded.

The older child who is predominantly flexed

There are some older children who are predominantly flexed when lying on their back or side, and because they move very little in their sleep, become very stiff. A few of such children are comfortable lying on their tummy during the day, and we occasionally suggest that they sleep in this position. However we would **not** do so until the child has sufficient head control to lift and turn his head when in this position and, even then, **only** when he first goes to bed, so that he can be carefully monitored to ensure that he does not get into any difficulties.

Note: Before putting your child to sleep on his tummy, do first speak to your therapist.

The older child with severe spasticity

Figure 14.6(a,b) illustrates two typical asymmetrical postures of a child with severe spasticity which give the impression that he is lying on his side when, in fact, he is not doing so. The excessive turning out and flexion of the hip of the lower leg pulls the pelvis over, the top leg turning in at the hip and pressing against the under-leg.

Figure 14.6(c) illustrates how, by having the child's head on a firm pillow, it is easier for him to keep his head, shoulders and arms forward. The T positioning roll previously described prevents the upper leg from pressing against the under-leg. As soon as he can lie comfortably on his other side during the day, he should sleep in this position.

Handling and play activities that will help a baby or young child adjust to new sleeping positions

As our aim is to enable the baby to sleep in different positions and be able to change position during sleep, we must first encourage and enable him to do this during his wakeful daytime hours. The best way to achieve this is through handling and while he plays.

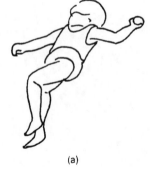 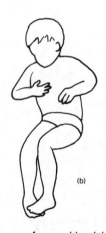 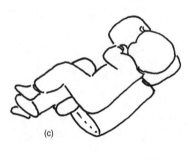

(a) (b) (c)

Figure 14.6 (a, b) Habitual asymmetrical postures of some older children with severe spasticity when lying on their backs
  (c) Illustrates the use of a T positioning roll, firm head pillow with back support if required

To illustrate how we might do this, we will take as our example a baby who prefers to sleep on his back but, when he does so, has a tendency to extend and adopt an assymetrical position of his head, trunk and limbs. It would therefore be better for him to sleep in side-lying.

Handling

Carrying is an excellent way of getting a baby used to being in a position that he finds uncomfortable, as he does not have the stimulation of lying on a supporting surface. It is always important to remember that, as well as getting your baby used to lying on his side, he **also** needs the experience of moving in and away from this position. Ways of doing this are illustrated in Chapter 19.

Playing on his side

One of the best ways to start playing with a baby when he lies on his side is on your lap with his back against you – supporting his head on your forearm or on your thigh by crossing your ankle over your knee or, perhaps, by having one foot on a small box so that he is lying on a slope with his head and upper body higher than his pelvis and legs. In this position it is easier to control his upper trunk and get his shoulders and arms forward, while at the same time controlling the position of his pelvis and legs, gradually introducing rotation and movement while he plays, as illustrated in Figure 14.7(a,b).

To enable you to appreciate why it is so important to have your baby well supported in side-lying when showing him toys to look at and play with,

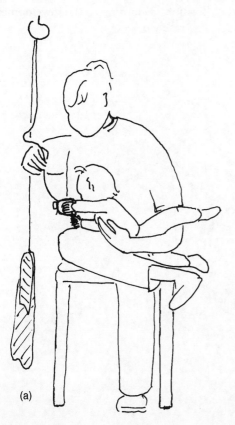

(a)

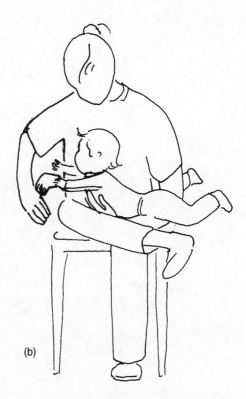

(b)

Figure 14.7 (a) Able to lie on his side, the baby is encouraged to reach forward, rotating his trunk while his mother controls the position of his pelvis and legs
(b) Finally rolling him from his side onto his tummy

try reading a book without a pillow under your head. After a few seconds you will be uncomfortable and find it difficult to read and soon you will have to prop yourself on an elbow, supporting your head with your hand.

If you have difficulty in keeping a young child, who is only moderately involved, on his side when he plays on the floor, it is worth trying a draught excluder as a means of support. They are malleable and firm. The present trend is to make them in the form of an animal, which is fun for the child. They can be purchased at any large department store.

Playing on his own

The baby

Until a baby feels comfortable lying on his side, when playing on his own we need to find ways in which we can minimize his problem of extension and asymmetry when lying on his back.

Because of their shape, a hammock (see Figure 8.14), a hollowed-out piece of foam (Figure 14.8) or a cylindrical pillow (Figure 14.9) will all provide the baby with good postural support when lying on his back, enabling him to maintain a symmetrical position, stabilize his shoulders and pelvis, and bring both his arms forward, to play in mid-line. When he has developed a full range of movement of his pelvis, i.e. he can round the lower part of his spine, he will then be able to reach forward and play with his feet.

Once a baby is happy playing with his mother when lying on his side, it is worth while seeing if he can play in this position on his own by using a wedge with a simple side-lyer (Figure 14.10).

Although our aim is to get the baby used to lying on his side, he should of course also play in other positions according to the developmental stage he has reached.

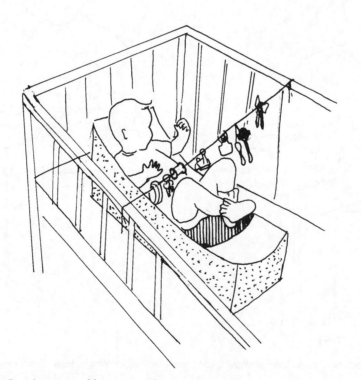

Figure 14.8   Using a hollowed out piece of foam to provide postural support

The older child

For the older child who is more severely involved, your therapist may advise a side-lying board for short periods (see Chapter 8 for side-lying boards and the important points regarding positioning the child).

The toys that will interest him will be those that he can operate by touch or simple switches – cause-and-effect toys, such as rewarding boxes that light up and respond by making animal noises, speak or play a tune or Bubble Tubes that change colour. A child's cassette player, including a variety of games that can be played on a sloping magnetic board, are among the many toys available.

To be completely independent

Before he is completely independent at bedtime, a child with cerebral palsy who is mobile will need to be taught, step by step, how to manage on his own, and have plenty of time to practice. It is therefore essential to get him to help himself as

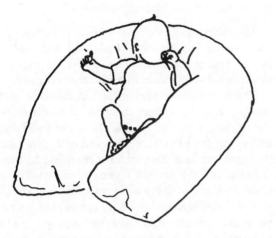

Figure 14.9 Using a cylindrical pillow

Toys

Toys that a baby can play with when lying on his side that are visually stimulating, easy to handle, presenting him with tactile experience, are discussed in Chapter 7.

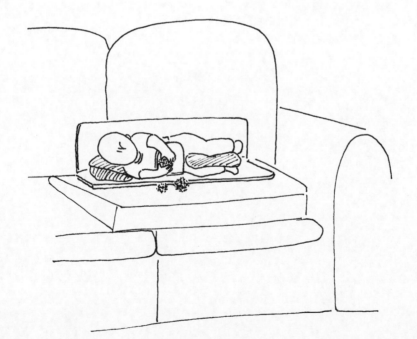

Figure 14.10 Placing a simple side lyer on a sofa gives some small children a greater sense of security, and also makes eye contact with an adult easier

soon as you can, however little he is able to do. Choose times to teach your child when there is least demand on your time, perhaps at weekends. It is usually easier to get a child to cooperate in the morning when he gets up, rather than at night when he has to go to bed!

With the guidance of your therapist, you will know how much your child is capable of managing on his own and how you can help him practice and reinforce some of the basic skills he has mastered in other activities. These will include dressing and undressing himself, and putting on his pyjamas. He will also need, for example, to:

- cover and uncover himself with his sheet, blankets or duvet
- move and adjust his position when covered
- sit up from lying down, and from there get himself to the edge of the bed and his legs over the side of the bed

- get on and off the bed by himself.

All of these basic skills are the building blocks of the tasks he has to learn. Repetition and practice are the bridge to the next task, or the same task he has learned to perform in a different position.

Children with cerebral palsy, in common with many children, pass through the phase of demanding attention during the night by crying, asking for drinks of water or wanting to come into their parents bed. Beware of responding to these appeals, as they are the most common way that children know of demanding attention and should not be encouraged. If you have already committed yourselves by becoming involved and are unable to break the habit or cannot understand why your child behaves in this way, do seek professional advice.

In cases of persistent sleeplessness and restlessness it is advisable to consult your doctor.

Chapter 15

Toilet training

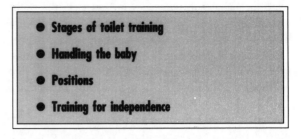

● Stages of toilet training

● Handling the baby

● Positions

● Training for independence

It is important to bear in mind that the time taken to toilet train a child varies considerably and that the whole process is by no means easy with many children. The age at which parents decide to start toilet training varies from one family to another; therefore the suggestions made here are only general guidelines.

Normally a child is around 1 year of age before he associates his pot with its function and begins to have some idea of the purpose of 'potting', and starts to indicate his needs by gesture. When he begins to walk independently, he becomes so absorbed in what he is doing that he often makes his needs known too late. Nevertheless, he is gradually becoming independent, and eventually reaches the stage, at around 2 years of age, when he is partially toilet trained, and he can manage to restrain himself until he has finished playing or whatever else he is doing. Generally at this time one sees him wriggling and jumping about until the last moment. He will be around 4 years of age before he starts to take himself to the lavatory and has the skills needed to pull his trousers up and down and coping finally with buttons or a zip.

So we can see that the process of toilet training takes time, and that lapses may occur when a child gets excited, distracted, or when his attention is focused on mastering a new skill such as walking.

The child with cerebral palsy, with his many physical problems, will probably take longer to become clean and dry than other children, so do **not** be tempted to compare notes with your friends, or expect him to match up with any brothers or sisters. The **length of time** it takes to achieve success is of only **secondary** importance; what **is** important is that he is encouraged to try, and given the opportunity to do so **in his own time**. It will take a child with cerebral palsy, for example, longer to maintain his balance and therefore relax when sitting on his potty and to understand what is expected of him.

If all your efforts to toilet train your child meet with complete failure, do not be despondent. In addition to any physical problems your child might have, there may be other underlying causes. For example, the arrival of a new baby may have made him feel that he is not getting enough attention, or he may have come to realize that when you change his diaper (nappy) he gets more of your time than if he uses his pot.

Clothing

Diapers/waterproof pants

Choose those that fit comfortably, have firm wide tapes, ultra-absorbent padding, with additional leak guards which provide an extra wall of protection. For a baby who has an umbilical hernia, Pampers 4 micro-nappies are recommended, as they have a special cut-out notch which leaves the baby's tummy button free.

For babies with sensitive skins, diaper liners or padded soft cellular cotton placed inside the diaper will prevent the skin from chafing. Most parents have found it more satisfactory to use waterproof pants that tie than the popper type.

Some babies with low tone are restricted in their movements because of excessive flexion, abduction and outward rotation in their lower limbs. This pattern is accentuated by the bulk of the diaper, which affects the baby's ability to sit, roll, get onto all fours and crawl. It is therefore important, before the baby starts to develop compensatory patterns of movement, that the hips are brought into a more neutral position. Your therapist will show you how to do this by folding a square of light cotton material over the outside of the diaper.

Although there is the additional work of washing, soft terry towelling squares have the advantage that they can be folded in a variety of ways, to control either excessive outward rotation or asymmetry at the hips.

Trainer waterproof pants with a PVC outer covering and soft terry towelling inside have been found to be the most satisfactory by parents. Pampers Junior diapers which have extra absorbency and are designed so that they are narrow between the legs will allow the baby who is mobile greater freedom of movement.

Briefs and pants

When the toddler has become continent and independent, regular briefs on the market are the best. For the older more handicapped child, elastic top pants with a dropped front attached to the waistband with Velcro can be used.

Handling

There is one **golden rule** to follow when changing your baby's diaper, whether putting on a clean one or taking off a soiled one, which applies especially to the baby who is predominantly extended: **never lift** the baby up by **both legs,** as this immediately throws his weight back onto his shoulders and head. This will result in increased spasticity, in one or both legs. Rather, lift him by one leg, turning his pelvis forward as you do so.

The majority of children with cerebral palsy adopt an asymmetrical posture when lying on their backs. This asymmetry develops particularly early in babies with spastic hemiplegia (involvement of one side of the body). A good way of controlling this asymmetry when changing a diaper is by making use of the padded surrounds on the baby's contoured changing mat. You can do this by putting the baby on the mat, with the side he retracts against one of the padded surrounds (Figure 15.1).

In some instances, changing the baby's diaper on a wedge, or at a slight incline, may help you keep him in a more symmetrical position and moderate any extensor spasticity or retraction present.

Let us now look at the four phases of toilet training:

● beginning of control
● volitional control
● learning to be independent
● independence.

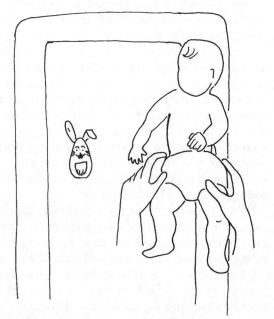

Figure 15.1 Illustrates how you can use the padded surrounds of a changing mat to control any assymetry or retraction of the shoulder and pelvis on one side when changing a baby's diaper

The beginning of control

Many children with cerebral palsy, because they feel insecure when sitting on their potty, find it difficult to relax and sit forward so that they can push with their abdominal muscles to empty their bowels.

Choice of position for the potty

Choice of position in which the potty is placed is therefore important in order to promote the feeling of security and encourage the child to relax. For a baby with no sitting balance, this means being in a position where his mother can give him maximum support, and is able to keep his hips bent, legs apart, shoulders and arms forward (Figure 15.2).

Choice of potty

Mothercare potty

This potty is highly recommended as it is stable, has a firm base and good back support, enabling the child to sit comfortably and securely with both feet flat on the ground (Figure 15.3).

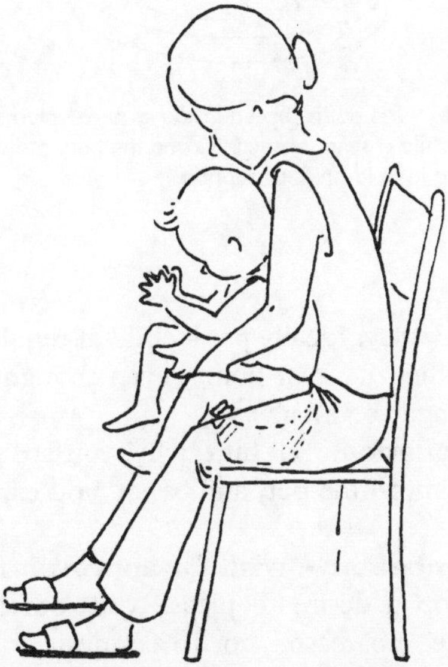

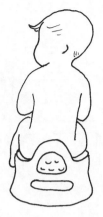

Figure 15.3   Mothercare potty

Musical potty

Some mothers have found a potty which plays a tune when their baby performs successfully to be a good way of motivating their baby to use his potty. A boy's potty with a splash-guard is usually most popular with parents regardless of their child's sex.

Mothercare potty chair and removable safety bar

For the child who can sit with support, we recommend this easily cleaned plastic potty chair with a detachable wooden bar in front. The chair has a wide base and is therefore very stable (Figure 15.4a). The Smirthwaite adjustable potty chair is recommended for the older child. An adjustable foot-rest can also be supplied if required (Figure 15.4b).

Two simple ideas we have used successfully with older children who have adequate sitting balance, but unless they have something to hold onto find it difficult to relax when sitting on their potty, are illustrated in Figures 15.5 and 15.6. They show the potty placed in a strong cardboard box with a bar to hold onto (Figure 15.5) and an upturned stool (Figure 15.6). A potty in the corner of the room with a stool or chair placed in front is another way of enabling a child to feel secure and relaxed.

Figure 15.2   Placing a potty on a chair will simetimes make it easier to keep the baby's weight forward, hips flexed, legs apart

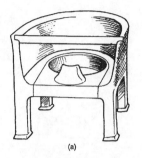

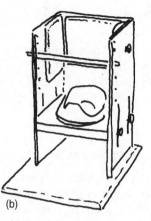

Figure 15.4   (a) Mothercare potty chair and adjustable bar; (b) Smirthwaite adjustable potty chair

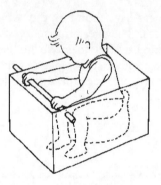

Figure 15.5   Potty fitted into a cardboard or wooden box with wooden bar to hold onto

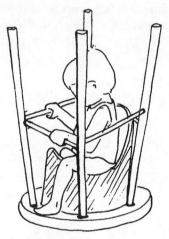

Figure 15.6   The pot is placed inside a large upturned stool, giving the child a sense of security, and the bars are well placed for the child to hold onto for support

Volitional control

The subject of potty training is one that has occupied paediatricians, child psychologists and others over the many decades of interest in child care and development. It is also an aspect that is well documented in the many texts available on the 'How to do parenting', each text reflecting current thinking or fashion. Parents of children with cerebral palsy will inevitably make their own decisions on the 'when' and 'how'. This text is only intended to highlight the special needs of the child which result from his movement disorder. However it will be useful to recapitulate the following:

- **Regularity**. Ideally pot a child at regular intervals when he is at home, even though he may no longer be a baby.
- **Explanation**. Tell him 'why' you are going to put him on the pot, and 'what' you expect him to do.
- **Approbation – wish for approval.** He must develop a desire to please you, otherwise he will see no reason not to continue to soil his diapers.

In turn you must give:

- **Security**. Always be within calling distance, giving him a sense of security in the knowledge that help is readily available.
- **Praise**. Always praise your child when he is clean and dry, but just as important do **not** make a fuss, become cross or withhold affection when he does not succeed. The latter will only serve to make him apprehensive or become stubborn.

Learning to be independent

Stage 1

The first stage towards independence in toilet training is reached when your child is able to let you know when he needs his potty. Always be sure that the gesture or word he uses to indicate his needs **is not only** familiar to yourself, but known to anyone else who might spend time with him during the day. Praise and encouragement are important at this time.

It is worth remembering that normally bowel control is achieved around 19 months before bladder control, as it is obviously easier to anticipate the child's needs. Bladder control by day is achieved at around 21 months. As a general rule boys take longer to train than girls; both, however, will be dry and clean during the day before training brings success at night.

Stage 2

The second stage of independence is reached when a child can:

- collect his potty and replace it
- sit down and get off his potty himself
- pull his pants up and down.

You can help him by

- Choosing a potty that enables your child to sit comfortably with both feet flat on the floor.
- Placing his potty in a position where he feels secure, with sufficient support to compensate for any lack of balance.

- Provide him with some form of support to hold onto, so that he can lower himself to sit and pull himself up to stand.
- Help him to master the skill of moving from sitting to standing, grasping and fixing with one hand, and so forth, during different activities thoughout the day.

Your therapist will show you how to break down the task of helping your child pull his pants up and down, i.e. letting him do the first and last part of the movement himself and then lower himself to sit. Figure 15.7 illustrates a child using a solid chair to support herself while learning to pull her trousers down.

When a child reaches the stage of getting his potty when asked, always put it away in the same place within easy reach for him, and tell anyone who is looking after your child during the day that he is able to get his potty on his own.

For a boy who is anxious to be independent but has difficulties in the standing position, using the kneeling position for a **short time** may give him this independence (Figure 15.8).

Toilet support systems

When your child reaches the stage of using the toilet, it is important that the system used enables

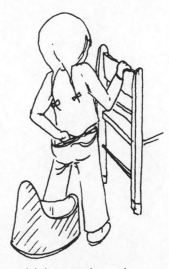

Figure 15.7   A solid chair provides good support when a child starts learning to pull her pants up and down

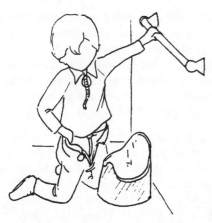

Figure 15.8 With the help of a bar to hold onto, a boy can often manage on his own in this position

him to sit securely with his tummy muscles relaxed. His feet should be supported either on a foot-rest, or a box with a non-slip surface. Arm-rests or a grab-rail may also be required.

As a toilet support system is one that has to be chosen to fit the specific needs of the individual child, we will just mention one which parents have found satisfactory from the many that are available. For the older child who needs additional support the Columbia (junior model) Toilet Support which has a moulded plastic backrest that can be positioned at a height suitable for maximum

comfort for the child and is easily removed when not required, is recommended (Figure 15.9). The child is supported by wide bands of webbing which are adjustable in length. A ring reducer, an all-plastic ring with integral splash-guard, reduces the size of the toilet aperture. Arm- and foot-rests can be purchased separately for use in conjunction with the toilet system. The height of the plastic foot-rest can be adjusted.

An excellent toilet trainer for the child who has good head and trunk control is the Adaptor Toilet Seat. The seat is made of moulded plastic, has a raised backrest and flush-guard at the front. It fits under a standard toilet seat, is easily removed and requires no extra fittings (Figure 15.10).

Independence

To be completely independent a child needs:

- to be mobile, either independently or using a wheelchair
- to be able to sit and come to standing and have some standing balance
- to have the ability to grasp, release and have fine motor skills
- to be able to cope with fastenings such as buttons or zips
- to be able to clean himself
- to be able to flush the toilet
- to be able to wash and dry his hands.

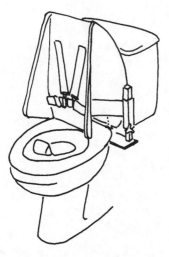

Figure 15.9 Columbia (junior model) Toilet Support

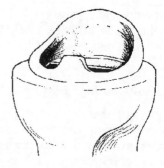

Figure 15.10 The Adaptor Toilet Seat

In the list of training tasks involved in achieving total independence in toileting, some of the essential skills that the child will need are given. Throughout this book we have tried to show how one motor accomplishment builds on or derives from another and also the importance of transferring the motor task learned in one position to another or a different situation. This is the basis of becoming functional in everyday life. Independence in toileting is a classic example of this progression because it requires the integration of many motor achievements.

Do remember from earlier chapters that the acquisition of a motor skill does not come at once, but in small sub-components. Therefore, once a child has reached the stage of taking himself to the toilet he should be provided with any outside help that will enable him to be completely independent; for example, a foldaway support or grab-rail to hold onto, a non-slip mat, foot-rest or box to provide a stable base for his feet. It is also important to see that the toilet roll is within easy reach and adjustments made to the flush handle if necessary.

Finally, do seek professional advice if you have worries regarding your child's bladder or bowel control, or need further advice in toilet training your child (see Chapter 2).

Chapter 16

Bathing

● Bathing aids

● Interactive play

● Tasks of washing

● Speech to reinforce learning

● Working towards independence

Bathing a child with cerebral palsy and teaching him to cooperate and eventually bath himself, often presents parents with problems, especially when their child grows older and heavier.

The difficulties one is faced with, particularly when bathing the more severely involved child, arises because of his inability to sit or use his hands. Although the mildly affected child who can sit when supported is easier to manage, he will not be able to cooperate and learn to bath himself until he has sitting balance and he no longer needs to rely on his hands for support.

To appreciate the difficulties a child with an unstable sitting base and inadequate sitting balance has to cope with when he attempts to bath himself, one has only to think how much we rely on our ability to balance when we have a bath. For example, when lifting a leg to wash a foot, or adjusting our position when washing our back. It becomes even more difficult if we hurt a hand or fracture a wrist and have to bath with one hand.

In this chapter we will discuss some of the problems and suggest ways that might make it easier to bath a baby and young child with cerebral palsy; suitable types of bathing seats and ways of helping the older child to start bathing himself will also be discussed.

Bath time is one of the daily routines that most babies and young children usually enjoy. It only starts to lose its appeal when it means interrupting their play time, or when they reach the stage of being responsible for bathing themselves.

Some problems and possible solutions

Bathing a baby with cerebral palsy is usually comparatively easy while he is small, as long as the base of the bath has an anti-slip surface so that the baby feels secure. If the surface should be slippery, a small towel placed under him will often be perfectly adequate or, if preferred, a small-sized bathmat which adheres to the bottom of the bath.

The care and attention you give to preparing the baby or young child's posture by the way you hand him **before** you put him in the bath **or take him out** is very important.

Some babies are difficult to handle when lifting them in and out of the bath, either because they throw their head and arms backwards (into extension) or they have poor head control and low truncal tone and often tend to 'slip through' one's hands. If this should be a problem, rather than putting your baby in and out of the bath in a semi-lying position, you may find him easier to control if you flex him first, seeing that his hips are bent, his trunk and arms brought well forward (Figure 16.1). If in the early months you find your baby difficult to flex, as a temporary measure you might try washing him as illustrated Figure 16.2.

Some babies push their head back when they have their face washed and ears cleaned. This can sometimes be prevented by bringing both the baby's arms forward and wrapping a towel

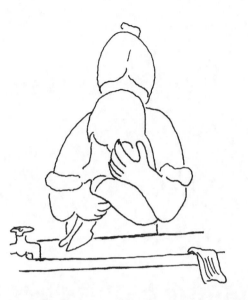

stand should be firm and stable and the bath at a manageable height (Figure 16.3). If you feel your baby needs more head support, a self-absorbent foam pillow held in place by Velcro strips can be attached to the top end of the bath.

When their baby outgrows his first baby bath, parents often find that it is difficult to bath him in a regular-sized bath. At this 'in-between stage' it may be worth while to look at the new concept in baby baths called the Eezi Bath (Figure 16.4). In the UK this bath can be purchased at Mothercare stores. The bath fits over most regular baths and is, therefore, at a convenient and manageable height. It can be filled directly from the taps and has a drainage plug to allow the water to run away, making it possible to wrap a dry towel around your baby before lifting him out of the bath.

For a young child who has poor head control and predominantly low tone, it is worth discussing with your therapist some of the versatile and easy to use pool aids, which have excellent buoyancy characteristics, such as Hi-comfort child's collar, or you might even try an adult's Hi-comfort Saddle Float for a small baby (both supplied by Nottingham Rehab).

Figure 16.1 Flexing a baby before putting him in and out of the bath

firmly around his shoulders and across his chest to maintain this position and give him a sense of stability and security.

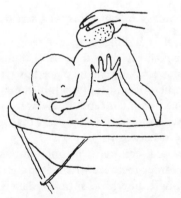

Figure 16.2 A simple way of holding a *young* baby who is excessively extended

Choosing a baby bath

The best type of baby bath is one that has a slight slope that supports the baby's back. The bath

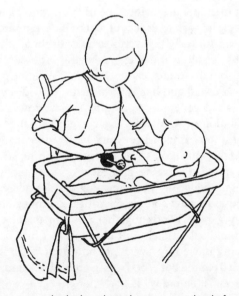

Figure 16.3 This bath and stand are a correct height for the mother, and an excellent shape for the baby

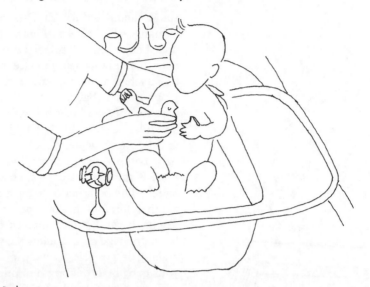

Figure 16.4   The Eezi Bath

Interactive play at bath time

Baby's bath time for you will undoubtedly be just another daily routine, but for your baby it will be a real opportunity to learn through play. Where better to share this experience of learning with you than at bath time. I appreciate that this means setting aside a fair amount of time, but it will be time very well spent.

As mentioned previously, early communication is a very important aspect of a baby's development that can so easily be overlooked. Bath time, when a baby is still at the stage of having little control over his movements, cannot use his hands for play and is relaxed and happy in his bath, provides you with an excellent opportunity to lay down the foundation of what will develop into verbal communication. Encourage your baby to focus on your face while you speak to him. When he starts to respond by cooing and kicking, keep up the dialogue between you, repeating his sounds and introducing new sounds from time to time. Gradually get his hands together for him to look at them and splash them in the water. Get him used to being moved by 'swishing' him backwards and forwards in the bath, both lying on his back and on his front, if he enjoys it.

If you look through any toy catalogue you will find a wide range of toys especially designed for a baby and young child to play with in the bath. Those that can be attached to the side of the bath, and toys with a suction base, are particularly good. A later section discusses the bath time learning situation for the young child.

Problems in handling at bath time

Problems in handling may increase as a child grows older and he is bathed in a standard-sized bath. Whereas a baby can be placed in a baby bath at a convenient height for an adult to manage, the normal-sized bath is deep and awkward in shape. The following suggestions are ideas that you might try at this in-between stage.

Many young children with moderate spasticity often feel rather insecure when sitting in a regular bath although they have sitting balance. If your bath does not have an anti-slip base, a regular mat with suction caps that adheres to the base of the bath will make him feel more secure. Some small children often feel happier if, in addition to a bathmat, they sit inside two rubber rings (Figure 16.5). Although this only provides the child with minimal support, it leaves him free to move while at the same time giving him a sense of security. Another way of helping a baby feel more confident, and at the same time enabling him to play

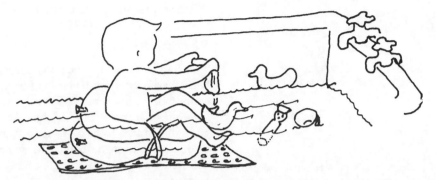

Figure 16.5   Two rubber rings tied together are a simple way of giving a young child minimal support

when in the bath, is by bathing him in a plastic laundry basket with a non-slip mat at the bottom. Depending on his degree of sitting balance, it may or may not be helpful to use a suction handrail threaded through the basket and attached to the side of the bath, for him to hold on to (Figure 16.6).

One of our mothers whose young child was severely handicapped found it easier to bath her child if she put him on his tummy on a half-inflated ball placed in the bath. This example is mentioned to illustrate how all parents can effectively handle their child in everyday situations, to reinforce the learning process in a therapeutic but creative way, if they have a clear understanding of his basic problems.

Choosing a bath seat

Although the first priority when choosing a bathing aid is to provide your child with a comfortable seat and a means of restraint that will enable him to feel secure when in the bath, it is also important

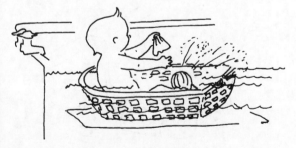

Figure 16.6   A laundry basket placed in the bath provides a secure confined space and minimal support

to make sure that the bath seat you choose makes it easy for **you** to bath your child.

This can be difficult, as it is not often possible to have a bath seat out on temporary loan. It is in this sort of situation that support groups are so useful because there will almost certainly be another mother who has faced the same problem, or even already has a similar bath seat to the one you have been recommended. She will be able to tell you if she has had any difficulty adjusting the seat or restraints, getting her child in and out, or washing him all over, i.e. his back and bottom, and for example whether she can wash his hair while he is in the seat.

Before purchasing a bath seat the following should be checked:

● that the angle of the bath rest and height of the seat are easily adjustable
● that the material of the seat is comfortable and keeps its shape. Avoid vinyl and plastic materials as they are cold and slippery
● the length of warranty and the availability of replacement parts.

The young child

With moderate sitting balance

Plastic-moulded bath support and bath handrails

For the young child who has good head and trunk control but only moderate balance, we would recommend G. & S. Smirthwaite plastic-moulded bath support and bath handrails. These adjust to the width of a regular-sized bath and are attached

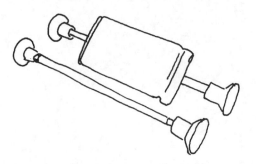

Figure 16.7 G. & S. Smirthwaite Plastic-Moulded Bath Support and Bath Hand Rail with suction grips

by suction panels. The plastic-moulded back support fits onto one of the rails and pivots to take up the natural angle of the back (Figure 16.7). Smirthwaite's slatted bath stool can also be used with their handrail, as in the sketch, or the plastic-moulded back support. This company also supply a plastic corner chair for children from 6 months to over 5 years (Figure 16.8). The chair is supplied with Velcro strap and buckle strap if requested, and a plastic abduction block is an accessory.

With inadequate sitting balance who cannot long sit

Safa bath seat

The Safa bath seat which fits across a standard bath, has been found helpful for the child who cannot bend his hips sufficiently to sit with his legs out in front of him (Figure 16.9). The seat gives the child a feeling of security, as his feet are on the bottom of the bath, and he can hold onto the metal bar surrounding the seat if and when he wants to.

This product has a plastic sling seat with holes for the legs to fit through and a plastic sling-type backrest. It is an inexpensive bath seat and has the advantage that it can also be used as a seat out of the bath.

With no sitting balance

The Rifton bath chair

The Rifton bath chair E.53 is suitable for small children who have no sitting balance and push back into extension when sitting, therefore needing more support. The angle of the back and seat support, which are both separately adjustable, are made of vinyl-coated fibre. Also supplied are pelvic and individual leg straps and lateral head supports that can be adjusted for height and width.

The older child

There are a wide variety of bathing aids available for the older child, but they are expensive so do consult your therapist before buying one. She will assess the level of your child's sitting ability and

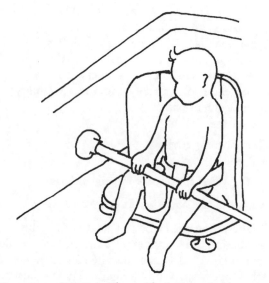

Figure 16.8 G. & S. Smirthwaite Plastic Corner Seat

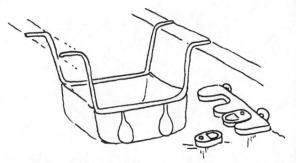

Figure 16.9 'Safa' Bath Seat

then advise you on the bathing aid that will meet his needs. The following are a few of the bath sets we would recommend.

With inadequate sitting balance but can long sit

Two bathing aids that enable the older child who has good head and trunk control, is able to sit with his legs out in front of him, but has inadequate sitting balance are the Columbia bathing aid with Hi-Back or Wrap Around bath support, with a height-adjustable yoke, and the Joncare paediatric bath and positioning aid.

Columbia bathing aid with Hi-Back and Wrap Around bath support

The upright plastic back support is adjustable and the nylon mesh seat base is attached to a stable plastic tubular frame, the child being supported by a harness that holds him around his chest and waist and which is held in place in front by a buckle (Figure 16.10). The Wrap Around bath support has a similar wide support frame and can be used with children who need less truncal support (Figure 16.11).

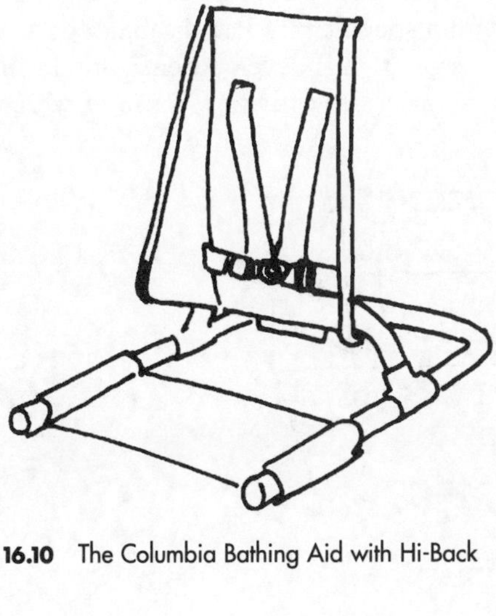

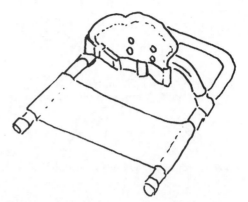

Figure 16.11   The Columbia Wrap Around Bath Support

Joncare paediatric bath and positioning aid

In the Joncare paediatric bath and positioning aid the child sits on a 10mm (½in) thick foam cushion held in place by vinyl mesh, restrained by a pelvic strap attached to the frame's tubes. The back-rest is a foam pad. This is suspended by webbing straps from the frame uprights. Two belts fasten around the chest, the top one around the armpits.

With no sitting balance

James Leckey multi-adjustable bath chair – nursery size

Until a child is able to sit independently, he will need a bathing seat that will restrain him in a semi-reclining position. Parents speak most highly of the James Leckey multi-adjustable chair. The backrest can be adjusted at any angle between 0 and 90° from the horizontal, and the front and back legs are also adjustable to give a variable seat height and set angle. The edges of the seat are padded, the material of the seat is made from blue woven nylon material, and the child secured by deep woven nylon mesh belts that have Velcro closures and are easy to wrap around the child. Four slim foam cylinders are provided which attach to the seat surface and can be used where extra postural support is needed (Figure 16.12).

The severely handicapped child

Sunflower Shallow Bath

For the older, more severely handicapped child who cannot sit, the best type of bathing aid is

Figure 16.10   The Columbia Bathing Aid with Hi-Back

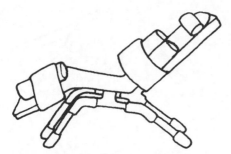

Figure 16.12   James Leckey Multi-Adjustable Bath Chair – nursery size

the Sunflower shallow bath. It is made of a thermoplastic material which is slip resistant. The effective length of the bath can be shortened by the insertion of a sloping backrest, but this has to be purchased separately. This bath also has similar advantages to the Eezi Bath described earlier, because it is designed to fit into a standard bath and therefore is a convenient height (Figure 16.13).

It is light and easy to move from the bath, can be filled from the bath taps and has a large outlet so that the child can remain in the bath and a towel wrapped around him before lifting him out. As the width of the bath is similar to that of the standard bath, the child can be rolled onto his side which makes washing him much easier. A hand shower attached to the bath taps, may also be helpful.

You may find, as your child gets heavier, that the only way you can manage is by giving him a shower. This older age group is really beyond the remit of this book and therefore I would only com-

ment that it is essential to seek expert advice before embarking on major home adaptations.

Preventative back care for parents

One of the problems that often arise when bathing a child as he grows and becomes heavier is that it puts a strain on the mother's back, which may predispose her to developing back problems. To avoid this happening it is worth while experimenting to see if kneeling on a cushion or sitting on a stool reduces the strain on your back. There are many leaflets and videos on preventative back care available and parents would be well advised to use them.

Bath time – a learning situation

The young child with sitting balance

When reading the following sections, please do not think that we are suggesting that you should do all the activities described every time you bath your child. We are conscious of the fact that bathing a child with cerebral palsy can take a long time and therefore the time you spend playing with him may be limited, plus the fact that other members of the family may want a bath!

No attempt has been made in this section to discuss which activities would be suitable for a child with a specific physical disability or at a particular stage in his development, but rather we suggest a variety of activities, some of which may

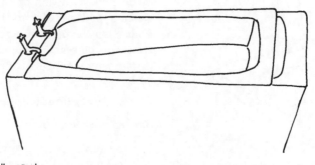

Figure 16.13   Sunflower Shallow Bath

be familiar to you while others may be new. We leave you to choose those that are applicable to your child.

If your child is to feel safe and enjoy his bath time, the way to encourage his confidence is to tell him what you are going to do. Start off by touching and naming the taps, explaining that one is for hot water, the other for cold, showing him how you turn the water on and off, and demonstrating the difference in sound between a heavy or light flow of water and letting him feel the difference. Let him see you test the temperature of the water and explain to him why you do this. In this way you will not only make a game out of bath time, but also create a very valuable learning experience in a situation in which you will most likely find it very much easier to secure your child's attention and cooperation.

Increasing sensory awareness and reinforcing motor learning

If you have a shower attached to the bath taps, a good way of helping a child who has good sitting balance develop an awareness of his own body image is by soaping him all over and then direct a light spray of water at various parts of his body, encouraging him to look, touch and, if possible, name them as you do so. Naturally you should carefully monitor his response to these games and, depending on his type of involvement, if you observe any unwanted activity, e.g. an increase in tone, you should avoid or modify the intensity of the game.

Drying your child with a rough towel sometimes firmly, sometimes lightly, can be made into a game for him and is another way of increasing his awareness of the part rubbed. While he is in the bath, let him feel the difference between a dry, wet, soapy sponge or flannel and encourage him to squeeze the water out.

Bath time is an excellent opportunity for letting your child practise any new abilities he has acquired, **especially** those of **hand function**. Place floating toys/objects in the bath which are easy for him to handle. These could include such household objects as empty 'Squeezy' bottles, yoghurt containers, corks and so on, not all

at once of course. Let him see the many ways in which they act in the water, linking words associated with his actions, i.e. how some float, others sink, are lighter when empty but heavier when filled with water, and so forth. Learning to fill and pour water form one container to another, for example, is a way of helping a child learn to time and grade his movements and develop eye–hand coordination, and he will make much less mess in the bath than playing in this way out of it!

Getting your child to give you the soap, his flannel or sponge while you wash him, and his toys before he gets out of the bath, are ways of encouraging him to practise grasping and releasing a number of different objects. It also extends his vocabulary.

A time to bring speech and movement together

As adults we often like to sing in the bath, so if you find your child likes to make a lot of noise as he splashes about in the water, encourage him to do so. Speech reinforces movement and control of movement as it links intention with action, so as your child develops language and speech skills get him to join in singing nursery rhymes with you or play games that incorporate actions with words such as 'This is the way we wash our hands ... our face ... our ears', and so on.

Working towards independence

Washing hands and face

It is especially important that, in preparation for going to nursery school, your child learns how to wash and dry his own hands and face. Consider the tasks he has to achieve to be independent:

● put plug in basin, or operate plunger
● turn taps on and off
● pick up soap
● put soap on flannel
● wash and dry hands/face
● replace towel on handrail.

To achieve these tasks he needs mobility, stability and hand function. All of these skills will not necessarily be available to him immediately, but you will soon appreciate that many of the movements he needs to perform the task are also used in other daily activities. It is only that he must learn to put them together from a different starting position.

The central message in making progress towards independence in functional tasks is to break the task down into manageable blocks. Use as much carry over of learning as you can from one task to another and most of all, while stimulating and challenging your child to greater independence, never frustrate him with a task beyond his capability.

So that he does not have to concentrate on too many things at once, start teaching your child to wash his hands and face in sitting. For a toddler, as a standard hand basin is too high give him a basin of water placed on a table; in this situation he will be able to concentrate on the task of washing. If he has good balance, then give him a high chair, or a box to stand on placed in front of the hand basin. At this stage he can also practise manipulating the taps which will involve reaching and grasping while maintaining a standing position (Figure 16.14).

Bathing

When a child reaches the stage of bathing himself he may still be unable to get in and out of the bath alone, unless he has some means of support. Help him by giving him a non-slip bathmat, a box or a stool of the right height on which he can sit before

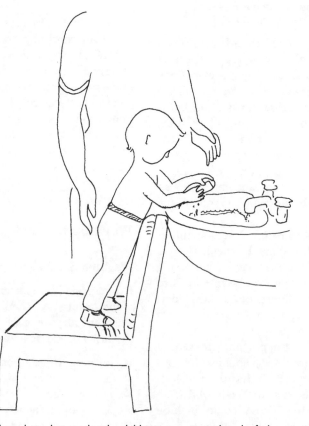

Figure 16.14   When learning to be independent see that the child is in a position where he feels secure and can support himself if necessary

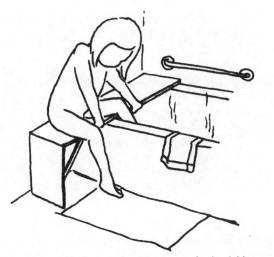

Figure 16.15 A simple way of making it easier for the child to get in and out of the bath and to manage on his own

The following items of equipment will help a child when he reaches the stage of bathing himself:

- a glove- or mitt-type flannel
- a mitt-type loofah
- a wooden nail brush with indented sides which make it easier to grip, or a piece of webbing over the top of the brush through which he can slip his hand
- a long-handled back brush
- a liquid soap container
- soap and nail brush with suction caps
- if a shower spray is not a permanent attachment, a hand spray attached to the taps for rinsing
- a large bath towel with a hole in the middle which can be slipped over the head, a terry towelling wrap, or a towel with a tape which can be tied to the wall
- a stool or chair nearby for his clothes, and a towel rail within easy reach.

We have tried to stress in this chapter, as we have in dealing with **all** everyday activities, the importance of working with your child towards independence, and getting his cooperation as early on as possible.

stepping in. Make sure he has something to hold onto: grab bars for this purpose can be purchased from most stores (Figure 16.15). To begin with, see that the bath contains a few inches of water only.

Chapter 17

Dressing

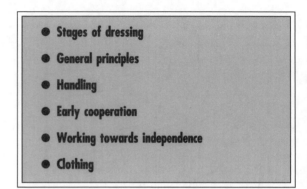

- Stages of dressing
- General principles
- Handling
- Early cooperation
- Working towards independence
- Clothing

In this chapter we will discuss some of the problems that might arise when dressing and undressing your child, ways of encouraging him to cooperate with his own dressing and, towards the end of the chapter, ideas on suitable clothing.

Before moving on to the practical aspects of handling, I think it is important to remind the reader what a complicated task dressing and undressing is for a child to learn. Not only does he need to have sitting balance, good coordination between his eyes and hands, the ability to reach, grasp and release, fix with one hand while moving the other, and have developed the fine motor skills necessary to cope with buttons, zips and laces. He also needs to understand the difference between front and back, top and bottom, inside and outside, be able to distinguish between large and small openings on various garments and to plan his movements in readiness for the task in hand. It is therefore not surprising that the majority of children are at least 5 years old or more before they are able to dress themselves without help.

A child normally starts to cooperate with his dressing when he is about 12 months, holding out a foot for his shoe, an arm for his sleeve, and so on. At about 18 months, with good sitting balance and no longer needing to rely on his hands for support, he deliberately pulls off his socks, shoes and hat. Previously he would have snatched them off unintentionally.

Between 18 months and 2 years, he starts to cooperate more, both with dressing and undressing, and is able to take off all his clothes by the time he is 3 years. He will be at least 4 years old

before he is able to put most of his clothes on himself.

Between 4 and 5 years he can dress and undress himself except for buttons, zips and laces. Whereas previously he could only manage to lace his shoes, he now starts to appreciate which holes to lace in and out of, and in which direction. Although able at this age to push his feet into his shoes, it does not become apparent to him which shoe goes on which foot until some time later.

Dressing and undressing the child with cerebral palsy

General principles

- Choose a position for dressing your child that minimizes unwanted movements or spasticity that create a block to your handling.
- Check to see that your child is lying or sitting **symmetrically** both before and while you are dressing him.
- A priority when dressing any child who is difficult to handle is to see that all his clothes are within easy reach.
- While your child is dependent on you dressing and undressing him, see that he is lying or sitting at a height which makes handling easier for you.
- A child should always be given every opportunity to help himself when being dressed and undressed, practising and using those skills he has, however limited these may be.

Handling the child with cerebral palsy

Dressing the young child who tends to push backwards into extension

If dressed lying on his back, the supporting surface should be inclined so that his head is slightly higher than his feet. This will make it easier for you to bend (flex) his head and bring his shoulders and arms forward and to bend his hips, knees and ankles.

If dressed on your lap, see that he is in a good stable sitting position, hips flexed, and his legs not too widely apart (abducted) as this will increase the turning in (internal rotation) of his hips. By handling him in this way, you will be able to turn his trunk, making it easier for you to bring his shoulders forward and keep his hips flexed. Alternatively you could try dressing the child in side-lying.

Dressing the young child who sits with semi-extended hips with a rounded (flexed) spine, chin poked forward, shoulders pulled forward, arms flexed against his side

It will facilitate your handling if you check to see that the child has a good stable sitting position, then bend him forwards at the hips, bringing both arms forward with straight elbows, palm facing up, turn the arms out at the shoulders, as illustrated in Figure 6.5(c) of Chapter 6. This will also help your child actively straighten his back and lift his head with his chin in. By handling in this way you will find it easier to keep his back straight and his head up.

Dressing the baby/child who has involuntary movements and fluctuating tone – the athetoid type of cerebral palsy

A baby who later develops fluctuating tone and involuntary movements often has low truncal tone during the early months, and when on his back lies with his arms and legs in varying degrees of flexion/abduction and outward rotation. He may also have a tendency to turn his head pre-dominantly to one side, resulting in asymmetry of the trunk and pelvis.

If one dresses the baby on his back because he has no active anti-gravity tone, it is difficult to prevent his limbs falling back onto the supporting surface each time and so reinforcing this abnormal pattern. We would therefore suggest that you try, at least as an additional position, dressing your baby either on his side or sitting on your lap.

Some of these children as they grow older are apt to push their heads and shoulders back and kick continuously when being dressed. If this should be the case, and the child is still of a manageable size, you could try dressing him on his tummy across your knee, as illustrated in Figure 17.1.

An older child who because of poor postural control cannot sit and maintain his balance when using both hands to dress himself can be helped by giving him a point of **stability** by supporting him either at his hips, thighs, knees or feet. Where and how much stabilization you give will, of course, depend on his ability to control his own sitting posture (Figure 17.2a–c).

Sitting a child facing the back of a chair, as shown in Figure 17.3, is a good way of teaching him to stabilize himself, by grasping the chair with one hand while he lifts and helps to push his other

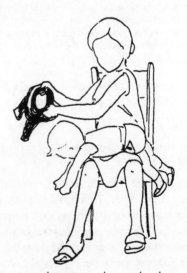

Figure 17.1 A good position to dress and undress a baby who has strong extensor spasm

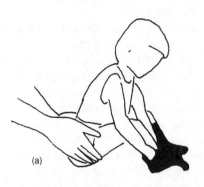

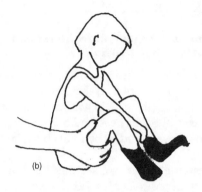

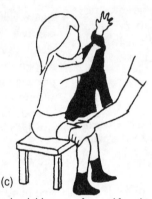

Figure 17.2   (a) Firm pressure over the pelvis enables the child to move forward from his hip joints, keeping his back straight as he bends his leg to take his sock off
(b) Holding the leg as illustrated with his weight taken through the right buttock helps the child transfer his weight while he lifts, the opposite leg to pull his sock up
(c) Some of these children when making an effort to speak, or when lifting their arms up to dress, lift their feet off the floor. If this should be a problem, apply firm pressure over the knees or on top of the feet

arm into his sleeve. The box under his feet provides him with another point of stability.

Dressing and undressing a baby who has moderate spasticity

When some babies with moderate spasticity reach the age of about 9 or 10 months, a number of patents have mentioned that, while dressing their baby, they find increasing resistance to certain movements, such as parting the legs to put on his diaper (nappy) or bringing his shoulders forward and straightening his arms to put through sleeves.

Figure 17.4(a) shows the incorrect way to dress a baby who has a tendency to turn his head to one side, with an increase in flexion of the arm on the skull side. Figure 17.4(b), however, shows that by rolling her baby towards herself his mother can encourage his participation, bring his shoulder forward, arm in extension, and talk to her baby while she dresses him. As a baby at this age is still too young to cooperate, I think problems sometimes arise because our method of handling becomes too **static**. Figure 17.5(a) illustrates the problem while Figure 17.5(b) shows how, by introducing movement, you can minimize abnormal patterns of movement while **at the same**

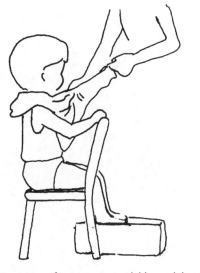

Figure 17.3 A way of encouraging a child to stabilize himself while being dressed

time facilitating the automatic reactions, in this instance, righting his head, as he props himself on his arm.

Putting the older child's arms in and out of sleeves, and taking off socks and shoes, are two of the most common problems parents have to cope with. The former because of an increase in

flexor tone in the arms, the latter because of increase in extensor tone in the legs. The following practical advice may help to overcome these difficulties.

Arms in and out of sleeves

Check to see that your child is sitting symmetrically, weight evenly distributed, **hips flexed, his feet flat on the floor**. It is very difficult to bring an arm forward, while the shoulders and trunk remain back, hips extended.

Do **not** take hold of his arm and pull, as this will only result in an **increase** in flexor tone. Straighten the arm **first**, with outward rotation at the shoulder, being sure that the **elbow is extended**, then put the sleeve on. Do the same when taking the sleeve off.

Shoes and socks

Check sitting position as above. Do **not** try to put your child's foot into socks or shoes while his leg is extended and foot plantar flexed, as this will result in an increase of extensor tone, i.e. his ankle will be harder to bend up and toes will curl under.

Flex (bend) his leg **first**, seeing that his hip is outwardly rotated (turned out). You will then find

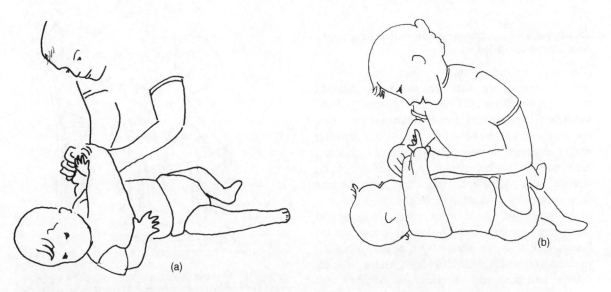

Figure 17.4   (a) By handling her baby from the wrong side, his mother has a problem, extending his arm to take his vest off
(b) By rolling him towards herself as she dresses and undresses him, handling is easier and she is able to interact with her baby

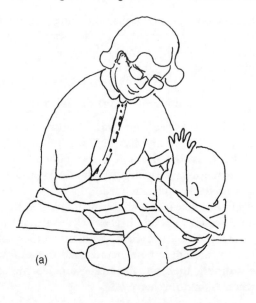

(a)

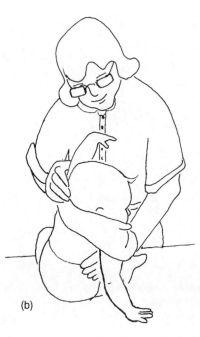

(b)

Figure 17.5 (a) Illustrates problems arising from too static a method of handling
(b) His grandmother, by rotating the baby's upper trunk is able to keep his hips flexed, at the same time encouraging him to right his head and take weight on an extended arm

it easier to bring his foot up. When doing up shoes, **always** see that his foot is **flat** on a support (Figure 17.6).

Dressing and undressing the more severely handicapped child

Dressing and undressing a child with cerebral palsy is never easy, and becomes more difficult as he grows older and heavier, especially if involuntary movements or fluctuations in tone increase at the same time that the child is growing and becoming heavier. Because these children have no sitting balance they will need to be dressed and undressed lying either on a bed or firm surface at a convenient height.

As abnormal patterns of postural tone and movement are strongest when the child lies on his back, it is worth while trying at least partially to dress and undress the child lying on his side. By rolling him from side to side, both before and while you dress him, he will not be in a position long enough to become stiff or push back into

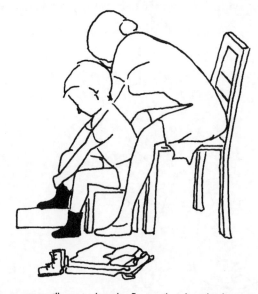

Figure 17.6 Illustrates how by flexing (bending) his leg **first** seeing that his hip is outwardly rotated (turned out). You will then find it easier to bring his foot up. When doing up shoes, *always* see that his foot is **flat** on a support

extension. It will make it easier to put clothes over his head, arms in sleeves, bend his hip and leg to put pants and trousers on, and do up clothes that fasten down the back.

Sitting on the floor/table/chair

Although in this chapter many of the illustrations show a mother sitting behind her child, we feel it is important to point out that this should **ONLY** be done while a child needs some support when you are dressing him, or perhaps when he starts to dress and undress himself the fact that you are behind him **at this stage** gives him confidence. Always be sure that there is **space** between you, as this will stop him leaning backwards against you and encourage him to move forward from his hips.

Figure 17.7(a) shows a child in a good position to see what his mother is doing – his hands are in the same position as his mother's as he completes the final stages of taking off his tee-shirt or, in Figure 17.7(b), his socks. By keeping his **hips flexed and his trunk well forward**, when he lifts and brings his arms forward, or lifts and bends his leg, there will be less danger of him losing his balance.

As soon as your child can sit on his own, move to the side or to the front of him.

Common problems and solutions

Early cooperation

We have only to watch a baby being dressed and undressed to realize how a mother chatters spontaneously to him and how, even before he can talk, he babbles in response, later asking for help immediately he needs it. Many children with cerebral palsy are unable to respond in this way, and in time it may become easier for a mother not to bother to talk to her child and unfortunately to dress him in silence.

There will be many occasions when, because of the extra time it takes to dress and undress your child, it will not be possible to take the time to talk to him; do however try to do so whenever you can. I assure you it is well worth the effort. For if we always dress a child in silence, almost as if he were a doll, we cannot blame him if he becomes detached and passive, showing little interest in what we are doing.

Ways to encourage your child to dress and undress himself

Never miss an opportunity of encouraging your child to be independent. Immediately it becomes obvious that he wants to try to learn and help himself, give all the encouragement you can. At

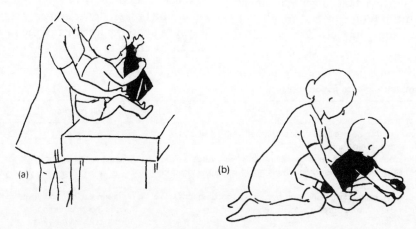

Figure 17.7 Shows a child in a good position to see what his mother is doing – his hands in the same position as his mother's as he completes the final stages of taking off (a) his tee-shirt (b) his socks

first, an enormous amount of effort will be needed on his part for little achievement, and in fact your patience will often run out long before that of your child, but do try to make it a golden rule **never to interfere** when he **does try**, unless of course he really gets into difficulties. You can do this by watching carefully to see how much he can manage on his own and at which point he needs minimal help.

Skills needed

Before looking at ways in which you might encourage and teach your child to dress and undress himself, let us look in greater detail at the abilities he will need before dressing can become an intentional, purposeful, goal-related activity. He will need to:

- sit unsupported, have full hip mobility, keeping both feet flat on the floor
- look at what he is doing and be able to scan, his eyes guiding his hands
- be able to adjust and maintain his balance when moving his arms in different positions, i.e. lift an arm without his feet coming off the floor, or without falling backwards
- have sufficient stability (fixation) at his shoulders so that he can perform skilled movements of his arms and hands, towards the midline and crossing the midline
- grasp, release and use fine finger movements regardless of the position of his arm, i.e. to hold with one hand while pushing or pulling with the other

- understand the relationship of the opening of his clothes in relation to parts of his body, i.e. the difference between large and small openings
- know the difference between up and down, over and under, back and front, inside and outside, left and right
- have the ability to sequence, i.e. know that socks go on before shoes, his shirt before his sweater
- speak, or make an effort, without an overflow of movements taking place in other parts of his body.

You will quickly appreciate from the list of skills needed that they not only encompass motor or movement achievements, but require maturation of other aspects of development, such as perception. Recognizing this if, for example, a child is unable to put on his socks we would need to ask ourselves what is stopping him doing so (Table 17.1). These and many more problems may prevent him from putting on his socks, i.e. not one difficulty but a number of difficulties interacting with one another.

With such a diverse range of abilities necessary before a child is able to dress and undress himself, I am sure you will realize that it would be a waste of time to concentrate solely on a child's manipulative skills without first having an understanding of his overall developmental level, i.e. physical (fine and gross motor), visual, sensory, and perceptual and intellectual abilities.

When a child starts to dress himself, each task should be broken down into easy stages, the child learning to do the last part of the movement first. Watch carefully to see exactly how much he can

Table 17.1   When a child struggles to put on socks

Question	Function required
Is his balance inadequate so that he needs to support himself with one hand?	
Can he bend forward far enough to reach his feet?	
When he bends one leg does the other extend so that he falls backwards?	Gross motor control
Is he able to grasp with straight arms, and maintain his grasp when pulling up his socks?	
Does he have the necessary manipulative skills, and eye–hand coordination?	Fine motor control, visual focus and following
Does he have difficulty in using the appropriate movements for the task.	Poor motor planning
Is he able to cross the mid-line?	Poor body awareness
Does he lack an understanding of what he has been asked to do?	Intellectual ability

manage to do on his own, and at which point he needs minimal help.

Some common motor problems

A few of the more common motor problems are as follows:

- having to hold and lift his clothes, especially pulling them over his head, without falling back; opening his clothes, for which he will need both hands
- starting to put on his sock and reaching down to his foot to pull it over the heel
- starting to pull down his pants; putting the second arm in the sleeve of his coat; doing up and undoing fasteners, especially those at the back.

A child with a spastic hemiplegia, for example, often has an associated grasping on the affected side when using his unaffected hand, making it difficult for him to use both hands together. Therefore, when learning for example to take off his socks, he will sometimes find this easier if he supports himself on his affected hand, inhibiting (stopping) this reaction, and later using the affected hand as a 'holding hand' (Figure 17.8a–d).

Supplementing, timing and sequencing his efforts

In many cases, adaptations to seating or clothing, or the use of splinting, may be necessary to facil-

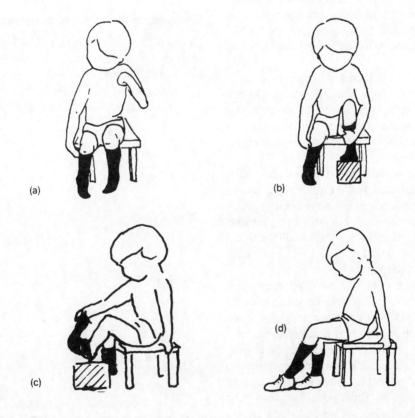

Figure 17.8 (a) The difficulty the hemiplegic child has to pull off his socks, and the effect that using the good hand has on the affected arm and hand
(b) By placing his affected leg on a box and bringing his arm forward, the child inhibits his own 'associated reactions'
(c,d) Ways requiring less effort to take off socks and shoes. The child should sit on a box or stool so that his feet are flat on the floor

itate function or, for example, the provision of spectacles for a child who has difficulty in seeing what he is doing.

If you always bear in mind that your child's functional level will be determined by his developmental level not by his chronological age, you will avoid asking or expecting him to achieve something that is beyond his capabilities. There is nothing more depressing for any of us than to tackle a difficult task with no reward at the end.

When playing with your child it is a good idea to get him to dress and undress his teddy bear to get the general idea of dressing. However, when teaching him to dress and undress himself, **always** do so at a time when you would normally be dressing him, rather than teaching him as a separate 'exercise'. This will, of course, involve a considerable amount of input on your part, as little can be achieved in a rush, and your child will **need time and a lot of repetition** to learn each new task.

Fortunately a child learns to undress himself before he learns to dress himself, which has the advantage that undressing is usually done in the evening when hopefully there is less of a rush. If pressure on your time is a problem, the weekend is a good time to start.

Training for gross and fine motor skills, which include acquiring head and trunk control, sitting balance, hip mobility, grasp and release, speech and language development, has only one purpose, namely, to allow your child to become functional in the activities of daily living that will ultimately allow him to be independent.

Dressing is not only an essential functional activity but because it requires the integration of so many of the skills he is being taught it is an excellent situation in which to practise these.

When helping your child, remember the important of vision, verbal instruction and vocalization of intention. For example, you can help him to relate such phrases as 'Push your foot into your shoe', 'Pull your arm out of your sleeve', as you perform the movement with him, and if he is beginning to talk, he should be asked to say the words at the same time as he does the actions. Later, colour can be included in the conversation, by comparing the colour of his clothes with other

things around him. This can be followed, when he has reached the stage of understanding such things, by showing him which is the top and bottom, which is the left and right, which is inside and which is outside. In this way he will not only be learning how to dress himself, but also accumulating knowledge that can be used in other activities.

Some of the ways I like to encourage young children to learn the basic movements of grasp, pull and push that they will use later when dressing and undressing themselves are illustrated in Figures 17.9 and 17.10(a–d), with a young child, and in Figures 17.11 and 17.12(a–d), with an older child.

Choosing a position for dressing

The position in which your child learns to dress himself will be determined by his ability to maintain a stable sitting base and balance when sitting.

Positions that will make it easier for the child who has only moderate sitting balance when he

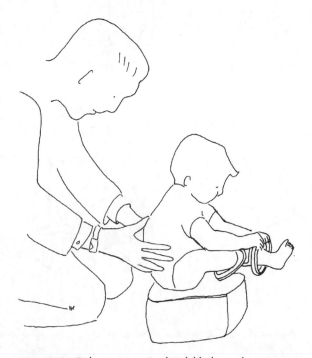

Figure 17.9 Father puts rings on his child's leg and encourages him to grasp a ring and pull it off

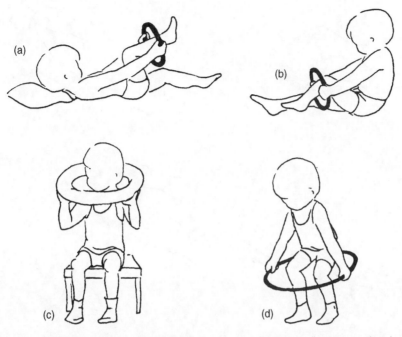

Figure 17.10   (a,b) First in lying then in sitting, the child grasps the ring with both hands, pulling it up and pushing it off his leg – a movement he will use when putting on and taking off his socks

(c) Sitting on a stool and pushing a 'swimming ring' over and above his head and pulling it down again, finally as far as his waist. This is preparation for taking off and pulling on clothes over his head

(d) Pulling a hoop from his feet up to his waist and pushing it down again; preparation for putting on trousers, pants, etc.

starts to dress himself are illustrated in Figures 17.13(a–c) and 17.14(a–c). Ways of giving a child who is mobile confidence when dressing are illustrated in Figures 17.15, 17.16(a–e) and 17.17(a,b).

These are general points of advice and obviously they may need adapting to meet the specific difficulties of each child. **Do not** continue to dress and undress your child from habit or just because it is quicker. If he is ever going to learn to be independent, he must **first be taught what to do and how to do it**, and then be encouraged to try for himself, first with guidance and then on his own.

If you think that he should be doing more for himself, leave him alone one day, while you carry

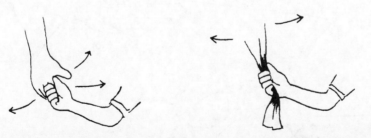

Figure 17.11   By grasping your fingers and later by holding a towel in his hand, the child's arm can be moved in all directions while he tries to retain his grasp. This can be followed by the child moving **your** arm in all directions while **you** hold the towel. The child should only practise the movements in a position in which he has good balance and does not need an arm to support himself

Note: Your finger and the towel are placed across the palm and then out between the thumb and index finger

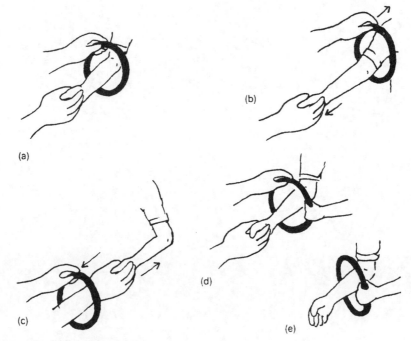

Figure 17.12 (a) Grasp the child's hand and the ring
   (b) Pull the child's arm through the ring, taking the ring up his shoulder while he says 'push'
   (c) Pushing the child's arm out of the ring while he says 'pull'
   (d) The child holds the ring and your hand, and he pulls and pushes with your help
   (e) Finally he holds the ring on his own and repeats the same movements

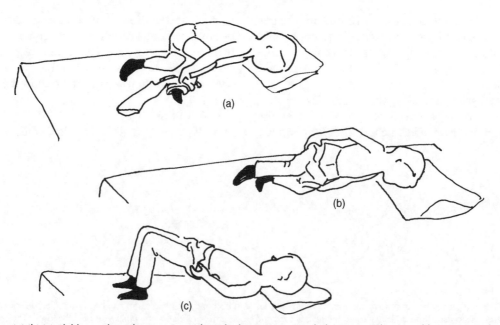

Figure 17.13 (a) (b) (c) Children with moderate spasticity but who have poor sitting balance, once they are able to grasp with extended arms may find learning to take their clothes off easier when they are lying

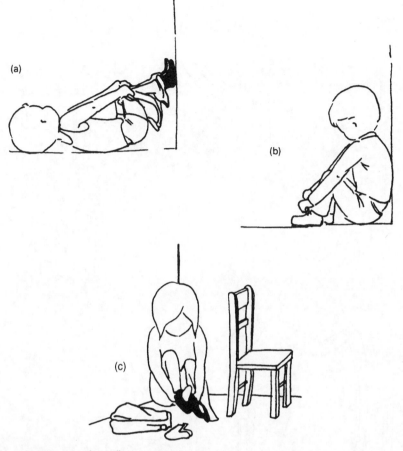

Figure 17.14 Two ways of making use of a wall

(a) By pressing his feet against the wall the child is able to lift his hips while he pulls up his trousers. This is a good position for the child who lacks stability

(b) Supporting himself against the wall the child can keep his hips and legs bent as he leans forward to do up his shoes

(c) Where balance in sitting is still not good enough to allow the child to have both hands free to dress himself and he has the tendency to fall backwards, use the corner of the wall to give him support. See that his clothes are within reach by his side, and if necessary have a stool or chair for him to hold

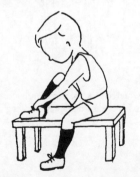

Figure 17.15 By turning sideways when sitting on a box or stool, the child with spasticity may find it easier to bend one leg without straightening the other and to reach his foot. Balance also will be better in this position

on with your work, and on your return you may be surprised. Children can be very crafty; we have known cases where a mother has been called to the front door or telephone to find, on her return, that her often bored and apparently helpless child has dressed himself, something which up to that moment no one believed he could possibly do!

Clothing

As the choice of clothes is a very personal thing for parents when their child is young, and for the

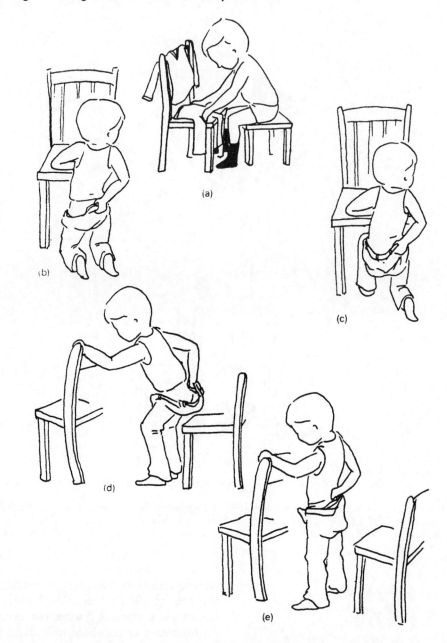

Figure 17.16 These five drawings indicate positions in which a child gains confidence when he starts to dress and undress himself. Place a chair or table in front of him so that he can use it for support when necessary; place his clothes out for him to begin with

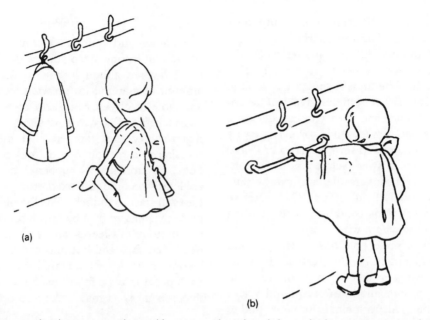

(a)

(b)

Figure 17.17 Dressing and undressing means being able to cope with outdoor clothes and, when starting nursery school, hanging them up

(a) Kneeling on their knees gives some children a wider and firmer base than when standing, making it easier for them to take their coat off without over-balancing

(b) A bathroom rail provides a useful support for the child to hold on to when taking off a cape or coat

child himself as he grows older, we will discuss clothing in general terms.

Materials

Whenever possible, choose clothes that are made of natural fibres such as cotton, wool or a blend of natural and man-made fibres: cotton 80% + polyester 20%, or cotton 80% + Bri-nylon 20% (soft stretched terry material). Other than for linings, avoid materials that have a slippery surface.

For waterproof garments, choose those made of Goretex or similar products whose linings are made of breathable fabrics and are light and windproof. When choosing outer garments for winter wear, thermo-insulated materials or those with 100% polyester padding in the jackets are good, because they are warm, light and can easily be machine washed.

Some babies and young children with cerebral palsy have sensitive skins and are apt to sweat and, because of this, often become hypersensitive to certain fabrics.

Warning

Always check to see that the materials used for all garments **CONFORM TO SAFETY REGULATIONS AND ARE FULLY FIREPROOF OR FIRE RETARDANT**.

Sleeves

All sleeves should be as loose as possible. The raglan or dolman sleeve provides the largest opening for the arm, which is important because it reduces the degree of accuracy or precise localization that the child has to use.

It is also important to have a wide opening at the bottom of the sleeve, large enough through which to slip your fingers and pull the child's arm through, if this should be necessary. If a cuff is tight, the seam can be opened and edged with Velcro.

Fastenings

The most difficult part of dressing or undressing for any child to cope with are fastenings. While it might be quite simple for him to open and close fastenings on clothes laid out in front of him for practice, it is quite a different matter when the fastenings are on the clothes he is wearing. This is particularly so if he finds it difficult to look at what he is doing. Try out different types of fastenings with your child, and then you can decide if shank buttons, large press studs, or even sewing up some button holes and sewing a strip of Velcro underneath, is the answer. Velcro has the advantage of being the most versatile, and can be purchased in 20 mm (7/8 in) strips. The secret of keeping Velcro in mint condition is to brush it from time to time with a wire brush.

Some parents prefer buttons sewn on with elastic, whereas others lift the buttons from the material by sewing a small button underneath; large buttons, or loop and button, zips and Velcro tape can also be used. Your aim is for your child to be independent and it is therefore worth while taking extra time and trouble choosing fasteners that he can manage.

Suitable types of clothing

Body suits

A body suit is a warm and comfortable garment for a baby – made in either pure cotton or a mix of cotton 80% and polyester 20%, sleeveless or with short sleeves, envelope neck and crutch popper openings. My reason for being so enthusiastic about this garment is that it allows the baby maximum freedom of movement and is excellent for any active movement session with your baby.

Vests

The most suitable are those which have the largest openings for the head – the 'envelope crossover' opening for the younger child, and a 'scoop neck' with shoulder straps for the older child. Where a wide shoulder strap is preferred, the seam can, if you wish, be opened and Velcro fastening used. Parents report favourably on thermolactyl vests when used for children who feel the cold.

Pyjamas

For babies and toddlers I would suggest Baby Stretch all-in-one sleep suits with popper fasteners. However, although they do allow a generous amount of material for growing feet, it is **always** advisable to **check regularly** to see if shrinkage has occurred. The **warning signs** come when the material becomes taut, so that the child's foot remains in a plantar flexed (toes pointing to the floor) position. If this happens, movement at the ankle will become restricted or impossible and the toes will start to 'bunch'. For the older child, two-piece pyjamas with ribbed neck bands and cuffs at the bottom of sleeves and legs are suitable. If necessary, tops and bottoms can be held together by buttons and, for the more handicapped child, a back panel may be found useful, or as an alternative, a night shirt may make handling easier.

Socks

Good-fitting socks are as important as well-fitting shoes and are one item of clothing that **should never be passed down through the family**.

Buy socks with as high a content of cotton as possible, as the feet of children with cerebral palsy are apt to be sweaty, and this is especially so if shoes do not allow sufficient air to circulate for the feet to breathe.

While socks are comparatively easy for a child to take off, putting them on can present quite a problem. Tubular socks with no heel shaping are therefore a good type of sock until he becomes more proficient.

Shirts and jumpers

Children's tee-shirts with short or long sleeves, sweat shirts with or without hoods, and jumpers are generously and loosely cut, with a large variety of neck openings – roll, crew, scooped with ribbed collars and cuffs – so that no special adaptations are necessary.

It is only when a child becomes older that difficulties may arise if he wears a long-sleeved shirt. Keeping his shirt tucked into his trousers, for example, may present a problem. This can be remedied by buttoning the shirt onto the trousers or pants, or by means of a tape sewn to the bottom of the shirt. If cuff buttons pose a problem, use two buttons connected by elastic. To save buttoning and unbuttoning the front of the shirt, edge each side of the front of the shirt with a strip of Velcro and sew up the buttonholes, or sew on extra large press studs.

Trousers/jog suits

Boys' and girls' pull-on trousers, jog pants with elastic tops and denims are all generously cut and are designed to stand up to hard wear. Dungarees with either long or short trousers are also an excellent buy.

One of the most useful garments on the market for children of all sizes, is the jog suit, either knitted or in cotton or polyester fabrics. Its great advantage is that the neck opening is simple, there are no fastenings to cope with and the trousers have elastic tops. It is a warm and comfortable garment for the child to wear and highly recommended.

Not recommended are the shiny nylon shell suits.

Dresses

Shifts or pinafore dresses are most practical; they are simple to put on and have no fastenings. Some designs have buttons on the shoulders and these can be replaced with Velcro if you wish. You may find it easier to dress your child if you buy the type of pinafore dress that has buttons on the shoulders and down one side.

Shifts and pinafore dresses can be made in a variety of materials and can be worn with a tee-shirt, blouse of jersey underneath. For the older child who **cannot** dress herself, a dress will be easier to put on if the fastener is down the back, so that both arms can be put through the sleeves first.

Overalls

PVC and allied materials are the best for overalls, as they can be washed down without being taken off. If overalls are used at mealtimes, be sure that they are the type with deep pockets around the hem, to catch falling pieces of food. Back fasteners will be found the most satisfactory.

Bibs

Absorbent terry bibs with PVC backing provide the best protection for babies and very young children. These come with simple ties at the back, or the poncho-style bib which goes over the head and ties at the side. For the messy eater just starting to feed himself, overalls with long sleeves or terry bibs with PVC backing have been found to be the answer by some parents. For the older child, a long life 'Dikki bib' might be tried. This has an adjustable neck fastening, moulded front to catch spills and has the advantage that it can be easily rinsed and wiped clean.

Note

Some mothers whose children dribble constantly find that a piece of terry towelling or similar absorbent material placed under the child's dress or top helps to absorb excessive moisture. There are also now available scarfs of absorbent material that are worth trying.

Capes and jackets

Capes with and without hoods (for wet and fine weather) and ponchos come in a variety of colours and as they have no sleeves are much easier and quicker to put on while a child is small. If required, a loop of elastic can be inserted for the shoulder, and one for the arm to prevent them slipping off. The design of the poncho is so simple that it can easily be made up in any material. Padded jackets can be difficult to put on and take off, but fortunately there is quite a large range to choose from these days and I would advise you to try a number before making a final decision.

For added warmth under a coat, a simple idea is to knit, or make in warm material, a sleeveless coat or waistcoat which is warm but not bulky, and is easy to put on and take off.

Mittens

Mittens are sometimes easier to get on than gloves. To prevent the child losing them, attach a piece of elastic or tape for the wrist.

Hats

As hats are often difficult to keep on, a hood with a band under the chin and snap-fastener, or a combined hood and scarf, are the most serviceable. Many jackets and coats have detachable hoods which are much easier to manage.

Shoes

Before discussing the various types of shoes available, let us first look at the important role our feet play, both for balance and walking. To illustrate the point try the following experiment:

Stand on one leg and feel the amount of movement in your foot and toes. Now stand with your weight on the inner side of your foot and try to balance on one leg – you will find that it is impossible. Claw your toes and get someone to push you, and you will immediately fall backwards and lose your balance. Walk with your weight first on the inner, then on the outer edges of your feet, and see the effect this has on your whole walking pattern and general posture of your body.

These are some of the problems your child may be experiencing when he tries to walk.

If you have ever suffered from a pair of shoes that were the wrong size, I am sure you will remember the discomfort and blisters that you got as a result, and how this affected the way you walked. This I think highlights the importance of always seeing that your child wears a well-fitting, supportive pair of shoes that can easily be modified if necessary. Otherwise his ability to balance, and the way he stands and walks, can only deteriorate.

Obviously it is not possible to give any specific advice regarding footwear, as not only are the needs of any two children not alike, but the type of shoes most suitable will change according to the problems presented at various times.

Some children may need to have a pair of boots or shoes specially prescribed, an additional support provided to build up his shoe on the inner or outer side, or for alterations to be made to the height of the heel. These will all be done by the orthotist. It is therefore important **always** to discuss the subject of footwear for your child with your therapist **before** going to buy shoes, as well as when buying subsequent pairs.

Some general comments regarding footwear

The first pair of shoes is just as important as subsequent pairs, and even at an early age size is very important. Each foot must be measured for length and width and the results compared to see whether one foot is longer or wider than the other. Differences are more likely to found in children with the hemiplegic type of cerebral palsy, where there may be a discrepancy in bony growth resulting from the unequal pull of the muscles. It is also necessary to see how the child's weight is distributed when he stands, **both in and out of his shoes**, and that his shoes are easy to put on and take off.

A shoe that opens down the front will make it easier to get the child's heel and foot well down into the shoe.

When a child can walk, he should be encouraged to do so **in** the shop, before deciding which shoes to buy. Even though he cannot talk, he will soon let you know which pair of shoes he likes the best by the fuss he makes when you try to take them off! Most children are very proud of their shoes, so if your child shows a preference for a certain colour, let him choose the ones he likes. This is doubly important with a child who is capable of walking but reluctant to do so!

When a child has reached the stage of taking off and putting on his own shoes, while in the shop satisfy yourself that he can manage them himself. Fortunately, these days it is no longer a problem, as a large number of shoes and boots have Velcro fastenings. Later, slip-on models, elastic-sided shoes, and elastic laces and eyelets that can be adapted to make lacing easier, are now available. It may seem an obvious point, but remember the thickness of a sock can make the difference to the fit of a shoe.

Children in general, and children with cerebral palsy in particular, are very hard on their shoes. In the UK, Shoe Goo, a polyester resin, Devcan Flexare, a rubber-like urethane which forms a glossy coat, or acrylic cement cap application which is evolved from dental and model plastic are materials that can be purchased for protecting shoes. New products for reinforcing shoes are frequently being introduced, so watch out for them!

Immediately your child's shoes show signs of wear ask your therapist to reinforce the toecaps, or advise you how this can be done. Do not wait until a hold appears. Many mothers, as an added precaution, have a protective material put on a new pair of shoes before they are worn. Children's shoes are such an expensive item, it is worth thinking about.

When special alterations have been made to shoes it is **essential to check** the way your child walks in them for the first two or three weeks to see if the alterations made have been beneficial so that, if necessary, further changes can be made without delay.

If your child is not able to tell you that his shoes are uncomfortable, look regularly to see if he has any areas of skin that look red or any pressure sores on his feet. Keep an eye on the heels and soles of his shoes to see if they are being worn evenly.

Note: However attached your child might become to his first pair of shoes, when at home, **do not** let him wear them **all** the time.

The following are shoes that parents have found the most suitable for their child and in the UK can be purchased in most good shoe shops.

For the younger child

● Elefanten which have a continental narrow heel and arch support (Figure 17.18).

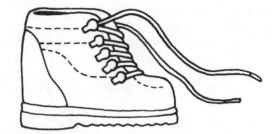

Figure 17.19 Richte boot

● Baby Botte and Superior Baby Botte both have narrow fittings.
● Richte is a good sports boot (Figure 17.19)

For the older child

● trainers which have soft, padded tongues and arch supports
● good-quality sandals
● for the child who cannot keep shoes on, knitted socks with leather soles or a Norway-type boot have been found useful
● Pedro boots (Figure 17.20), covering a wide range of sizes – on prescription in the UK
● Wellingtons – these are now in PVC and come in all sizes, short or long with warm linings.

Note

Unfortunately I have to end this section with a word of warning. The shoes that we have mentioned are expensive, but as far as your child is concerned they are an article of clothing that should always have **top** priority; inexpensive

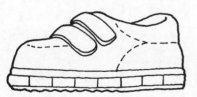

Figure 17.18 Elefanten shoe

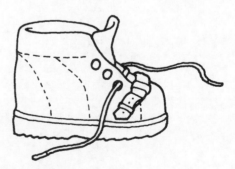
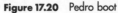

Figure 17.20 Pedro boot

shoes will **not provide** the child with the adequate support that he needs.

All children enjoy being told how nice they look and should be encouraged to take pride in their appearance. When old enough and within reasonable limits, they should be allowed to choose the colour and type of clothes and shoes they prefer to wear.

Chapter 18

Feeding

Helen A. Mueller

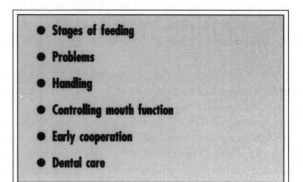

- Stages of feeding
- Problems
- Handling
- Controlling mouth function
- Early cooperation
- Dental care

From birth and through the early years, feeding presents problems for most children with cerebral palsy. We need hardly stress the importance of proper food intake for the child's physical, emotional, social and dental development. A good feeding pattern is essential for future speech.

Early stages of feeding

The following outlines the early stages of development of feeding, so that a comparison can be made with the problems experienced by a child who has cerebral palsy.

During the first few months a baby takes food in by what is known as a 'sucking–swallowing reflex'.

As this reflex is insufficient from birth in some babies with cerebral palsy, mealtimes can present real difficulties for him and for his mother, either because he will become impatient and tense and start crying or else he escapes by falling asleep for most, if not all, of the feeding time; sometimes the mother will then enlarge the hole in the nipple, tilt the baby back and let the liquid trickle down. This is passive feeding and while it may help to get the food down, it usually causes choking and certainly does nothing to help to develop better mouth functioning and sensation.

After the first few weeks, a mother starts to give her child juice with a small spoon and he will suck the liquid in; after about 6 months and when he begins to sit, he is ready to learn to take the liquid or food from a spoon with his lips and transfer it for swallowing, a process which generally takes about a month or more before he is proficient.

During this time the baby with cerebral palsy may appear also to be sucking by opening and closing motions of his mouth, but his attempts are ineffectual, so once again the liquid food has to be poured down the back of his throat. If you offer him semi-solid liquids, such as yoghurt, he is very likely to manage earlier and more easily to swallow it taking it with his lips.

At six to seven months a baby normally begins to munch – in effect he is getting ready to be able to bite off and to chew solids; gagging occurs much less frequently now and dribbling will generally be noticed only during the teething period. These are signs that oral control is developing. The child with cerebral palsy is often unable to chew and instead makes forward motions with his tongue, pushing the food back out or glueing it to the roof of his mouth; the food may get squashed but it is not chewed and when it reaches the back of the mouth it is uncontrolled, generally leading to gagging and choking.

About one month, after a baby has learned to take food from a spoon, he will, while in a sitting position, be ready to drink liquids from a cup or a glass. In the early stage there is bound to be some incoordination, resulting in the liquids leaking out on the side of the mouth together with some coughing and gulping; these effects will continue to be seen until his oral control has become efficient enough to enable him to deal adequately even with wholly liquid foods. The child with cerebral palsy, however, will probably be unable to get his lips 'attached' to the cup or glass, while his tongue will very likely protrude over or under the rim of the cup or glass; you may already have noticed these abnormalities while he was having his bottle. The mouth makes the same unsuccessful opening and closing motions, the tongue pushing forward as the child tries to drink. These abnormalities are similar to those described when we were speaking of chewing; this results once again in the child's head having to be tilted backwards, letting the liquid run in and down passively which provokes choking, coughing and air-gulping.

As drinking through a straw usually calls for good oral control, the use of straws for drinking by children is not adopted until they are 3–4 years old. The type of sucking used when drinking through a straw requires much finer coordination of the lips than is necessary for reflex sucking by the infant. Drinking through straws is something the child with cerebral palsy can seldom manage as instead of holding the straw and sucking it with his lips, he puts the straw into his mouth like a nipple and bites it or holds it up so that the liquid flows in passively. This lack of coordination will show itself by the irregular flow and by coughing, choking and air-gulping.

Feeding the child with cerebral palsy

What are the major feeding problems of the child with cerebral palsy? They are lack of mouth, head and trunk control, lack of sitting balance, and inability to bend his hips sufficiently to enable him to stretch his arms forward to grasp and to maintain that grasp irrespective of the position of his arms; finally, his inability to bring his hands to his mouth and his lack of eye–hand coordination.

It must be stressed that it is only by careful observation and analysis of the child's disabilities and abilities can we hope to help him. We must not expect improvement in the child's feeding abilities until we have helped him to acquire the fundamental abilities which will make self-feeding possible – that is, the ability to move his head, jaw, lips and tongue independently from the body and hands while having good sitting balance. Stability in the pelvis and trunk are the prerequisite.

Some positions for feeding

We continue to stress that adequate control of the 'whole' child is essential while he is being fed. Unless this control is secured he will become more spastic or will have increased involuntary movements, even before the bottle or spoon is placed in his mouth, thus making it harder for him to suck or to use his lips; whenever possible do avoid placing your hand on the back of the child's head for support as this will immediately cause him to push back.

A good feeding position for the young infant and the severely handicapped baby is shown in (Figure 18.1a–c). The baby's legs are kept apart and scissoring is made impossible by your body, his arms and head are brought forward from the shoulders, and kept in this position by placing your hand flat and with pressure on his lower chest Figure 18.2(a–c). If you need that hand for oral control, use your forearm to apply pressure on the child's chest. Have his food at your side so that the child can see it and not on the table where he would have to stretch backwards to find out where each spoonful is coming from. This is a position which allows good overall control as well as good eye contact and is especially useful for those children who have a tendency towards asymmetry; by sitting closer to the table and placing the wedge at a steeper angle (Figure 8.3a,b) you will gradually be able to get the child into a more upright position.

A good feeding position for the baby who has some sitting balance is on your lap, controlling him as shown in Figure 18.4. You can keep him from throwing himself into extension by flexing his hips and placing your leg under his knees

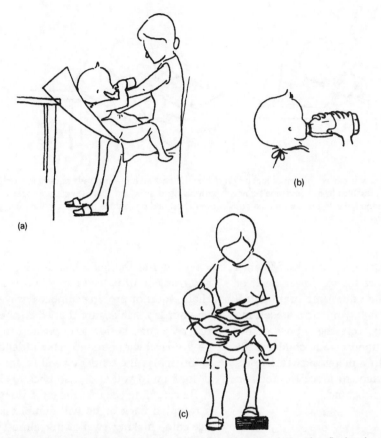

Figure 18.1 (a) Bottle feeding. When needed, mother applies pressure to the chest with a flat hand and oral control during sucking
(b) The baby puts his hands around the bottle
(c) *Correct.* Feeding of a baby in half-sitting position with head and both arms forward

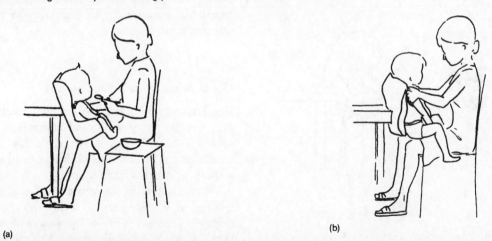

Figure 18.2 (a) Half-sitting position for the child with some sitting balance. Remember to put the food in front of him. If the child still needs support, an 'infant seat' can be used, resting against the table edge
(b) When sitting balance improves, sit the baby up straight with his legs abducted and his hips will flexed. You may still have to control him from the shoulders

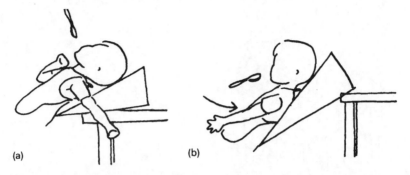

Figure 18.3 (a) *Wrong.* The baby is placed in front of mother on a foam-rubber wedge, which rests against the table edge. Without control and when the spoon is presented from above, the baby will push his head back and cannot swallow properly

(b) *Correct.* If you put your hand flat with pressure on the baby's lower chest and present the spoon from the front, you help him to control his head and to swallow

higher than the leg under his buttocks. When a child needs extra support for his lower back or his shoulder, while at the same time oral control is necessary, you may find your arm becoming over-tired; to avoid this, rest the elbow of the arm you are using to support your child on the table and cushion it with a pillow. As stated previously, it is very important to place the food in front of the child and not behind.

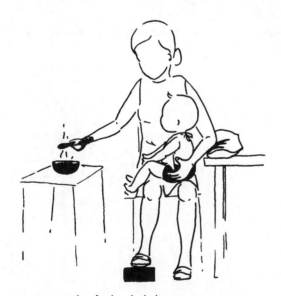

Figure 18.4 When feeding the baby in a sitting position on your lap, you can prevent hyperextension by putting your leg under his knees on a stool to give him more hip flexion. If he needs support on his lower back or shoulders, put your arm on a pillow on the table. The food must be in front of the child

As soon as the child has developed some head and trunk control, feed him while he is sitting on a chair – do not prolong unnecessarily feeding him on your lap. Make sure that when the child is sitting on a chair beside or opposite you that you are on eye-level with him or even a little lower than he is, otherwise the tendency will be for him to have to look up to you and push back his head.

Be careful to see that the child does not sit with a rounded back or he will compensate by lifting his chin, making swallowing almost impossible. Have **you** ever tried to swallow with your head tilted back? See also that his hips and knees are at a right angle and his legs are slightly apart; groin straps will occasionally be necessary to maintain this position.

Controlling mouth functioning

Besides controlling the 'whole' child during feeding, we can apply additional control in the oral area which will help to improve his sucking–swallowing reflex and his ability both to eat from a spoon and drink from a cup.

When control of the muscles of the mouth is lacking, it is necessary to apply oral control to improve feeding. This is applied with two fingers – index and middle finger. The middle finger is the most important and must be placed just behind the chin and firm pressure of the finger must continue to be applied; this pressure by the

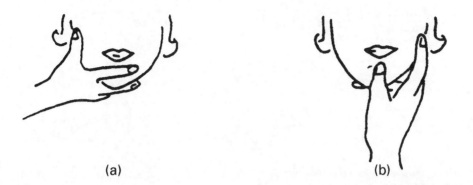

(a)   (b)

Figure 18.5   (a) Oral control as applied when the child is on your right side with your arm around his head: thumb off his jaw joint, index finger on chin, middle finger behind chin applying constant firm pressure
(b) Oral control as applied from the front: thumb on jaw chin, index finger off jaw joint, middle finger applied firmly just behind the chin

middle finger enables tongue functioning to be indirectly controlled thus helping swallowing to be more normal. Figure 18.5(b) shows oral-control as applied from the front, while Figure 18.5(a) shows its application when the child is on your right side with your arm around the base of his head. The child will probably respond on the first occasion to oral control by pushing against it, but give him time to adjust; do not pull his head back but keep it upright with his neck straight and you will soon find that he accepts this help.

Before presenting the bottle, spoon or cup to the child, apply oral control, otherwise you will find that his efforts to reach them will often cause hyperextension of the whole body.

With the gradual improvement of oral functioning you will gradually be able to lessen and finally withdraw oral control.

The most common of all problems that make feeding of the child with cerebral palsy so difficult are tongue-thrust, prolonged and exaggerated bite reflex, abnormally strong gag reflex, tactile hypersensitivity in the oral area and dribbling. Good oral control is therefore a most important factor for children with oral dysfunction.

Remember: Good oral functioning, including coordinated swallowing, depends largely on a straight spine. Spontaneous mouth closure and swallowing can be facilitated by temporarily elongating the neck a little extra.

Hypersentitivity

Touch in the mouth will increase sensitivity and become exaggerated if there is over-stimulation by the use of a nipple, spoon, straw or teat or if a mother wipes a dribbling child's wet mouth and chin often during feeding and at other times during the day. Guard against hypersensitivity by avoiding such overactivity and where possible make use of oral-control. Where hypersensitivity has become very pronounced, consult your speech therapist.

Dribbling and open mouth

This is a common problem among children with cerebral palsy and will certainly not disappear when parents continue merely to remind the children throughout the day to close their mouths and to swallow. The obedient child will of course try to draw in the saliva but lacking the ability to swallow properly, his efforts will be of momentary effect only and the accumulated saliva will dribble out again just as soon as he reopens his mouth with an extensor spasm, when feeding, babbling or trying to speak. You will help your child more if occasionally during the day you place your finger across between his upper lip and nose, exercising firm and continuous pressure, back (not down) and do this without talking to him or interrupting

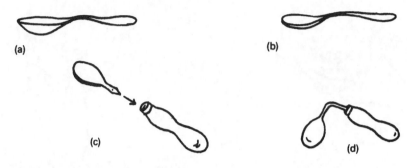

Figure 18.6 (a) *Wrong*. The spoon is too deep and pointed
(b) *Correct*. The spoon should be fairly flat and rounded
(c) To adapt the metal spoonhandle, it can be cut to a point and pushed firmly into a tool handle
(d) To adapt the metal spoon, bend it at an angle and tilt it according to the child's needs

his play; gradually you will find that spontaneous mouth-closure and spontaneous swallowing will take place. In addition, continue to use oral-control in feeding and drinking as this will establish a proper swallowing pattern.

Bottle-drinking

With babies who have an abnormal sucking–swallowing reflex, improvement can immediately be achieved by combined body, head and oral control. The old-fashioned round nipple is the easiest for the cerebral palsied infant. If he still has difficulties in sealing his lips around the nipple, bring his cheeks forward with two fingers of the hand you are using for oral control and, if you have enlarged the hole in the nipple, thicken the formula of the liquid which will stop if from trickling down into his throat uncontrolledly. If the child is so severely handicapped that he has no sucking–swallowing reflex and needs to be tube-fed, the only way to get him off the tube and to more normal feeding is by spoon-feeding.

Spoon-feeding

Here again oral control is very important, but often will not be sufficient to enable the cerebral palsied baby to start taking semi-solid foods from a spoon; here, firm pressure with the spoon flat on his tongue will prevent the tongue from pushing forward and will bring about spontaneous use of

lips and tongue. In these cases, use a metal or bone spoon, as a plastic spoon will break very easily and is generally too deep (Figure 18.6a).

Make sure that the spoon is not too deep, otherwise the food cannot easily be scraped out of it with the lips, or not one too long and pointed which might cause stimulation of the gag reflex (Figure 18.6b). The spoon should **always** be presented and placed **from midline, never** from the side when feeding children with cerebral palsy.

Having pressed the spoon on the tongue firmly, be sure to take it out without scraping it on the upper teeth or lip (Figure 18.7a,b); at the same time do let the child try to get the food off with his upper lip while you press with the spoon on his tongue. Feeding will be easier for him if, to begin with, you place only a small amount of food in the front of the spoon. As soon as you withdraw the spoon, see that the mouth is closed so as to keep the tongue inside for carrying the food around the mouth instead of letting the tongue push the food out.

If spoon-feeding presents real difficulty, as a last resort use your fingers but then only with such solids as meat, bread, fruit, etc.

When introducing spoon-feeding you will find that strained but fairly dry food is best to begin with, liquids and thinly strained foods are considerably more difficult, and those of a mixed texture such as thin vegetable soup will always remain the most difficult with which to cope.

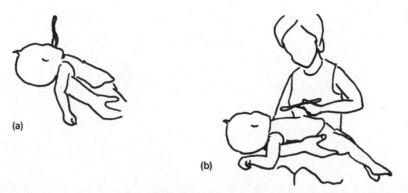

Figure 18.7 (a) *Wrong*. The child is fed while he is totally passive in hyperextension, food is scraped off on the upper teeth, causing gagging, coughing and choking
(b) The child can never develop good swallowing in hyperextension with one arm behind mother

Chewing

To develop chewing, it is best to place such food as particles of meat or crusts of brown bread by hand between his teeth on the side of his mouth, helping him to close his mouth by using oral control. Biting off the food can be stimulated by pulling slightly on the bread or by scraping the crusty food on the side of the teeth before putting it in between and helping the child to close his mouth firmly with oral control. Once the child has managed to bite, the jaws must stay closed and here again oral control is important and is secured by continuous firm pressure with the middle finger; this will lead to the chewing motions; do not move the child's jaw or try to get him to open or close his mouth as if he were biting and do **not** apply intermittent pressure – all this would only reinforce abnormal patterns.

If the child finds chewing difficult, try the following – take a small quantity of best quality raw meat, cut a 'finger-size' piece and sprinkle it with a small quantity of seasoning salt; this method has the advantage of being absolutely safe as a piece cannot be bitten off with the danger of it slipping back into the child's throat. While you hold onto one end of it, the child, with oral control, chews on the other end and while he is doing so chews out the nourishing juices of the meat and at the same time is practising swallowing and after a while he can start on the unchewed end of the finger of meat. It is much better to practise this

at the beginning of the main meal, as it is an effective preparation for chewing.

If during feeding a piece of food slips back into the child's throat and gets stuck, make sure to bring him well forward into good flexion at once and do not become nervous; if you react quickly and calmly there will be no danger, as the piece will come back out and the child will not be unduly frightened. **Do not** pat his back as this causes inhalation and may lead to aspiration.

Drinking

It is difficult for the small child with oral dysfunction to learn to drink liquids and help will be necessary for some time; here again, careful control of the whole body, the head and of the jaw, in particular, is of the utmost importance (Figure 18.8a,b). As already said, it is by no means enough merely to get the liquid down by some means or another, as then the child is forced into a totally passive role and will not learn, and you will be in an even worse situation than before as oral hypersensitivity is likely to increase, and with it choking and gagging or maybe even aspiration of liquid.

Start by using a plastic beaker and one with a projecting rim (Figure 18.9a). Cut out an opening on one side for the nose (Figure 18.9b), which will enable you to tilt the beaker until the last drops have gone and avoids the necessity of bending the

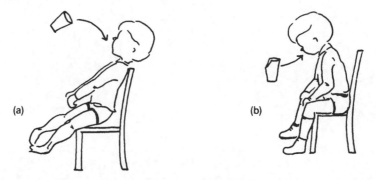

Figure 18.8   (a) *Wrong.* The cup is presented from above and the child is tilted back
(b) *Correct.* The child is in a sitting position for drinking, with the trunk and head well forward and the beaker is presented from the front

child's head back (Figure 18.9c); also you will be able to see and control what is happening at his mouth.

The most important single factor in learning to drink is the mouth closure, as it is only if the jaws remain closed and the rim of the beaker is resting between the child's lips, will he eventually be able to use his lips and be able to swallow without gulping air. Tilt the beaker to the point where the liquid touches the upper lip, leaving the child to do the rest. **Do not** remove the beaker after each swallow, but let it rest between the lips, as otherwise the strong stimulus which may result can lead to you losing head and oral control. To start with, slightly thickened liquids such as yoghurt will be found easier; acid liquids are the most difficult owing to their tendency to increase the flow of saliva.

Never give the child who has drinking difficulties a cup or a beaker which has a spout, as this

will only make him relapse to primitive and abnormal sucking.

Drinking with a polyester tube

If we observe the progress of a **normal** child towards the ability to feed, it will be seen that sucking through a straw or tube is difficult and only comes at a late stage in his development; with children with cerebral palsy, however, it should not be attempted until fairly well coordinated drinking ability has been reached and then only to improve lip mobility or to help the athetoid or ataxic child, who has difficulties in lifting the cup, to drink independently.

Use a thick-walled polythene or polyester tube and one with a small inner diameter, so that one suck allows a limited amount of liquid to come through and no air is gulped. The same method as that used in drinking from a cup should be

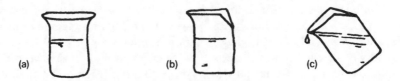

Figure 18.9   (a) A plastic beaker with a projecting rim is useful to start proper drinking
(b) The beaker can be cut out on one side for the child's nose
(c) Tilt the beaker this way for drinking

used – the tube should be held and sucked by the lips alone, the jaws remaining closed with oral control if it is needed. To keep the tube in place and to avoid spilling, a beaker with a lid and a spout, similar to those used for patients in hospital, **in which the tube can be inserted**, can be used. This will enable the child to put both his hands on the table round the beaker and help to stabilize him while he is sucking in the liquid through the tube.

The first steps towards self-feeding

Babies of a few weeks often rest a hand on their bottle while they are being fed. At about 5–6 months they hold the bottle with both hands, and gradually the hands are brought in front of the child's face and he beings to look at them.

At about 1 month he starts to put one hand to his mouth, without being conscious that he is doing so; this is then followed by both hands and he starts to suck them.

At about 6 months when he starts to reach out and grasp, he will take a rusk to his mouth and suck it, but he will quickly drop it. At about 9 months he will take a rusk to his mouth but now in a deliberate way and will drop it only when he has had enough or his attention is distracted.

Some children at about 8–9 months begin to 'understand' that the spoon and the food go together and will guide their mother's hand when she is feeding them with a spoon. Others at this stage will help to guide a cup to their mouth. Babies, of course, differ considerably and some will never bother to help or will do so only when they are hungry.

Between the age of 9 and 12 months a child will go through the stage of putting his hands into his food for the joy of squeezing it and will then smear it over his face and anything else that happens to be near. At this time the child will often snatch at the spoon when he is being fed, but will only use it to bang on the table or to plunge it into the food; he is still unable to use a spoon to feed himself.

At about 15 months he has the ability to grasp the spoon with his whole hand and to feed himself, for short periods however, and in a clumsy way. Finding difficulty in getting the food onto the spoon, he will use his other hand to push the food on, dropping a great deal and turning the spoon over in his mouth in his effort to get the food off.

From now on, through constant practice, his abilities commence to improve fairly rapidly and by the time he reaches the age of 2 years he has become proficient and most of the time usually insists on feeding himself.

The child with cerebral palsy

The athetoid child and the severely spastic quadriplegic child are often unable to reach the stage of being able to bring their hands before their face, much less to hold and to bring an object to their mouth; it must be appreciated that there is a clear difference between the problems of these two types of handicapped children. The athetoid child holds his arms away from his body, his head control and ability to focus his eyes are poor and his grasp is weak and ineffectual. The spastic quadriplegic child, whose whole body is involved, has both arms pressed against his side or over his chest with his hands clenched, usually with the thumbs tucked against the palms, and has great difficulty in opening his fingers.

On the other hand the spastic diplegic child – whose head, arms and hands are slightly affected – at the age of about 5 months has little difficulty in reaching the stage of being able to take things to his mouth while lying on his back or on his tummy while he is at play. His difficulties, however, will be seen when he is sitting, as having no sitting balance he has to rely on his arms and hands for support and if he lifts up an arm to take his hand to his mouth or leans his head slightly backwards, he is in danger of falling backwards.

The hemiplegic child will also be able, without much difficulty, to follow the normal developmental sequences leading to self-feeding. He, however, will only use and look at his unaffected good hand and if his sitting position is poor, there will be an increase of 'associated reactions' in his affected arm and hand and he will experience difficulty when he starts to try to use a knife and a fork.

There is little point in forcing this child to use his affected hand unless he has a good grasp and can move his arm freely; the problem is that when trying to use a knife and fork the effort of cutting with the unaffected good hand makes the affected arm and hand too stiff to handle the fork and to bring it to his mouth.

This is another example of an 'associated reaction' and it is one that can be overcome by allowing the child to eat in the manner adopted by some adults, that is to say, first cutting up the food, then laying down the knife and using the same hand to lift the fork to the mouth. The child, however, should gradually learn to hold a fork in the affected hand and to apply pressure with his index finger. This is an isolated movement and he will have to learn to point with his index finger, keeping his other fingers bent before he can be taught to press down with a straight index finger on the fork.

We must not forget that normally a child is not proficient in using a knife until he is about 5 years of age or more.

When your child is learning to feed himself, do not expect every mouthful to be a success and be prepared for a mess. A PVC overall with long sleeves and a deep pocket at the bottom, and one that fastens down the back, is a 'must' at this time. Give him plenty of time and do not stint praise for achievement, otherwise he will soon lose interest and be happy to let you continue to feed him.

Until a child has acquired adequate sitting balance he must be controlled in his chair so that he has both hands free; the first essential of course is a suitable chair, when necessary use groin straps or a simple belt around his middle. In the case of the athetoid or ataxic child, a strap over the feet provides adequate stability and keeps the feet down, but adopt this method only as a temporary measure.

Start to prepare the child for self-feeding while he is still a young infant by bringing his arms forward to the bottle – refer again to Figure 18.1(a,b). In play, encourage him to bring his hands to his mouth, i.e. mouthing, but **never** encourage thumb-sucking and later when you feed him with a spoon and a cup, try occasionally to open up his hands and put them on yours or around his beaker.

When your child has reached the stage where he wants to feed himself, analyse his difficulties carefully so that you will know exactly where he needs your help. Do not bother him unduly, and keep whatever help you feel you must give him to a minimum as this will lead to the maximum of effect, study Figures 18.10–18.16 and select whichever is most suitable. When the child manages increasingly well, then reduce your help gradually and quietly to let him become more and more independent.

Gadgets for use in feeding must be kept to an absolute minimum; some of the following may, however, prove to be of some use. For the child who has difficulty in getting the food onto a spoon, the steep side of a small bowl will be found more useful than a plate and by placing a non-slip mat underneath, it will be prevented from slipping; if a deep-sided plate can be managed, use the type that can have hot water put into the base to keep the food warm, as so many cerebral palsied children are slow eaters.

It should be remembered that an important part of self-feeding is to pick up your own knife, spoon and fork, cup or glass, no easy task for a cerebral palsied child; non-slip mats can now be bought in

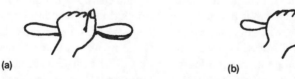

(a)   (b)

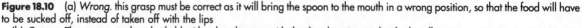

Figure 18.10 (a) *Wrong.* this grasp must be correct as it will bring the spoon to the mouth in a wrong position, so that the food will have to be sucked off, instead of taken off with the lips
(b) *Correct.* The spoon needs to be held with a hand-grasp with the thumb going under the handle

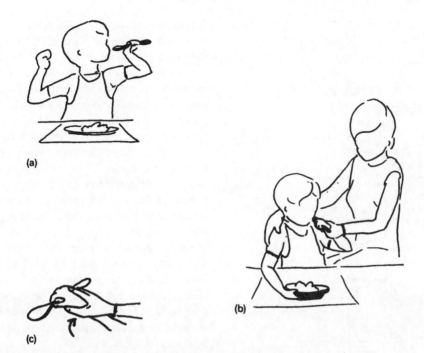

(a)

(c)

(b)

Figure 18.11 (a) *Wrong*. Self-feeding without control in hyperextension and in an asymmetrical pattern
  (b) *Correct*. Self-feeding at the table, with control at the shoulder and supination of the hand holding the spoon
  (c) Adding supination to the hand by turning it out lightly from the root of the thumb

large sizes and will give additional help. When a child reaches the stage of learning left, right, top and bottom, reinforce this by getting him to place his own knife, fork and spoon in the correct position. Encourage him later to lay the places for the rest of the family including putting the glasses in the correct position.

Spoons, forks and knives can be fitted with plastic handles; these can be obtained in many 'do-it-yourself shops' and are available in three sizes and they can be bent according to your needs, see Figure 18.6(c) and (d). Rubazote tubing (supplied by Nottingham Rehab) also makes a good temporary handle; do not forget to exchange the fitted spoon for a normal one just as soon as the child can hold it, in most cases a dessert spoon will usually be best.

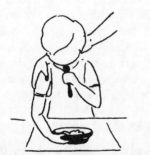

Figure 18.12 *Correct*. A self-feeding child needs very little shoulder control. The hand, which he does not use, is put around the plate or bowl to keep it in front and to avoid extensor pattern

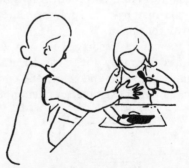

Figure 18.13 The self-feeding child sits across the corner of the table. You can help him with head control by putting your hand flat on his chest with pressure

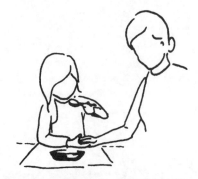

Figure 18.14   You can help your self-feeding child to avoid asymmetrical patterns by flexing his arm across him tummy on top or under the table, supinating his hand

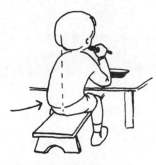

Figure 18.15   When trunk and head control are still difficult for the self-feeding child, sitting on a bench in riding fashion may be a good solution: if he tends to sit with a rounded back, he will need support at the lower part of his back

Sometimes it will be necessary to help the self-feeding child with supination to keep him from placing the spoon in his mouth sideways instead of straight from the front. To do this, place your hand lightly over the child's hand, turning the root of his thumb outwards with your own thumb (refer again to Figure 18.11b,c); if he still cannot manage you may have to apply pressure on this tongue with the spoon.

When the child is feeding, help him with your hand to feed normally and most certainly avoid telling him what to do and do not be continually correcting him. For example, an open mouth, or a

Figure 18.16   For support on lower back, attach a block to the bench

tongue thrust are part of a pattern of total extension (refer again to Figure 18.7a,b). A jaw and tongue that deviate to one side are part of a general pattern of asymmetry; lack of head control means that the child does not have the pelvis and trunk stability necessary for the jaw, lips and tongue to work in a coordinated manner. If your child has the added problem of a high palate, be very careful **not** to give him mushy or sticky foods such as bananas.

The early patterns of feeding are so closely linked to the development of future patterns of speech that any abnormal feeding patterns that are allowed to develop, or to persist, will certainly affect the child's attempts to babble and later to make articulate sounds. By working closely with your speech therapist in attempting to prevent faulty feeding patterns, you will also be helping the child to develop the movements of the mouth, tongue and lips which he will need when he starts to speak.

Despite the difficulties, mealtimes should be enjoyable times for the child and for his parents – try not to become over-anxious as if you are he too will become over-anxious or frustrated.

Remember that teaching your child to wash his hands before and after meals and to wipe his mouth and hands afterwards are important items in his programme of self-feeding and self-care.

Dental care

Children with cerebral palsy are usually very difficult to treat dentally; feeding problems, especially those of chewing, but also seizure-medication, make their teeth extremely susceptible to caries and the gums tend to become inflamed and swollen. Dental care is therefore all the more important. Teeth cleaning also presents a problem due to their hypersensitive mouth and gums.

Advice on cleaning teeth

Before the milk teeth appear, or for the child who has not had previous treatment for a hypersensitive mouth, a good way of cleaning the gums is to use cotton wool dabbed in bicarbonate-of-soda or saline or even water. When the first teeth are coming through use a small infant-sized toothbrush with water, gradually introducing toothpaste; remember that it is the mechanical brushing which keeps the child's mouth clean and healthy rather than the toothpaste.

When cleaning your child's teeth, place him in a sitting position that enables him to have good trunk and head control.

With the small baby you will find it easier if you sit on a stool in front of the washbasin, with the baby on your lap or astride your knee. For the older child who can clean his own teeth, a stool close to the washbasin will enable him to rest his arms, giving him added stability.

If your child has difficulties in closing his mouth or is hypersensitive, oral-control as used in feeding may be found helpful (refer again to Figure 18.5a,b). Remember that brushing the gums is just as important as brushing the teeth; always massage the gums towards the roots of the teeth. When you brush the outside of his gums and teeth, use a circular movement, keeping his jaws closed and the head slightly flexed.

In time, your child will learn to spit out the accumulated water, saliva and toothpaste. As a first stop in learning to do this – that is before you open his jaw half-way to brush the inside of his gums and teeth – allow the accumulated water and so forth just to dribble out. It is important that you take care when doing this to see that your child's head does not push back, otherwise choking and gagging will occur. Bringing the child's shoulders and head slightly forward will prevent this.

The electric toothbrush

For children with cerebral palsy an electric toothbrush has considerable advantages. Independent studies in the USA and in Switzerland have shown that children with cerebral palsy who use electric toothbrushes have much healthier mouths than those who use ordinary brushes. There are two main reasons for this. First, it is sometimes difficult for these children to make the correct brushing action with an ordinary toothbrush, whereas an electric toothbrush needing less manipulation is usually easier to use. Secondly, these children can never brush as intensively and precisely by hand, whereas the electric toothbrush automatically massages thoroughly the gums and supporting tissue of the teeth; the tissues of the teeth of many of these children are notoriously spongy and swollen due to lack of the massage, which takes place while chewing solid foods. It is important, however, that the electric toothbrush has fine, intensive vibration and is used without pressure.

Special instructions on dental care

As dental surgery is difficult for the child with cerebral palsy and for his dentist, it is very important that parents should be careful about cleaning the child's teeth after every meal.

Avoid sugary foods, sweets and confectionery and soft drinks containing sugar; if the child does have sticky foods they should be restricted to mealtimes only and the teeth should be cleaned immediately afterwards. The child should be encouraged to eat cleansing foods, for example, apples, cucumbers and so on, in preference to sugary foods.

It is important that the smallest toothbrush available be used, as this enables you to brush the child's gums all over. Dentists stress that brushing the gums is even more important than brushing the teeth, as the gums are the supporting structure of the teeth and it is essential that the gums remain healthy. Food particles do collect around the edge of the gums, with the result that bacteria multiply rapidly and the teeth start to decay, so use dental floss to prevent food collecting between the teeth.

How often and from what age should the child have his teeth seen by his dentist? The answer is that the child is never too young; preferably he should be seen at the same time as other members of his family. If he attends at a sufficiently early age, not only will he become accustomed to going to the dental check-up and will gradually become free from the fear which usually accompanies such visits, the chances are that no treatment will be necessary for the first few visits, but these visits will be extremely useful in gaining the child's confidence. Finally every child should be seen by his dentist at least at six-monthly intervals.

Chapter 19

Carrying

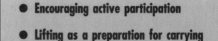

- Encouraging active participation
- Lifting as a preparation for carrying
- Handling and carrying
- Baby carriers

The way we carry a child can influence his motor behaviour and we should therefore make every attempt to ensure that carrying is a **dynamic** experience for the child and **not** a **passive** one and that it provides yet another learning opportunity. It is a subject, as I am sure the reader will appreciate, for which we can only present general guidelines because the specific details will be determined by the particular and unique difficulties of your child, his size and weight and of course your own physical build.

We will look at some of the problems that might arise when picking up and carrying the child inside and outside the home, discussing ways of handling which may help you correct any abnormal postural patterns present, stimulate head and trunk control and balance reactions. Thus encouraging your child, when possible, to adjust his position by himself and, should he lose his balance, hold on to you when necessary.

Lifting and carrying

The baby who has normal muscle tone

Until a baby has developed some means of locomotion he will be completely dependent on his mother to carry him from one place to another. He will be picked up, carried and put down many times a day while she sees to his needs of feeding, bathing, dressing, placing him in his cot or pram, or down to play.

Automatically, while he is small she will hold him close to her, supporting him firmly and completely. This is a soothing tactile experience for the baby who will enjoy the closeness, warmth and movement of his mother. From time to time she will smile, talk, or perhaps give him a kiss, reinforcing the bond between them.

At around 5 months, when she bends down to pick him up, he immediately anticipates her intention by lifting his head and reaching out towards her, often kicking his legs in excitement. When she puts him down he keeps his head, shoulders and arms forward until the last moment. She can carry her child in a variety of positions, moving him if he becomes too heavy, knowing that he will automatically hold on, for instance by putting his arms around her neck if he feels insecure.

Later, as his balance improves and he is able to adjust his position by himself, she will only need to give him minimal support.

So we can see that although a baby is dependent on his mother to pick him up and put him down, at no time is it a passive experience but rather a dynamic one, the mother reducing her support and encouraging his active participation. Figure 19.1 illustrates how we normally carry a young child who has good balance.

The baby with cerebral palsy

Often a baby with cerebral palsy will need to be picked up and carried for longer than a normal baby and of necessity be given much more support. It is, however, important that this extra sup-

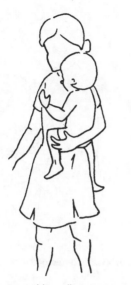

Figure 19.1 How one would usually carry a young child who has good balance

port is adjusted and withdrawn as early as possible. This gives the baby the opportunity of adjusting his own position; he learns to maintain and regain his balance himself, and look around and interact with the environment.

Although the basic principles of handling will remain the same whether you are carrying your child inside or outside the home, putting him into his high chair, pushchair or a car seat, the techniques of handling will need to be modified and changed according to the child's reactions in different situations and under different circumstances.

For example, carrying a child around the house when you have both hands free is very different from carrying him when you are out. Then you may have to hold the hand of a toddler, or perhaps a shopping bag at the same time. Again, putting your child into his high chair or pushchair is very much easier than, for example, putting him into his car seat.

The way you carry your child will be influenced by your own physique, i.e. your size and height, whether you have small or large hands, and so forth. I would therefore ask the reader to resist the temptation of just looking at the illustrations, but also to read carefully the reasons **why** certain

ways of carrying have been suggested. You can then modify your handling to suit your own needs and those of your baby, remembering that the techniques you use will change at different stages in his development.

The baby and young child who has moderate spasticity and is predominantly extended

Bringing the child up to sitting

Before sitting the child up, see that his weight is evenly distributed and that he is lying as symmetrically as possible, keeping this symmetry as you bring him up to sitting. If, when you go to pick him up, he gets excited, pushing himself backwards into extension and becoming stiff, making it difficult for you to bend his hips and bring his arms forward, try first rolling him onto his side. Then semi-flexing his hips and legs, bring his arms forward and get him up to sitting through side-lying.

Figure 19.2(a,b) illustrates a way of bringing baby up to sitting, who is predominantly extended, his arms flexed and retracted at the shoulders. It is important to note how your forearms keep his legs apart and turned out, leaving your hands free to control the shoulders by lifting and turning them in. Handled in this way will help to bring the head and arms forward and facilitate the bending of the hips and legs.

With the **older child** you may find it easier to control the position of his legs if you have them over the edge of a bed or table. This position should **not** be used if it causes the child to hollow his back and flex his hips.

Carrying

Figure 19.3 illustrates how, by holding the child **incorrectly**, one can reinforce any abnormal postural patterns present. His mother, by having the child's legs around her waist, has increased the internal rotation and adduction of his hips, and because she is supporting him under one buttock

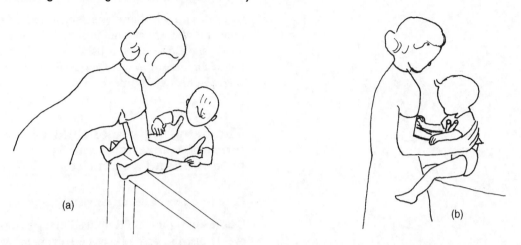

Figure 19.2 (a,b) A way of bringing a baby up to sitting, who is predominantly extended, his arms flexed and retracted at the shoulders

only, his pelvis is tilted up on this side accentuating the asymmetry of the trunk and legs. The fact that he is supported high up on his back and not under his armpits means that he is unable to extend his back or lift his head.

In order to make carrying a positive therapeutic influence you could try one of the following methods.

You will see in Figure 19.4 that, by holding the child on your hip, it is possible to flex his legs with less abduction while at the same time rotating his trunk. Supporting him under his armpit enables him to get his arms up and forward and lift his head. Carried in this way, the child has good eye contact with his mother and is able to make use of any ability he might have to grasp and balance.

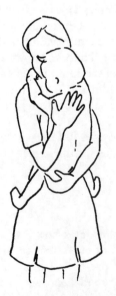

Figure 19.3 How, by holding the child **incorrectly**, one can reinforce any abnormal postural patterns present

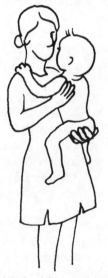

Figure 19.4 By holding the child on your hip, it is possible to flex his legs with less abduction while at the same time rotating his trunk

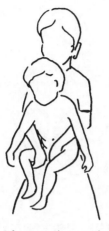

Figure 19.5 A way of carrying that a mother might use at home

Figure 19.5 illustrates a way of carrying that a mother might use in the home. The child is facing away from her, his legs flexed, abducted and outwardly rotated, the mother using her forearms to stop the child's shoulders from pushing down. Keeping his hips flexed, she has pulled his bottom towards her, his trunk leaning forwards. Carried

in this way stimulates the child to **lift his head** and **extend his back**.

The older child with severe spasticity who is predominantly extended

Bringing the child up to sitting

Lifting a child who is predominantly extended when he is lying often presents a problem, as shown in Figure 19.6(a). If he is lifted in this way it is then impossible to flex and abduct his hips or put his arms up over your shoulders (Figure 19.6b). The problem is dictated by the difficulty we have in bringing up to sitting, i.e. in bending him at the hips and bringing his shoulders forward. To help solve this, try rolling him onto his side first and then placing a hand on his chest at the same time as you bring his head and shoulders forward. It will then be easier to flex his hips and keep his legs apart (Figure 19.7).

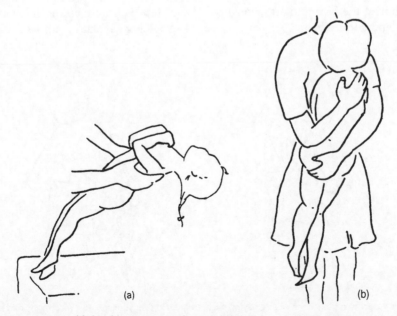

(a) (b)

Figure 19.6 (a) The incorrect way to lift the older more severely extended child from the lying position
(b) Illustrates the problems in carrying that result i.e. difficulty in bending his hips, bending and parting his legs, and bring his arms up over ones shoulders

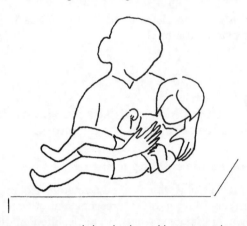

Figure 19.7 How to help solve the problem presented in Figure 19.6 by rolling the child onto his side first, and then placing a hand on his chest at the same time as you bring his head and shoulders forward

Carrying

Often the only way to carry a child as he gets heavier is over your shoulder. Figure 19.8(a) illustrates the problems that arise when this is done **incorrectly**. The child's head is hyperextended, with excessive flexion at the shoulders, his arms pulled together (adducted), which results in increased extension of the hips and legs, making it difficult to flex and abduct them.

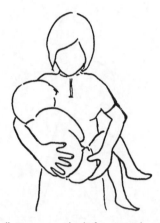

Figure 19.9 Illustrates a method of carrying that should **always be avoided**

Figure 19.8(b) illustrates how by keeping both the child's arms over your shoulder forward and away from his body, it enables him to lift his head and straighten his back. Now, with both hands free, his mother is able to keep her child's hips flexed, abducted and outwardly rotated.

Note

A method of carrying that should **always be avoided** with all children is illustrated in Figure 19.9. Being carried in this way, like a baby, is not

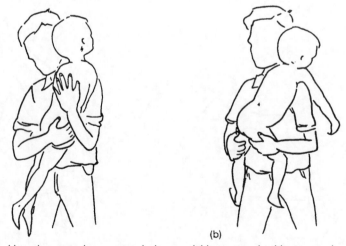

(a)   (b)

Figure 19.8 (a) Shows the problems that arise when carrying the heavier child over your shoulder *incorrectly*, and how it could be better done

(b) By keeping the arms over your shoulder and holding the legs high up on the thighs, if it is possible to keep the legs apart and turned out

only bad emotionally for the child, but denies him the opportunity to do anything to help himself and reinforces any asymmetry that may be present.

The young child with moderate/severe spasticity who is predominantly flexed

The young child who is predominantly flexed adopts a position in which he extends his head with a 'short neck', i.e. his chin poked forward, arms turned in at the shoulders, flexed against his body, one or both hands fisted, hips and legs turned in and partially extended.

Carrying

A good way of carrying the child at home is on his side, pressed against you, as illustrated in Figure 19.10(a,b). In this position you can keep the child's back extended, stop the pulling down and bending of his arms, while at the same time keeping his hips and legs extended, apart and turned out at the hips and, in addition, introducing rotation between the shoulders and pelvis.

An alternative and more active way of encouraging a child to lift his head, extend his back and hips, and reach out with both arms to explore his

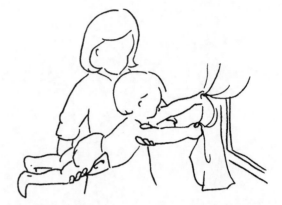

Figure 19.11   An alternative and more active way of getting a child to explore his surroundings as you carry him

surroundings as you carry him, is illustrated in Figure 19.11.

Figure 19.12 illustrates how, when both parents are available, an older, heavier child can be carried in a way that combines carrying with treatment. The child's legs are extended and outwardly rotated at the hips, his feet flat against one parent's body. When the tone in his muscles decreases sufficiently for you to straighten his hips, if you stabilize his pelvis and push your thumbs up from the bottom of his buttocks, you can stimulate him to actively lift his head and extend his back. We would **not** recommend carrying the child in

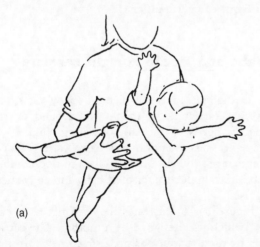

(a)

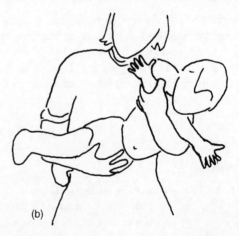

(b)

Figure 19.10   (a) A good way of carrying the child at home is on his side, pressed against you
(b) Introducing rotation i.e. between pelvis and shoulders

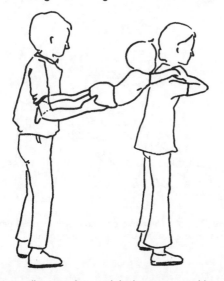

Figure 19.12 Illustrartes how, with both parents, an older, heavier child can be carried in a way that combines carrying with treatment

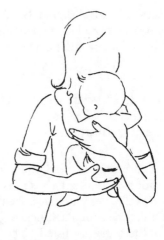

Figure 19.13 Illustrates the incorrect way to carry a baby who has low tone

this way if, when doing so, the child adducts and internally rotates his legs.

The baby/young child with low postural tone and/or fluctuating tone and involuntary movements

Bringing the baby up to sitting

I always find it easier before lifting a baby to 'gather him together'. I do this by bending and bringing his legs together over his abdomen, both arms forward hugging his legs. The baby then can be brought up to sitting by either rolling him onto his side or straight up, whichever is easier.

Carrying

Figure 19.13 illustrates the **incorrect** way to carry a baby who has low tone. He is completely passive; there is no eye-to-eye contact and, because of the lack of fixation at the hips and shoulders, the abnormal postural pattern of the limbs remains unchanged, his body flexed.

Figure 19.14(a–e) illustrates the **correct** ways to carry a baby and young child by giving pelvic and, when necessary, shoulder girdle stability to enable him to lift his head and shoulders, bring his arms forward, extend his back and interact with his parents and the environment.

Figure 19.15 illustrates an alternative method of carrying a baby or small child in the prone position which encourages head and trunk extension.

Note: When carrying a baby in this way care must be taken to see that his weight is taken **evenly** on his forearms and that his elbows are **in front** of his shoulders.

Baby and kiddie upright carriers

It is difficult to recommend a baby or kiddie upright carrier as so much will depend on the specific needs of the baby or young child. I will therefore just mention the baby carrier that a number of mothers I have spoken to find comfortable and supportive for their baby and convenient to use.

Figure 19.16 illustrates the Wilkinet baby carrier which was designed by a mother. The carrier can be used in four positions, from newborn to 2 kg (5 lb) in weight. It is recommended for the following reasons:

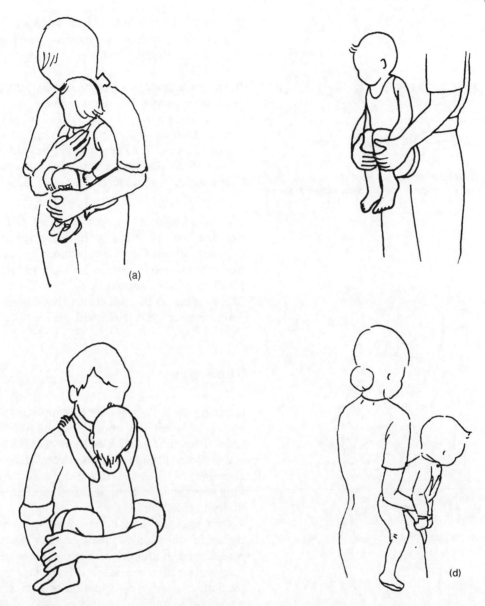

Figure 19.14   (a–e) Illustrates the various ways of carrying a baby and young child with low truncal tone, providing the necessary support to enable him to interact with his parents and the environment

(a) By stabilizing the pelvis and shoulder girdle the child with poor head control and low truncal tone is encouraged to lift her head

(b) A simple way of carrying a child at home – the child's bottom against his father might tilt forwards, is a good way of facilitating active extension of the head and trunk

(c) Introducing rotation and encouraging grasp

(d) One of the ways you might try carrying a child who has low truncal tone **combined** with slightly increased tone in the legs

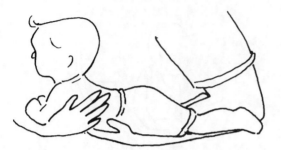

Figure 19.15   Illustrates an alternative method of carrying a baby or small child in the prone position which encourages head and trunk extension

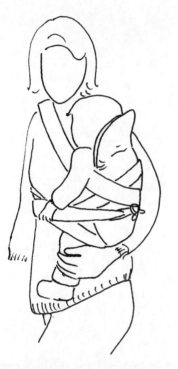

Figure 19.16   Illustrates the Wilkinet baby carrier

- the baby's head and back are supported by an all-in-one cushioned support, well-padded shoulder straps providing extra support for the head
- the lower spine is supported against the parent by **base** supports **under** the thigh and bottom
- long straps are used rather than buckle fasteners – these wrap around the parent **and** baby and tie over the baby's back, ensuring even weight distribution and putting no strain on the parent's shoulders or on the small of the back.

If you should decide on the type of kiddie carrier that rests on one's back, do remember that these are designed for the child who has head control and can actively extend his back and hold on. Ideally the frame should be light weight and also free standing, as this will ensure that it is easier for you to manage your child without help.

Summary

Carrying should always be kept to a minimum, especially when the child is at home. One is often tempted to carry a child, as it saves time or is done in response to his often vocal demand for attention, but it must be remembered that each time we carry a child he is deprived of an opportunity to move on his own.

Carrying should not be a passive experience and by careful attention to the position in which he is placed prior to lifting, which is the preparation for carrying (or the first stage of carrying), we can facilitate his active participation by inhibiting the unwanted movements or abnormal postural tone. Use of any equipment for carrying should be evaluated on the premise.

Chapter 20

Chairs, pushchairs and car seats

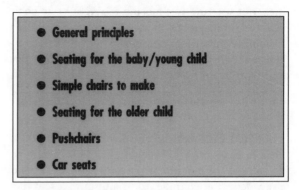

- General principles
- Seating for the baby/young child
- Simple chairs to make
- Seating for the older child
- Pushchairs
- Car seats

As the efficiency of the support provided by different types of chairs and pushchairs will depend on the problems and abilities of each child, we will confine ourselves to discussing just a few seating systems, giving a description of their use, followed by some simple types of seating you could make yourself, and ending the chapter with a selection of pushchairs and car seats.

Adaptive seating for the child with cerebral palsy aims to correct and control postural asymmetry, improve voluntary upper limb function, and enhance communication, feeding, and social skills and learning, in their widest sense.

Following the many clinical observations, research and publications on the subject of seating systems, it has now been established that a versatile seating system should:

- provide the child with a stable postural base (the position of the pelvis being a key factor)
- provide the child with postural trunk control and alignment
- be sufficiently adapted for growth and ability
- control the child's posture while at the same time enabling him to develop his own sitting ability.

However, owing to the variability of the cerebral palsied child's problems, opinions on the literature differ as regards the most efficient seating system that will meet **all** the above criteria. Aware of the problems involved in the design of both chairs and pushchairs, manufacturers using

the latest computerized technology and advances in design techniques, and working in close collaboration with orthotists and therapists, are continually modifying and redesigning their seating systems.

Because of the high cost of materials, chairs and pushchairs involve a considerable financial outlay for parents and are certainly not items that should be chosen directly from a catalogue. They should **only** be purchased after **discussion** with your physical or occupational therapist who, following an evaluation of your child's abilities in a number of positions and having noted any asymmetries of posture or movement present, will be in a position to give you advice regarding the most suitable seating for your child, whether any adaptations need to be made, and the minimal amount of support that will be necessary to stimulate postural control and hand function, and so forth.

Some general considerations

Sitting only becomes the most **functional position** for play when a baby is approximately 8–9 months. By this time he has good trunk control, balance and hip mobility. He can reach out in any direction to get his toys and no longer has to rely on his hands for support and therefore is able to develop and practise fine manipulative skills when sitting.

Obviously we cannot wait until a child with cerebral palsy has developed all these basic abilities, but we can, by choosing the right basic chair adapted for his needs, enable the child to maintain a stable symmetrical posture so that he can concentrate, when sitting, on using his hands for play and later when learning to eat and dress himself.

No child should spend prolonged periods of the day in a chair

The child with total involvement, for example, if he is to sit securely in his chair, will only be able to do so if he has maximum postural support. This is equivalent, for example, to us sitting in a seat in a cinema where there is no room to stretch our legs for 3 hours. Although we are able continually to adjust our position, when we do eventually get up we often feel rather stiff. It is therefore obvious that a child who is unable to move or adjust his position, will not only become very stiff but in time will be in danger of contractures developing. It is therefore important that children who are limited in their ability to move should spend part of the day in a variety of positions on the floor and be given every opportunity and encouragement to **move** freely. Whenever possible they should also spend time in an upright position, using one of the many standing systems available. The position a chair is placed in a room, and the occasions a child needs to sit in his chair will depend on his stage of development and his ability to use his hands.

At mealtimes, the best position for a baby who can sit in a high chair would be at the table with the family – a practical position for his mother while she feeds him, and later when helping him to eat by himself, or when playing **on his own** while **she** is **nearby**. But if he has brothers and sisters who prefer playing on the floor or at a low table, he will most likely become frustrated if he cannot play beside them. To avoid this happening, if the high chair is not the type that can be converted into a low one, it would be better to find another position for the baby, perhaps on the floor so that he could play at their level for at least some of the time.

It is worth remembering that, when you are playing with your baby, your lap or the corner of the sofa is softer and more comfortable than a chair!

To take another example: a child who has some sitting balance, although able to sit on a box seat and watch television when supporting himself on his hands may not have sufficient balance for activities where he needs to use both hands. But he **would** be able to use the **same** box seat if we placed it in the corner of the room with a chair or table in front of him to hold on to or lean against, and a non-slip mat for his feet. In this way, the child would have a sense of security and be able to develop sitting balance with minimal support when for example playing, and later when learning to dress and undress himself.

Some older children **even when they have good sitting balance**, often find dressing and undressing easier if they sit on a bench, rather than on a regular chair or their bed, as the width of the seat provides them with a good supporting surface.

Assessment

All seating needs to be continually evaluated, and **your observations** of your child's achievements or any difficulties he has when sitting in his chair are invaluable. You may have noticed, for example, that when using his hands your child slips down in his chair and it becomes impossible for him to see what he is doing, or when trying to reach for his toys he bends forward from his trunk rather than from his hip joints, and you wonder if there is some way of stabilizing his pelvis. On the other hand, you may feel that his sitting balance when he sits on the floor has improved so much that the minimal support previously suggested for his chair is no longer necessary. Rather than waiting for your child's next reassessment, make a note, or if you have a video camera a short sequence of any points you may wish to discuss with your therapist, so that she can assess and make any changes that are necessary.

It is also a good idea to check the chair itself to see if there is any **uneven** wear on the seat or armrests, as this will indicate that the postural support recommended may need to be reassessed.

As your therapist will recommend the chair most suitable for your child's needs, we have chosen just a few chairs of different designs, including those that you can make yourself for the age group covered in this book, to give an idea of the chairs that are available. We will also comment on their suitability or otherwise for children with varying disabilities.

Chairs

The Snug Seat

The Snug Seat has been specially designed to provide postural support and a stable sitting base for a baby and younger child (age range 6 months to 4 years) who has low truncal tone and poor head control. The modular seat comes with an extensive range of positional pads which can easily be adapted for the baby's changing needs, and the range of adjustments to the angle of the chair means that the baby can be placed in a more upright position at the appropriate time in the child's postural development. It is supported in a strong, lightweight steel frame, with a stable base and can easily be moved from room to room, enabling your child to interact with you in a different environment (Figure 20.1).

Note: Although this seating is a good supportive system for babies with poor head control and low truncal tone who flop forward when placed in sitting, **as soon as** the baby starts **actively** to extend his head and back he should be seated in a more upright seat with good pelvic stabilization.

Tumble Forms Deluxe Floor Sitter

This floor sitter, owing to its contour shape, is often the only type of seating that a young **severely involved** child because of his strong hypertonus (spasticity) and asymmetrical posture finds comfortable. The seat is made of soft washable material of firm-density foam that retains its shape and includes an integral abductor and positioning belt. A separate wedge holds the unit in an upright or inclining position. This chair (Figure 20.2) can also be used for feeding.

Note: The contour shape of this seating module is designed to fit the fleshy contours of the buttocks, and is therefore comfortable for the severely involved child. However, research has shown that this shape will not provide sufficient stabilization to counteract any asymmetry that may be present at the pelvis, and care must therefore be taken to see that **any** tendency to asymmetry is corrected by the hip positioning belt supplied with this model.

It has also been established that, as the centre of gravity is behind the sitting base, there is a tendency for the pelvis to tilt backwards and the child

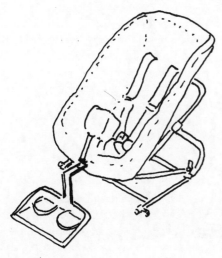

Figure 20.1 The Snug Seat

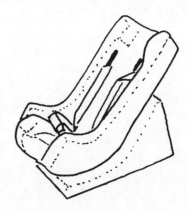

Figure 20.2 Tumble Forms Deluxe Floor Sitter

to slip down and forward in the chair. This should carefully be monitored.

Corner chairs/seats

Since the previous edition of this book, manufacturers have vastly improved the design and adaptability of these seats. They now offer:

- upholstered adjustable back and lateral wing supports
- padding that extends over the top of the seat for neck and head support
- wedge-shaped abductor pummel with positional changes
- seats that can be raised by locking in an extra sitting base
- trays that are adjustable in both height and angle.

Figure 20.3(a,b) illustrates the James Leckey Corner Sitter. The seat, back and side supports are padded, the padding extending over the back of the supports. The oblong reversible pommel is adjustable in depth. Adjustable trays in both height and angle are available as an accessory. Figure 20.4(a) shows G. & S. Smirthwaite's Variable Height Corner Chairs (model 516), suitable for children from 12 to 18 months upwards. The upholstered wings and back are adjustable. Accessories are a handrail and a 25 mm (1 in) thick seat cushion. Figure 20.4(b) illustrates the possibilities for raising a corner chair (design by G. & S. Smirthwaite Ltd).

Note: This type of seating is useful for the child with intermittent spasm and involuntary movements or moderate spasticity who can sit in long sitting, but lack sufficient sitting balance to use both hands in this position. It also has the added

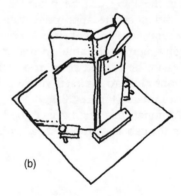

(a)

(b)

Figure 20.3　(a) James Leckey Corner Sitter – front view
(b) James Leckey Corner Sitter – back view

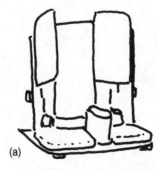

(a)

Figure 20.4　(a) G. & S. Smirthwaite's Variable Height Corner Chair (Model (516))

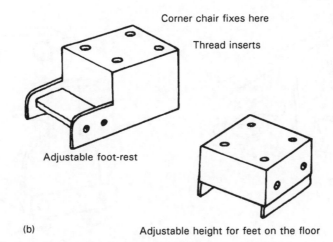

Corner chair fixes here

Thread inserts

Adjustable foot-rest

(b)

Adjustable height for feet on the floor

Figure 20.4 (b) The manufacturer's design for raising their corner chair

advantage that any additional support can easily be moved and adjusted as the child learns to sit on his own.

Children with extensor spasticity and tight hamstrings, whose pattern of sitting is back on their sacrum with a flexed spine, should **not** use a corner seat **unless** the sitting base is raised so that the child can sit with his legs flexed, feet flat on the floor.

The folding canvas corner seat

This seat was designed by the Cheyne Walk Spastic Centre and to meet the need for a foldable chair suitable for children with spasticity, age 2–8 years. The design of the seat encourages the legs to roll outwards, and when it is raised off the ground the child's feet can be flat on the ground. It slopes backwards to reduce the necessity of strapping. To prevent the seat being pushed backwards, there are two extensions at the back well behind the corner (Figure 20.5).

Note: We would **only** recommend this chair for the moderately involved child who can sit supported but lacks balance, but **not** the severely involved child. Its **main advantage** is that it is light and portable, and therefore can be used **outside** if, for example, you are visiting friends.

'Safa' bath seat

This seat was originally designed by a father as a bath seat for his child (Figure 20.6). We have also found it useful as a regular seat for young children who are just beginning to get sitting balance, and it is particularly good for the young child with spasticity involving one side of his body (hemiplegia). The seat gives the child a feeling of security as his feet are on the ground; it also has the advantage that if he feels he is losing his balance he can hold onto the metal bar in front of the seat and therefore no extra support is necessary. When needed, a table can be placed in front for play. We have found the most satisfactory way of suspending the seat is between two chairs (see Figure 13.7, Chapter 13).

Note: We do **not recommend** this type of seat for any child with strong extensor or flexor spasticity or intermittent spasms.

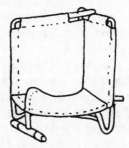

Figure 20.5 Folding canvas corner seat

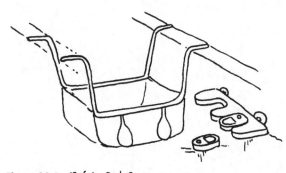

Figure 20.6   'Safa' – Bath Seat

The Roller chair

The Roller chair was originally designed by the author for children with extensor spasticity who were unable to achieve pelvic and trunk alignment or sit with their hips flexed, legs abducted and outwardly rotated with their feet flat on the floor, making it difficult or impossible for them to bring their arms forward, with the additional problem that as they brought their hands together towards the mid-line, adduction as well as extension of the legs was present. Groin straps and the round abduction pommels, which were once used, were found to be inadequate. A pommel, although it held the child's knees apart, did not solve the basic problem, i.e. the extension, adduction and internal rotation (turning in) at the hips. Thus the idea of the Roller chair, with help in the design from a parent, was born. I was later approached by Mr M.S. Wason of the Isle of Wight who amended the basic design, adding a back to the set and making its height and that of the roller itself adjustable, with a simple brake for the castors so that the child could push himself around (Figure 20.7a). The Engine Seat is very stable and can also be used as a walker, with a lightweight passenger on board to make it more fun (Figure 20.7a–d).

At present, a number of manufacturers using the same principle have improved the design and added many other useful features, such as that by Jenx Ltd for their Liora Roller Seat. Its suggested use is for children with mild to moderate seating needs, as it combines its function as a seat with a means of improving dynamic balanced by adjust-

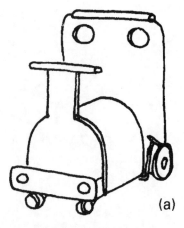

(a)

Figure 20.7   (a) The Engine Seat

ing the amount of freedom of the roller to roll. Another design feature is by G. & S. Smirthwaite Ltd in their adjustable height bolster chair (512) (Figure 20.8). The bolster is oval and can be turned 90° to give 225–300 mm (9–12 in) of abduction. The foot, arm and headrest wings are adjustable. A laminated plastic tray is supplied with the chair. It is recommended for the more severely involved child.

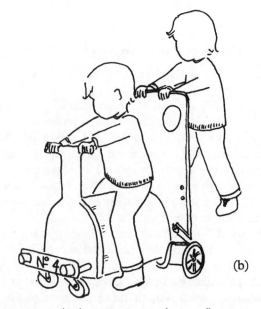

(b)

Figure 20.7   (b) The Engine Seat used as a walker

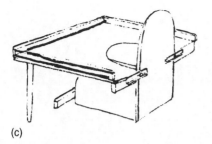

(c)

Figure 20.7 (c) Cut-out table showing the use of door bolts to attach table to the chair back

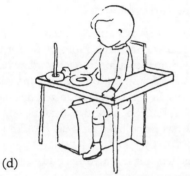

(d)

Figure 20.7 (d) Child sitting on **roller chair** with cut-out table in front. Note that height of roller is level with the knees. There should be a space of about 50 mm (2 in) between the child and table at the front and at the sides

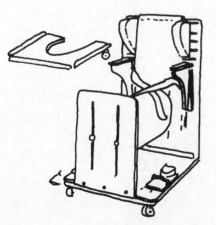

Figure 20.8 G. & S. Smirthwaite Adjustable Height Booster Chair (512)

The bean bag chair

It is always advisable in life to own up to one's mistakes, and the use of this chair for the severely involved child is one of mine. Hopefully, if any parent did take up the suggestion they also read the repeated warning – **only use for short periods**. The only excuse I have is that in 1974, when the second edition of this book was published, there was not the wide selection of seating systems available for these children that there is today. However, many houses do possess bean bag chairs, and I still think they make a comfortable chair for a mother to sit in when playing with her baby or young child. I also sometimes use a bean bag chair when teaching babies to roll, creep and crawl, as it is soft and can be pushed into various shapes. Babies feel secure on its wide surface and enjoy the movement of the polystyrene bead filling.

Complete seating systems

A large number of manufacturers have now designed complete seating systems which enable the child to have correct postural control in the sitting position, with external modifications that can be removed as the child grows and his abilities change. These chairs are very versatile and are supplied with a large number of adaptations. Seating systems have also been designed, where the child sits in a forward leaning position with an extended trunk, shoulders and arms forward, thus placing him in a functional position. An example of such systems are the Jenx prone angle chairs. The basic chair has chest and lateral supports, adjustable footplate, seat and abduction cushion. A variety of optional accessories are also available.

The Baby S.A.M. seating system illustrated in Figure 20.9(a,b) has been developed for the very young child with postural impairment, who either has or is at risk of developing spinal deformity. The child sits in a straddled, forward-leaning position. The seat provides a stable base for the pelvis and thighs, while a thoracic support maintains the alignment of the trunk over the pelvis. The child feels secure and is enabled to hold up his head,

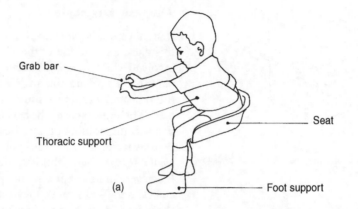

Grab bar

Thoracic support

Seat

(a)

Foot support

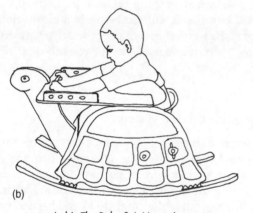

(b)

Figure 20.9   (a,b) The Baby S.A.M. seating system

develop sitting ability, and use his hands for play and function.

The Baby S.A.M. is a static seat. For the child of 3 years of age and above, the S.A.M. can be used as a powered and static system. Any enquiries about this seat should be made to the Mary Marlborough Disability Centre.

Inflatable chairs

If you look around the shops you will see the inflatable chairs in various shapes such as a triangle, or round seat for very small children. A word of warning when using an inflatable chair as they are generally rather light, for safety they should always be placed where there is additional stable support.

Triangle inflatable chair

We have found this chair, which is available from large department stores, most useful for the young child who pushes himself backwards when sitting, as the lack of stimulation on the buttocks, due to the hollow in the seat, minimizes this strong pattern of extension and the triangle-shaped back helps to keep the head up and shoulders forward (Figure 20.10).

Note: Do not leave your child unsupervised in an inflatable chair.

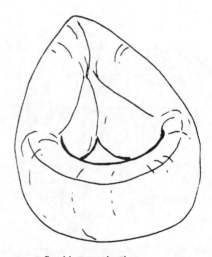

Figure 20.10   Inflatable Triangle Chair

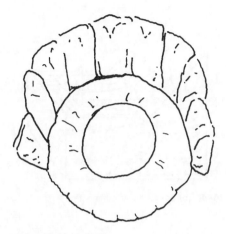

Figure 20.11   The Booster Seat

The Booster Seat

This seat should only be used for **small children**. It is small and light and can be placed in an armchair or pram, but not of course in a pushchair. Some parents have found the seat useful when feeding their child (Figure 20.11). It can be purchased from Mothercare and is in the UK Heinz Baby Catalogue.

Baby seats

Until a baby reaches the stage, when he is sitting, of being able to bring his trunk forward and support himself on his hands, regular baby seats that can be purchased from such stores as Mothercare will usually be found adequate for a baby's needs (Figure 20.12a,b).

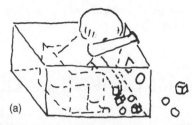

Figure 20.13   (a) 'Sit-at-Table' seat used in a cardboard box

For a young child who has just developed sitting balance, a regular child's seat such as the 'Sit-at-Table' seat is, when placed in a cardboard box, is an excellent way of giving him confidence (can be purchased from Mothercare). The fact that if he loses his balance he has the sides of the box to hold on to makes him feel safe, and this encourages him to lean forward automatically as he reaches to pick up his toys, or attempts to get those that have fallen outside (Figure 20.13a,b). It

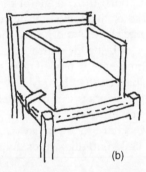

(b)

Figure 20.13   (b) 'Sit-at-Table' seat used attached to a solid chair

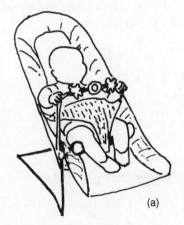

(a)

Figure 20.12   Regular Baby Seats

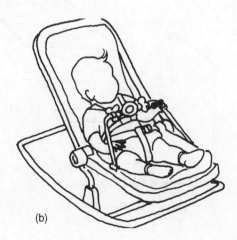

(b)

can also be used at mealtimes and when a child plays at a table.

Chairs you can make yourself

Box seat

This seat is made of wood, is simple to make and is designed so that a young child can sit with his legs straight out in front of him. The straight back of the box, in combination with the sloping angle of the blunt-ended wedge and the narrowness of the sides of the box, gives the child with poor sitting balance a stable base and a feeling of security, so that additional support is usually unnecessary (Figure 20.14a,b).

The correct angle of the seat is of the utmost importance, as the child's lower back must rest against the support. If the angle of the seat is too steep, the base of the spine will be rounded, his pelvis tilted backwards, and he will be unable to flex at his hips or bring his arms forward to play. If the child's arms have a tendency to press down when he sits, be sure that the tray is at chest height or tilted. Different trays can be slotted in to add variety to the child's play.

Mothers who have to apply 'jaw control' when feeding their child find this seat useful, as the child

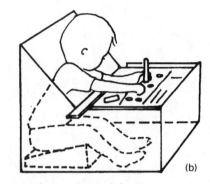

Figure 20.14 (b) Box Chair with fitment

is well supported leaving her hands comparatively free. Being small, the box seat has the added advantage that it can be placed on a table at mealtimes at a useful height for the mother.

Note: We do **not recommend** this seat for a child with poor head and trunk control, or those who are very flexed. A child with asymmetrical patterns of posture and movement may need additional support.

Simple wooden chair

This is a stable chair whose simple design is easy to make and has been found very successful. The different heights of the seating placements means that two seats can be interchangeable over a long period of time, using one as a chair the other as a table. This is a useful chair for the child with moderately increased tone. The child's feet should be flat on the floor (Figure 20.15).

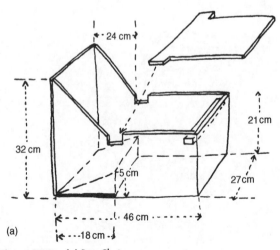

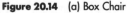

Figure 20.14 (a) Box Chair

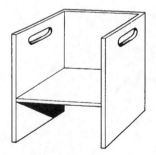

Figure 20.15 Simple wooden chair

Cardboard boxes

A young child with inadequate balance will often feel more secure when sitting in a confined space. For this reason we have lately, both for treatment and for play, made use of large cardboard boxes of varying sizes, which can usually be obtained from any department store or supermarket.

A strong cardboard box makes an excellent play area because toys can be attached across the top, to the sides, or laid on the floor of the box, and a smaller box can be placed inside to form a table (Figure 20.16). It is worth stressing again that **sitting need not be a passive or static function**, and when the child has reached the stage of moving in the sitting position and is starting to pull himself up to standing and so forth, a box makes an excellent practice area for such activities.

When playing in the box, obviously using a far bigger box than illustrated, a child often becomes quite adventurous, automatically practising the basic patterns necessary for getting up to standing. Having reached this milestone, he starts to try to walk sideways around the inside of the box. It is, in fact, **a mobile playpen** and being light can be taken into different rooms while mother does the housework without having to worry about her child's safety.

You can vary the make-up of the box to give the child varying sensations. Sometimes you could, for example, line the bottom and sides with pieces of carpet (display squares of carpets that are no longer in production make an excellent lining and can often be purchased from large stores), or perhaps squares of soft fluffy-type material, such as that which bedroom slippers are made of, which provide a good contrast. You can also vary the contents of the box by filling it with tissue paper, or newspaper, wrapping up some of his toys, or putting in odds and ends around the house that your child enjoys playing with, such as wooden spoons, empty cartons, 'squeezy' bottles and so forth, **always making sure that none of the articles is hazardous**.

Note: We do **not recommend** the use of a cardboard box for a child who has no sitting balance.

The cylinder chair

The cylinder used for this chair is made of thick reinforced cardboard – the cylinders themselves are used commercially. With the section cut out, it forms a useful seat. It can be covered in foam and then a washable material with a foam cushion added to the seat. The seat is a thick disc of reinforced cardboard and gives the necessary stability to the cylinder.

This seat has been found most useful at mealtimes for children who have fairly good sitting balance, but are still apprehensive when using both hands. The shape of the back of the cylinder keeps the shoulders forward and this makes it easier for the child to bring his arms forward, especially for those children who tend to fall backwards when they lift a spoon to take food to their mouths. The shape also gives good support, providing a sense of security for the child. For the young child, the seat can be placed on the floor as illustrated (Figure 20.17a–c).

Note: We do **note recommend** this chair unless a child has fairly good sitting balance. Its main function is to enable the child to get both arms forward for better hand function.

Chair inserts

Fortunately there is a wide variety of padded inserts for babies' chairs and pushchairs on the market that are made to provide comfort and support, some having eyelet holes for a safety harness. They are made in a variety of materials and fillings, e.g. 50% cotton, 50% polyester with 100%

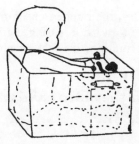

Figure 20.16   Card box as a play area for the moderately involved child

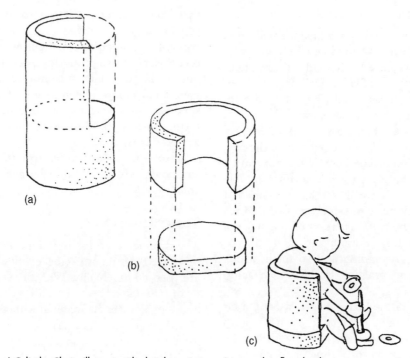

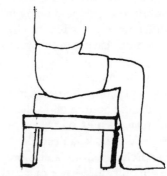

Figure 20.17   (a–c) Cylinder Chair. Illustrating the height variations. Seat used at floor level

polyester fillings, or padded foam with PVC coverings, and are particularly useful for a small baby.

For the older child the Bobath Centre, in collaboration with Tools for Living, have designed a Pommel seat to use as an insert into chairs, pushchairs, buggies and wheelchairs. The foam seat has a large semi-rigid pommel to provide good pelvic stability and excellent abduction (Figure 20.18).

Ramped cushions are invaluable in providing the child who tends to lean backwards because he has tight muscles behind the knees (hamstring muscles) with a stable sitting position. As shown

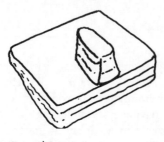

Figure 20.18   Pommel Seat

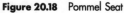

Figure 20.19   Ramped support cushion

in Figure 20.19, the ramped cushion enables the child to come forward in sitting, i.e. bend at the hips, without rounding his back because his thighs are supported.

Seating for the older child who can sit unsupported

When your child reaches the stage of no longer needing a back support, he requires seating that provides him with a good stable base, such as a box stool that can be adjusted to variable heights and enables him to get up from the sitting position to standing.

A variable height ladder back chair is also recommended. This type of seating is particularly good for the child with fluctuating tone and inter-mittent spasms, low truncal tone or moderate spasticity. The ladder back enables the child to reach forward and grasp the rungs and, by 'walk-ing' his hands up them, to get into an upright position (Figure 20.20). The stool can be fitted with removable skis, and provides a stable early walker.

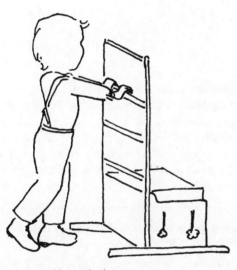

Figure 20.20 Ladder Back Chair

Tripp Trapp chair

This chair is popular with parents whose child has adequate balance, as it 'grows' with the child. It has a broad base with steel spacer bars for ade-quate strength and safety. The two platforms can be altered in height and depth, the foot-rest easily positioned.

For a young child with minimal problems a spe-cial backrest, deep front rail, activity rail and pom-mel can also be supplied (Figure 20.21).

Tables

Chair and table heights need to relate to one another. The table should be at elbow height, so that the upper trunk comes forward which in turn facilitates the forward movement at the hips, shoulders and arms. It also makes it possible for the child to weight-bear on his forearms, provid-ing him with a position of stability when needed. There are a wide range of versatile designs of tables on the market that can be adjusted for height, and angle from the horizontal to the ver-tical, making it easier for the child to use his hands under his own visual guidance, which is important as vision plays a major role in controlling the movements of young children.

Optional extras which encourage the develop-ment of basic hand skills, such as vertical and horizontal hand grabs, and a variety of play frame attachments for the younger child are also available.

Although it is important to have a washable table top surface this usually means that the sur-face will be slippery, and we would strongly advise the use of non-slip mats. These latter can also be purchased in sheets or strips.

Summary

In closing this section on the various types of seat-ing, we must emphasize that **your aim**, as soon as your child has developed adequate sitting balance, should be to have him sitting without any addi-tional support and, in time, in a variety of chairs in everyday use. Complete independence will only be achieved when the child has sufficient balance to use both hands for functional activities, can get his chair for himself, pull it up to the table and get on and off by himself.

Pushchairs

The principles and critical factors that I have dis-cussed in relation to chairs largely also apply to pushchairs. Naturally there are some differences. In a pushchair you are looking at a child who is

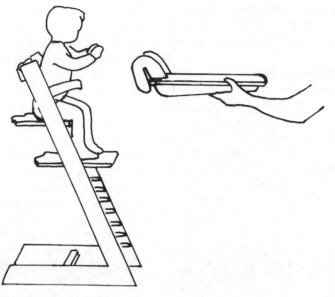

Figure 20.21   Tripp Trapp Chair

sitting but not actively involved in using his hands for skilled movements. With a chair our aim is to try to provide a structure that enables the child to function. The chair in these circumstances is a facilitator for daily activities such as eating, play and learning, as well as reinforcing the basic aims of symmetry, control and stability.

The developments in the design and manufacture that I have already alluded to in earlier paragraphs about chairs also apply to pushchairs.

Before buying a pushchair it is always advisable to get professional advice from your therapist, rather than choosing one that has been recommended or from a catalogue. If the shop will allow you to have the pushchair on approval, take advantage of this service, as this will not only give you an idea whether it meets the needs of your child, but also an opportunity to see how practical it is for yourself – to fold, carry, stack in a car boot or take on public transport – and whether it is easy to store.

You will also be able to see if your child sits as well in his pushchair when you are pushing it as he does when stationary. This is important because the occasions when he is out with you should be an active not a passive experience, rather an opportunity for him to interact with you as he experiences the stimulation of all that is going on around him, and to do this he needs to be in a secure, stable sitting position. Nothing can be more conducive to a child's mental inertia than lying back in a half-reclining position, gazing up at the sky.

Some general points to bear in mind when choosing a pushchair

- Choose a lightweight but stable pushchair with an attractive design, with padded or rubber hand grips, a good braking system, and one that is easy to manoeuvre.
- Pick a versatile system, preferably one that has a basic chassis that will take different-sized seats as the child grows.
- Where adjustments to the angle of the backrest, set height and angle of the foot-rest are available, see if they are simple and quick for you to manage.
- Check not only the age and weight range recommended, but also the height range.
- See that the backrest and seat are firm and that the sides high enough to give support.

- Accessories add to the cost of the pushchair, so check carefully to see if your child's ability to sit improves with additional support by trying them out first.
- Material used on the seat should be non-slip. Fabric covers can only be sponged clean, so choose removable covers that can be machine washed when possible. With a buggy, it will be found easier if you choose a model where the rain gear can remain in place, especially in the UK
- It is important to check, if the pushchair is an imported model, that spare parts are available, and whether the company provides service arrangements for repairs.
- Finally, check that the pushchair or buggy **meets furniture and fire regulations**, and the length of the guarantee.

Having chosen the most suitable pushchair, you might find that you need to purchase additional postural supports similar to those used by your child when sitting in his chair. Manufacturers vary as to the accessories they supply as standard features with their pushchairs. These are expensive items, and your therapist will tell you if she thinks your child would benefit by having any extra support.

Accessories that may be helpful
Groin straps

These help to stabilize the pelvis when taken in front of the pelvis and over the hip joints at an angle of 45° and pulled down and back tied under the seat.

Abduction pummel block

By keeping the legs apart these provide the child with a wide sitting base.

Lateral trunk supports

These stabilize the pelvis, keeping the trunk in mid-line.

Waistcoat (safety jacket) body support or chest pad

These items provides a better alignment of the head and trunk for the child whose upper trunk 'flops' forward.

Retention bar

This is a most useful addition to any pushchair and can be used by a child immediately he has learned to grasp, giving him a feeling of security and stability, enabling him to sit with minimal support.

Foot-rests

The foot-rests on some pushchairs are made in a solid piece, whereas others have a separate support for each foot. If your child should have an asymmetrical posture, his weight pushing down on one side may result in one foot-rest becoming lower than the other. It is easy not to notice this is happening, so check regularly to see that it has not occurred.

Designs of pushchairs

As there is currently such a wide choice and variety of pushchairs available, each aiming to provide postural control to a varying degree, it is now possible following your child's assessment for his therapist to choose a pushchair that is tailor-made for him, with postural components that can be reduced gradually as the child develops his own postural control.

For babies and young children who have only moderate involvement, we have found that the wide range of design and choice of pushchairs on the market for this age group can be used with little or no modification, such as the Be Be Comfort Automatic, Maclaren Shenelle, Britax Debut, and the Waks Rider which accommodates one or two children, all of which can be purchased readily.

It is essential, as we mentioned when discussing chairs, that a child should at all times be given every opportunity to use whatever potential abilities he has to control and adjust his position by himself whenever possible, in this way learning to get his own balance. Therefore, the outside support given him and the adjustments made to a pushchair should be restricted to the absolute minimum, providing the child with a stable base, postural trunk control and alignment, and removing any outside support immediately it is no longer required.

The following are a few of the pushchairs for babies and young children that parents have found met the needs of their child, provide a wide range of optional accessories, and are easy to store, fold, push and steer. All the pushchairs listed come in a wide range of sizes, but we have only mentioned the smallest size in each case.

- The Snug Seat discussed earlier and shown in Figure 20.1 can easily be mounted on the collapsible wheeled chassis which is made of light steel tubing and painted dark red. The nursery model is for children from approximately 9 months to 4 years of age.
- The Alvema 110 is in a wide range of sizes, starting at 18 months of age.
- The Convaid Cruiser Buggy, Model 4J, is suitable for infants up to 5 years of age.
- The Jan Pushchair 325 (model 3250M) is suitable for children who are moderately or minimally involved; age range approximately 1–4 years of age. The seat can be removed and placed facing away from or towards the person pushing the chair.
- The Buggy Major. Parents find this lightweight pushchair useful when travelling by car or public transport, although we do not feel that it is ideal for long-term use. Additional support is provided by a Rehab Waistcoat Harness and an intermediate seat can be purchased that slips over the existing seat.

Car seats

If your baby is in a carry cot during the early months we would suggest that you use the Britax Carrycot Restraint. The majority of our parents have found the Britax Cruiser the most satisfac-

tory car seat for the weight range 9–25 kg (20–55 lb) (Figure 20.22).

The Britax Babysure is a rearward-facing seat which is stable with a fully adjustable built-in harness and a recommended weight range built up to approximately 10 kg (22 lb). For extra support and safety, a head support cushion is recommended.

Both these car seats are approved to European Standard R4402 – Universal.

In order to ensure your child's safety when travelling in a car, do ask for advice. There is a wide range of car seats available and constant production innovations being made. The same safety rules regarding car seats apply to all children, which is to say that the seat must provide adequate restraint and protection, with harness straps that fit properly and are easily adjusted. To provide maximum protection, it is extremely important when buying a car seat that you get the **correct** restraint for your child's weight, as the ages given by the manufacturers are **only** an approximate guide. It is also important to bear in mind that if the passenger seats in your car have an air bag, **rearward-facing** car seats **must not be used**.

Note: When travelling by air, it is always a good idea to check with your airline to be sure that the car seat you have is accepted by the Civil Aviation Authority.

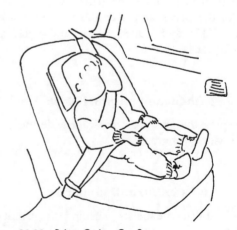

Figure 20.22 Britax Cruiser Car Seat

Chapter 21

Aids to mobility

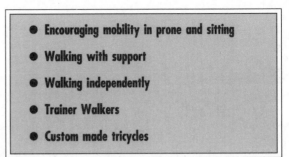

- Encouraging mobility in prone and sitting
- Walking with support
- Walking independently
- Trainer Walkers
- Custom made tricycles

For many parents, freedom of independent mobility for their child is one of their main goals. This may be totally free independent mobility or with the assistance of an aid to mobility.

The choice of mobility will be dependent on many factors, such as the age of the child, his level of impairment and the situation in which independent mobility is attempted, e.g. at home across the sitting room floor, or outside in the garden. The important points when choosing an aid that will enable the child to be mobile are that:

- it should increase the child's potential for independent exploration of his environment with safety
- it should challenge his ability to improve his independence
- in seeking these aims it should not increase abnormal postural tone or potentially harmful poor patterns of movement.

Once a child has mastered the skill of crawling and walking independently, he is able to learn more about the world around him both inside and outside the home. He finds his way into cupboards and drawers, opening and closing doors, inspecting and experimenting with and promptly discarding the contents – no place in the house is left undisturbed. As his play becomes more energetic, his favourite toys are those he can push and pull, a trike without pedals or one of the sturdy toys on wheels that he can sit astride and propel himself around. It will, however, be quite a time before he has the coordination needed to manage a tricycle with pedals.

Because of this lack of mobility, many children with cerebral palsy are denied the freedom of exploring and playing in this way. The sketches in this chapter (Figures 21.1–21.13) illustrate various ideas that might help a child be mobile both inside and outside the home, using toys found in department stores that can easily be adapted and mobility equipment designed especially to meet the needs of the child with cerebral palsy. Ways of helping a child achieve balance in standing and walking, with minimal support and independently, are illustrated.

We have also included two types of walkers as mobility aids, but your therapist will of course select the walker that she feels is the most appropriate for your child.

Note: The suggestions we have made in Figures 21.4(a,b) we would **not recommend** be used by children where spasticity increases with the effort of standing and walking, or those who have a flexor posture of their trunk and lower limbs.

Mobility in sitting

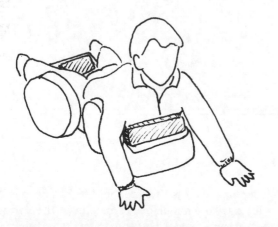

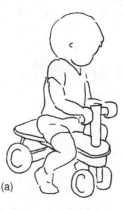

(a)

Figure 21.1   A scooter board enables a child who can creep but finds it difficult to take weight on mobile extended arms with an alternative method of being mobile, while maintaining an extended position. The Jettmobile illustrated is made of a material that is soft for the child to lie on, and includes three positioning shapes and abductor wedge. The amount of support a child will need will, of course, depend on his specific physical difficulties

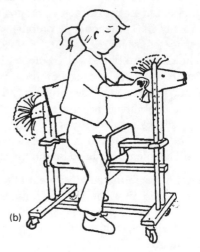

(b)

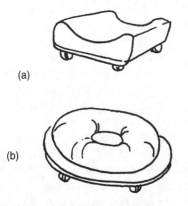

(a)

(b)

Figure 21.2   (a) Small scooped out wooden stool
(b) Rubber ring with padded cushion. Both can be used as an alternative means of locomotion by a child who moves by 'bunny-hopping' – encouraging him to push with his legs rather than relying on his arms

Figure 21.3   (a) James Galt wooden tricycle – a popular stable first tricycle
(b) Munster Horse. A wooden mobile horse, with head, tail and seat adjustable by wooden pegs. The width of the seat is altered by the cushions. By encouraging grasp with extended arms, the child's weight is brought forward over her sitting base

'Walking' with support

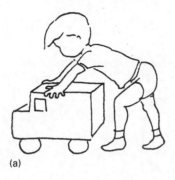

(a)

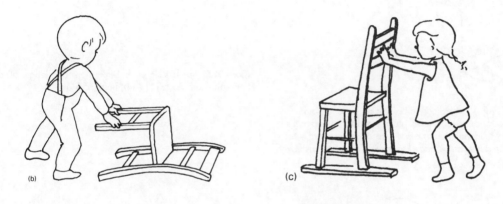

(b)

(c)

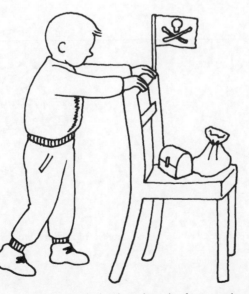

Figure 21.4 (a–d) These sketches illustrate how by varying the height and weight of a toy or chair pushed, we can also vary the degree of hip flexion

Sturdy trucks used as 'walkers' for young children.

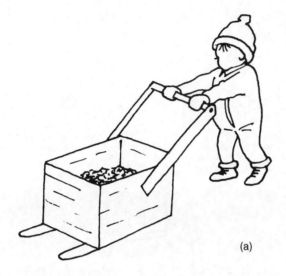

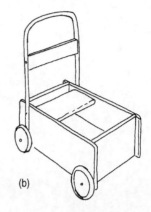

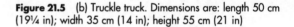

(a)

(b)

Figure 21.5   (b) Truckle truck. Dimensions are: length 50 cm (19¼ in); width 35 cm (14 in); height 55 cm (21 in)

Figure 21.5   (a) A large wooden box makes a good home-walker. The additional stability will provide resistance and make it easier for the child with the arthetoid type of cerebral palsy to push Wooden skids can be added to make it easier to push over carpets

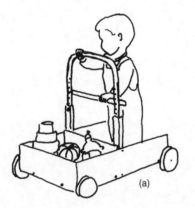

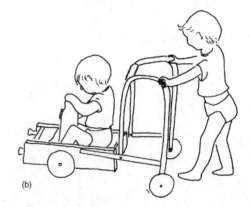

(a)

(b)

Figure 21.6   (a) Kaye walker
(b)   Baby-walker with a frame which gives it added weight and security. The child can progress from holding the horizontal bars to the side bars

Providing minimal support

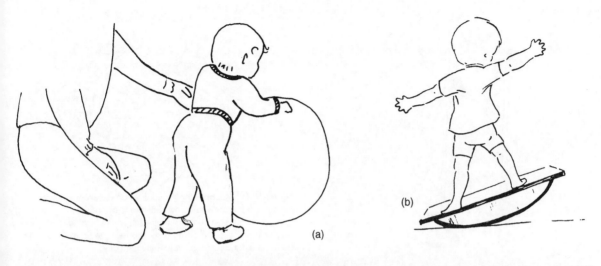

Figure 21.7   (a) Walking with a large ball which only provides minimal support
  (b)   The balance board illustrated is a good way of getting an older child to balance and transfer his weight from one leg to the other
The child must learn to tilt the board slowly from side to side, so that he has to work both to maintain and regain his balance. For a small
child, a home-made balance board can be made by nailing a large rolling pin to a flat piece of wood

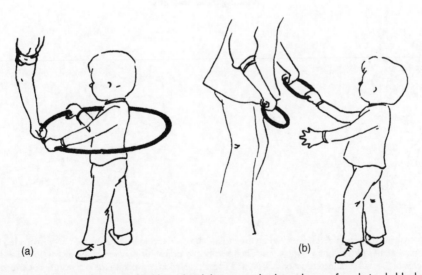

Figure 21.8   Hoops and quoit rings make a useful stable and mobile support, bridging the gap from being held when walking to
independent walking
  (a) A hoop gives the most support
  (b) The child first learns to grasp the quoit rings in *pronation* as illustrated, but should progress as soon as possible to grasping them in
supination as this will help to inhibit any flexor spasticity which causes the pulling of the arms. Finally the child walks holding both quoit
rings himself

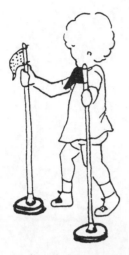

Figure 21.9   Two poles with discs are ideal for the child who has some standing balance and is starting to walk on her own. While they provide some support, she will be unable to lean on them and therefore has to work to remain upright. Start by holding the top of the sticks, but as soon as possible, let the child manage on her own

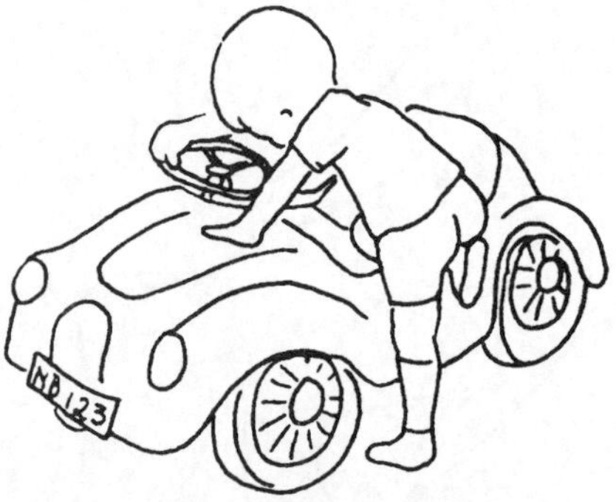

Figure 21.11   A car without pedals is an excellent way of encouraging a child to be mobile who is apprehensive of moving around on his own. A car with pedals, as illustrated, is a good way of training a child with a spastic hemiplegia to grasp with both hands and move his legs symmetrically

Walking independently

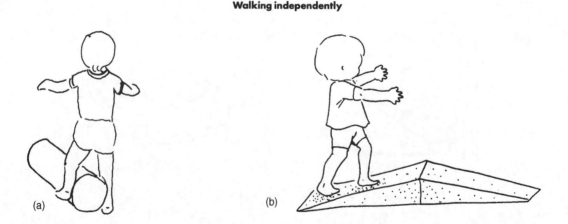

(a)

(b)

Figure 21.10 (a) By walking the length of a roll placed on the ground the child has to transfer his weight onto one leg before taking a step (b) Walking on foam wedges placed in this way is fun. The child has to adjust his position to the incline, and the softness of the foam facilitates movements of the feet (balance reactions). Vary the speed, direction of walking, i.e. forwards, backwards or sideways, and finally get the child to stop on command – to begin with the child could have a pole in each hand for support to give him confidence

Walking trainers

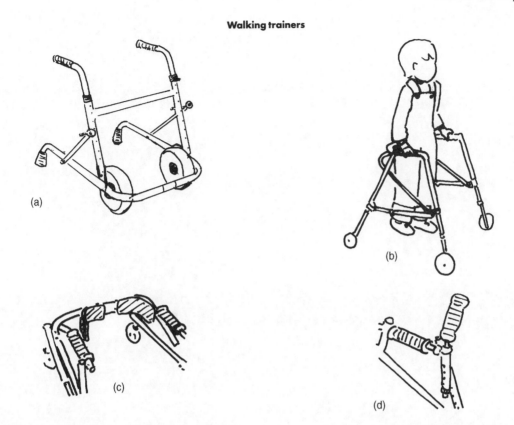

Figure 21.12   (a) Folding Rolator. (Also recommended is the DMA Children's Folding Adjustable Walker 246 from Days Medical Aids Ltd.)
(b) Kaye Postural Control Walker, available in six sizes with a new range of posture-related accessories
(c) Hip symmetry/location pads.
(d) Vertical hand holds

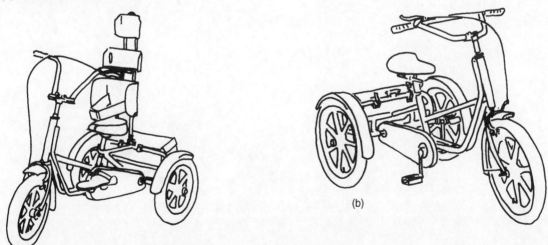

Figure 21.13   The two custom-made tricycles illustrated are from a range of well-designed tricycles. After personal assessment the company will also provide customized accessories and power-assisted models if required
(a) The Kitten Series 3, illustrating hip and thoracic supports, head pad and adjustable footplates
(b) Colt Series Mark 4

Part V
Additional information

Chapter 22

The management of contractures and deformities

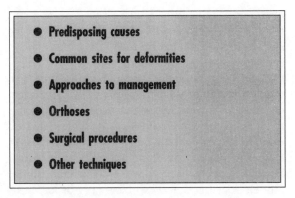

- Predisposing causes
- Common sites for deformities
- Approaches to management
- Orthoses
- Surgical procedures
- Other techniques

The central theme of this book is how you as parents can help your child achieve his optimal function; that is, to enable him to perform purposeful tasks that allow him to interact with his environment as he grows and his life experience expands towards adulthood. A key point of emphasis from birth has been the importance of symmetry and weight-bearing both in **position** and **movement**. Indeed, we have stressed that the former is only a prelude to the latter.

Although the purpose of this book is to provide practical guidance for parents on what to do, and how to do it, underpinning this has been the importance of understanding your child's difficulties and the cause of the difficulties. Understanding, as we have said earlier, not only makes it easier to comply with treatment priorities, but empowers parents to ask pertinent questions and, by being prepared with some information, to make the most of clinic visits.

The following paragraphs provide some simple and basic information about the management of contractures and deformities more commonly seen as a secondary problem to cerebral palsy.

The basis of contractures and deformity

As we have said in earlier sections, development is a series of events and changes in the central nervous system that take place over time, none having a discrete beginning or end but simply melding together to provide the platform for the next step in maturation – an evolution of activity. Growth of the muscles and bones is also taking place as part of the maturational process and in health these take place in harmony; indeed, bones depend on the pull of the muscles which attach to them for the stimulus to grow.

We move or stand still, perform complex tasks and graded movements because the muscles of our limbs and trunk are precisely and sensitively controlled by the central nervous system, but the muscles themselves must be capable of producing force. For example, when we bend our knee the muscles passing over the front of our thigh encompassing the knee cap (patella) and attaching to our shin bone must lengthen, whereas those muscles on the back of the thigh contract or shorten. This can only happen because muscles, their tendons (specialized parts of the muscle that attach to bone) and the ligaments and joint capsules have elasticity and are flexible. The strength of the muscle and their angle of pull is normally perfectly balanced. The force is applied through a finely designed series of cantilevers, where the bones provide the lever arms, the joints the fulcrum of movement and the muscles the force to execute the movement.

In cerebral palsy, where patterns of spasticity or changed tone exists, unusual forces are applied over some joints and the increased tone of some muscle groups means that those muscles are never stretched or elongated by their antagonists and a state of imbalance is created.

Over a period of time those muscles and their tendons which are hypertonic (spastic) lose their elasticity, as indeed does the tissue surrounding the joint over which they work. These factors used to be thought to be the only predisposing elements of the development of contractures. However, more recent research using animal models suggests that a key factor predisposing to the development of contractures is the failure of the affected muscles to grow normally in relation to bone.

Bony deformity at the hip

Deformities occurring at the hip have another component of which we should be aware. The hip joint is a ball-and-socket joint. The socket (acetabulum) lies in the pelvic bone and is flatter in shape during the infant's early months and only truly becomes a socket as the child begins to take weight through the joint. The ball is the head of the femur (thigh) and as the child grows and begins to accept weight through the joint, the position in which the femur is carried in relation to the pelvis changes. You will probably have noticed that toddlers taking their early steps tend to walk with their legs more widely apart and their feet in the 'quarter to three' position, then as they adopt a more mature walking pattern their legs come together and the feet face forward. This change is in part due to the migration of the head of the femur (the ball) to a less anteverted position.

In children with spasticity these bony changes may not occur as normal with growth because of the spasticity and delay or failure to accept weight through the joint. The child with cerebral palsy may therefore have a predisposition to subluxation (partial dislocation) or even full dislocation of the hip as a result of the unusual and unopposed pull of some hypertonic muscles and the delayed maturational changes in the bony structure.

Where do contractures occur?

Common sites for deformity in cerebral palsy are in the lower limbs and spine, although in the more involved child or in the child with spastic hemiplegia, the hand, wrist and elbow may be affected. To generalize is always dangerous when one is writing about such a complex problem. You must remember that there are many provisos to the eventual pattern of the contractures and the likelihood of their occurrence in a particular child – your child.

How may contractures affect the child's function?

In order to stand and therefore by implication to move we need a stable base – our feet. In children with hypertonicity (spasticity), the foot is thrust into an extended position, so that only the toe is on the ground; in order to try to achieve some balance or stability the hip and knee must be bent (flexed). Any attempt to put the foot flat on the ground results in the knee being over-extended, or snapping back. Clearly such a child has no stability in standing or walking, and consequently because balance is then lacking, purposeful hand and arm function is in disarray. Further, achieving a good fit of footwear is compromised.

Contractures and/or deformity at the hip make the achievement of a stable sitting position difficult because if one hip is flexed, adducted or drawn back, it is impossible for the pelvis to be in correct alignment and the weight of the trunk will be shifted to one side. In turn, this will affect arm and hand function.

What can be done?

There are broadly two approaches to the management of deformity – the conservation approach and the surgical approach. The conservation approach comprises physiotherapy and the use of orthotic appliances, while the surgical approach involves an operation or a series of operations, usually to release tight muscle tendons, to alter their angle of pull or to stabilize joints

It is important to recognize that these two approaches are not mutually exclusive, nor should the surgical approach be regarded as a last resort, only to be embarked upon when other methods have failed.

From the historical perspective the use of surgical procedures in the management of cerebral palsy has waxed and waned in popularity and has not always enjoyed success or earned the acclaim of patients. However, as in most specialities within medicine, tremendous advances have been made in the very recent past, not only with surgical techniques but in the understanding of the fundamental problems underlying the deformities.

The advances in surgical technique have been supported by, and occurred in parallel with, the technological advances that now permit greater accuracy in determining the precise cause of the mechanical problem that the child presents with at the hip, knee or ankle; for example, modern methods of gait analysis, which allow each phase of the child's walking pattern to be recorded and analysed, and more sensitive electromyographic recordings. The latter provide accurate information on which muscles are working at any point in the normal walking cycle, so helping the professional staff to associate which aberrant firing of a muscle is responsible for disturbances in the child's gait.

Hemiplegia

In hemiplegia, the more commonly performed surgical release is at the ankle, where a procedure to elongate the Tendo Achilles (heel cord) may be performed, with the objective of allowing the child to place the foot flat on the ground and provide a stable ankle. The difficulty for the surgeon is to ensure that he does not over-lengthen the tendon.

Spastic diplegia

Nearly all children with spastic diplegia have achieved independent walking by around 4 years of age, and the extent to which they need to use walking aids will depend upon the severity of the condition.

Typically your child may walk in one of three ways, dictated by the pattern of spasticity and its severity, these are:

- with the hips and knees bent (flexed) and the hips turned inwards
- with the hips bent and turned inwards, but with the knees over-straightened (hyperextended)
- with the hips bent and turned in, but with the knee in a more neutral or balanced position.

In each of these three walking patterns the child will have to adopt a different posture of the spine, in order to remain upright and compensate for the spastic patterns in the legs.

It can readily be observed that any attempt to correct one contracture surgically will immediately have a marked effect on the mechanical forces acting at all other joints. For this reason, surgery to ameliorate spastic diplegia must be carefully planned and staged, in order to avoid the situation where in correcting one deformity the child's functional status deteriorates because of the altered biomechanical status at all other joints and the spine.

It would be inappropriate in this book to attempt to discuss the many surgical procedures that can be undertaken, partly because your child has his own unique set of problems. Suffice to say that in some children operative intervention does offer considerable benefit, **particularly when a holistic view of the child's difficulties has been taken**.

It is essential that the **surgery is planned and coordinated and that the aims and objectives of the surgery are carefully discussed and understood**.

Orthoses (calipers or braces)

Ankle–knee–foot orthosis (AFO)

An AFO is a type of splint or brace that is used to control the ankle and the knee, its name is derived from the fact that it covers the posterior (back) of the foot, ankle and lower leg.

They are made of lightweight materials, such as polypropylene, and are worn inside regular shoes, therefore having the additional advantage of being unobtrusive and cosmetically acceptable.

AFOs may be used to control the ankle and foot and to prevent the knee from snapping back in an exaggerated way during standing or walking.

The purpose of the AFO must always be very precisely described and defined, so that when it is made, it is easy to see if it fulfils the prescription and it can then be evaluated to see if it has improved the child's function.

Who may benefit from an AFO?

The child with hypotonia (low tone)

The young child with low tone may show considerable degrees of joint laxity and in standing the foot may be forced into a valgus position as a result of weight-bearing, i.e. the weight is taken on the inner side of the foot. In such a child there may well be instability at the knee due to an inadequacy of the knee extensor muscles, that is the group of muscles lying along the front of the thigh and responsible for straightening the knee. Wearing an AFO will control the foot and ankle, preventing the development of a 'rocker bottom' foot deformity, and will induce some stability at the knee.

The child with increased tone

The child whose increased tone pushes the foot into an equinus position on weight-bearing, i.e. a position where the toe points downwards, will benefit from an AFO, gaining improved standing ability. An uncorrected equinus position of the ankle forces the knee into full extension during weight-bearing, which if allowed to continue will, over a period of time, cause the knee to become lax. The AFO will bring the knee into slight flexion.

Cautions on wearing an AFO

A child wearing an AFO may find crawling difficult because, of course, the splint is there to prevent plantar flexion (the foot pushing down), so that the only way for the child to progress forward in crawling is to bend the knees more, or to increase the degree of hip abduction with rotation. If, therefore, the child is at the stage where crawling is his main/only method of movement and free exploration, it is **better to remove** the AFO during periods of play.

Similarly wearing an AFO may make sitting on the floor problematical because the child will tend to adopt the 'W' sitting position, and in long sitting they will be unstable and tend to fall backwards. The child should therefore be encouraged to use a chair or remove the AFO.

Surgical correction of deformities

Deformities of the hip

There are a number of surgical procedures that may be performed to correct deformity at the hip and the procedure of choice will depend on the predominating cause of the deformity. The surgical procedures available range from simple release of tendons of muscles whose spastic pull is causing the hip problem, through to bony correction, for example where the head of the femur is not lying within the acetabular socket. The key questions are:

- What is the objective of surgery – is it to allow greater potential for standing, or is it to enable the child to achieve a better sitting position, or is it to pre-empt the possibility of a scoliosis (curvature of the spine)?
- What effect will surgery have on other joints of the lower limb and how will it affect function?

Deformities of the hand and wrist

Deformities of the hand and wrist occur for the same reasons as those occurring in the lower extremity, but because we do not use our hands primarily for weight-bearing and the architecture of the joints is different, the bony structural considerations are less evident. We essentially use our hands for grasp, release and manipulation, and in health we are able to generate enormous strength through our hands, converting them into powerful tools. We are also able to use them to protect ourselves if we should fall.

In children with cerebral palsy, the abnormal pull of the spastic muscles results in the hand and wrist assuming an abnormal posture and therefore any attempt at volitional movement is compromised. However, it is essential to recognize that the placement and direction of hand movement is determined by the shoulder and elbow. Therefore, a primary consideration when contemplating surgical correction at the wrist and hand must be the extent of control that the child has over the shoulder and elbow.

Other techniques

Reflex-inhibiting casts

The use of reflex-inhibiting casts is a technique which is advocated by some physiotherapists in order to reduce the degree of spasticity (hypertonus) of the muscles acting over the ankle and foot, namely those muscles responsible for the child pushing his foot downwards and turning it in, i.e. assuming a position known as equino varus.

The protagonists of this technique claim that it results in decreased tone of the co-contracting muscles and therefore facilitates increased postural stability, permitting improved weight-bearing in walking children.

The technique requires the application of plaster of Paris or fibre-based casts to the lower leg and foot, with these in the corrected position, in other words with the ankle plantigrade or at a right angle to the leg and the foot in neutral rotation. The casts are worn for periods of up to 3 weeks and during this time intensive rehabilitation is given.

The published results of this technique are somewhat controversial, with some researchers claiming excellent results with little recurrence of the increased tone and contracture, whereas others find the technique less beneficial and a high incidence of recurrence within 6 months of removal of the casts.

One finding about which there is a concordance of opinion is that the application of casts induces a degree of muscle wasting (atrophy); indeed some clinicians suggest that it is this wasting that is responsible for the apparent decrease in tone.

Selective posterior rhizotomy

This is a neurosurgical procedure that may help some patients with cerebral palsy. It has been found to be most beneficial in those patients who have good selective control of movement but whose function in daily activities is seriously impaired by spasticity. It is more frequently used in patients with spastic diplegia and those with total body involvement, and is not usually advocated in patients who have low tone, fluctuating tone or where there is obvious weakness. It must be clear that **careful, comprehensive and precise assessment is necessary** before the probable benefit to a particular child can be determined.

The anticipated benefits of the procedure are a reduction of spasticity in the selected muscles and an improvement in the range of motion possible at the joints over which those muscles work, the combination of these two factors resulting in improved functional capacity.

What is selective posterior rhizotomy and how does it work?

In order to answer these two questions it is necessary to explain a little of how we normally control muscle activity. Skeletal muscles have within them many muscle spindles, which are specialized sense organs whose role is to send back messages to the spinal cord about how much the muscle in which they are situated is being stretched. The messages pass along a nerve to the spinal cord and in turn stimulate another nerve. This nerve, the motor nerve, comes from the anterior horn cell in the spinal cord. The motor nerve sends messages to the muscle causing it to contract, so a loop is completed.

However, in order that muscles are not being stimulated to contract too much and inappropriately, the brain normally sends signals down to the anterior horn cell, through what are called descending nerve tracts or pathways, and these signals or messages serve to dampen, or inhibit, and set the threshold for the anterior horn cells.

A good analogy is a railway, where the passage of a train is controlled by a signal box. In cerebral palsy it is these descending tracts from the brain, the coordinating centre, that are not functioning well and therefore the control at the spinal cord level is less efficient, so that the signal coming in from the muscle is largely uncontrolled, with the result that the stimulus for the muscle to contract is unopposed. Hence the muscle exhibits increased tone and is said to be spastic.

In selective posterior rhizotomy, those posterior rootlets that serve the muscles which exhibit abnormal responses are identified by electrical stimulation and then selectively cut so that their influence is decreased, and hence the spasticity is decreased. In order for the surgeon to gain access to the spinal cord, small pieces of bone must be removed from the vertebrae of the spinal column.

Selective posterior rhizotomy is a technique which has been used for many years, although early reports provided mixed findings. More recently, the technique has seen a resurgence of interest in some centres around the world and in some well-selected children the results reported are good.

It must be emphasized that this procedure is not suitable for all children with cerebral palsy and very stringent assessment must be undertaken before children who will potentially benefit from the procedure can be identified.

Summary

In the preceding paragraphs I have tried to introduce some of the current thinking in relation to the use of orthoses and some other techniques as they apply to the management of the child with cerebral palsy. I have intentionally not described specific techniques because these are appropriately the province of other professionals. Indeed, this chapter is only included in this book for parents in response to their comments to me made over the years since the last edition, and is primarily intended to help them prepare for discussions with the various professional staff involved in giving the specialist advice and treatment. I have consciously refrained from discussing management of spinal deformity (scoliosis), other than to indicate how abnormal postures and movements at the hips provide a platform for the development of spinal curves. Problems of spinal deformity are not usually seen in children with cerebral palsy within the age range for whom this book has been written, namely 0–5 years.

Clearly, everything that has been advocated in this book on how to handle your child has been reinforcing ways of achieving movement and the acquisition of skills in a way that reduces spasticity, or seeks to establish a more normal balance of tone. However, it is of paramount importance to recognize that although the objective has been to help you help your child towards achieving his maximal potential, the responsibility for this task is shared with the many professionals as well. The presence of contractures and/or deformities should not be seen as a failure of management but rather as a secondary or consequent problem.

Chapter 23

Going into hospital

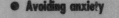

- Avoiding anxiety
- Explanation of basic problems
- Role of the play leader

Research has shown that up to the age of around 3–4 years of age the greatest anxiety for children going into hospital is that of being separated from their mother. After this age it seems that it is the fear of what is going to happen to them that is the most worrying.

It is therefore always a good idea with a young child, once a date has been fixed for him to go into hospital, to make an appointment for you and your child to meet with the head nurse of the unit. She will arrange for you both to visit the ward, see the playroom and meet the nurses and play leader. If arrangements have been made for you to sleep in the hospital, seeing where your room is will also reassure your child that you will be with him both during the day and at night. Meeting the nurse in charge will also give you the opportunity to tell her if your child has special needs, for example a particular type of chair, or a piece of equipment that he uses, then if it is not available you can find out whether you should bring it in with you.

To give your child an idea of the people he is going to meet and what goes on in a hospital, I would suggest that you buy one of the many well-illustrated books written for children of all ages on 'Going into Hospital', so that you can look at them together.

If an older child has to go into hospital for surgery, some of his worries and anxieties can be avoided if you can explain in simple terms what is going to be done and how the operation is going to help him. It is also important that a child knows that if he feels sore or uncomfortable after the operation that he will be given medicines that will make him feel better.

As it is most likely that a child following surgery will be put into plaster or a cast after his operation, it is important that he is told beforehand, and given a reason why this is being done. Otherwise, if he is told for example that he is going to have an operation that will help him walk, and then he wakes up and finds one or both of his legs are in plaster and that he cannot take weight on his legs for a couple of days, he will have every reason to feel let down and frustrated.

A short explanation of your child's basic problems and special needs will always be welcomed by the nursing staff, including any additional help you can give them that will make it easier for them to handle your child. This is especially important if he is difficult to feed, bath or dress. If he can for example only communicate by gesture, be sure to let the staff know how he indicates that he is uncomfortable, hungry, thirsty or needs to go to the toilet, and the gesture he uses for 'yes' or 'no'.

Although there will always be plenty of toys on the unit, be sure your child also has the comfort of having his own favourite toy(s) with him. If he is limited in his ability to use his hands or finds it easier to play in a certain position, let the nurses and play leader know, so that they can select the toys he can manage and enjoy.

Once in hospital, play leaders as well as helping him to settle down and cope with hospital life, will also prepare him through play activities for some of the treatments or procedures that he might have to experience. Naturally the way they accomplish this will depend on the child's intellectual age, but for a young child for example, his teddy might find himself being bandaged or having his heart listened to, and he may even go off to the X-ray department for photographs! All of these simple 'games' will help reduce the child's anxiety. This type of play should not be confused with dressing up and playing 'doctors and nurses', as the games he plays will relate to those events he will be experiencing himself.

Fortunately most hospitals now encourage parents' full participation in the care of their child in hospital and from the child's perspective hospitals provide a more friendly environment.

Chapter 24

Recreational activities

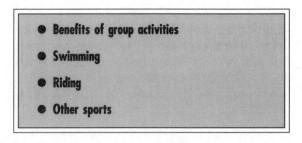

- ● **Benefits of group activities**
- ● **Swimming**
- ● **Riding**
- ● **Other sports**

Swimming and riding

I am frequently asked by parents if I think it would be a good idea if they took their child swimming and/or riding. My answer is always a very enthusiastic 'yes', but with two provisos, namely, that they should first speak to their paediatrician or GP to make sure that he agrees, and secondly that their child must be taught by a **qualified instructor** under close supervision. Obviously, it is also important that your child enjoys being in the water and, in the case of riding, is not frightened of horses.

Both activities are an excellent form of recreation, which in many instances may be shared and enjoyed with other members of the family. In addition, as the child grows older he will have the opportunity of joining a club, and later entering for competitions and galas, if he should choose to do so.

By taking part in group activities, the child's social skills will be greatly enhanced as he learns to share and to take his turn, appreciating the significance of learning and working as a member of a team. Previously he may have only experienced working in a one-to-one relationship, e.g. with his therapist, or may have found himself the central focus of attention for much of the time.

Some benefits of recreational activities

- ● Both swimming and riding provide the child with an atmosphere and experience that is enjoyable and fun.

- ● For many children it is their first opportunity to move freely and with greater confidence.
- ● The child finds himself in a situation where, by using his own initiative and with minimal assistance, it is possible for him to experiment with different ways of accomplishing a new set of skills, in this way discovering his own capabilities. This provides an opportunity he might not otherwise have.
- ● As with any programme of rehabilitation, the goals in recreational activities can be broken down into simple components, gradually increasing in complexity as his skills and confidence grow this way, enabling the child to do well. He will perform on a par with, or at times even better than, his peers. This enables him to enjoy a sense of achievement and a feeling of success which is so important for his self-image.
- ● The freedom of mobility that the child achieves when he becomes independent in either sport minimizes the difference between himself and those more able-bodied, such as friends and other siblings, so that he is able to compete with them on equal terms.

I always think the most important spin-off for children taking part in either sport is that eventually the child is able to experience what it feels like to be in complete control of his **own space**, to understand how **his** body works and to be responsible for it and be independent.

Both sports are excellent adjuncts to the child's total programme, helping to improve symmetry, trunk control, overall mobility and balance. They also increase the child's ability to perceive movement, spatial relationships such as up and down, left and right, visual and auditory discrimination, eye–hand coordination and fine motor skills, all in an environment far removed from a treatment centre, classroom or nursery.

Swimming

If there are no contra-indications, the best time to start swimming with babies is between 9 and 12 months, as at this age they have no fear of water. To begin with we would recommend joining a small group, run for mothers and babies, that takes place in a special teaching or therapy pool where the water is kept at a minimum of 30°C (86°F). The best person to introduce the baby to the water is his mother. However, if for some reason she is not happy or does not feel relaxed in a pool, the baby's father or another adult member of the family may accompany the baby. In any event, a **qualified instructor** is **always present** to give guidance and support.

When working in the Child Development Centre at Charing Cross Hospital, together with a colleague I formed a mother and baby group, which we called the 'Aquatots'. Although the essence of our session was informality, we incorporated the approach of 'Teach your Baby to Swim' by Claire Timmermans and the Halliwick method for teaching the disabled to swim, evolved by James McMillan.

We used the water to:

- encourage mother and baby interaction
- teach handling techniques
- help with symmetry, trunk control and balance
- encourage a greater degree of physical organization
- help develop self-confidence
- facilitate sensorimotor integration
- practise the beginning of breath control to encourage the making of sounds and communication.

Each session started with us working individually with mother and often father with their baby. We finished with group activities with a selection of nursery rhymes which incorporated the goals set for that session. I must admit, we did at times take a liberty with some very well-known nursery rhymes, as the majority seem to end with everyone falling down!

Our group proved not only to be beneficial for the babies, but great fun for us all. The sketch of a baby enjoying his new-found independence in Figure 24.1 has been drawn from a photograph of a member of our Aquatot group – an important day for him, his parents and all of us!

Figure 24.2 illustrates the Simdyna swimming float produced by Swedish Rolo Plastics. This float is recommended, as it enables the child to lie on his back with his legs horizontal in the water, and if the float is repositioned to do the same when on his tummy.

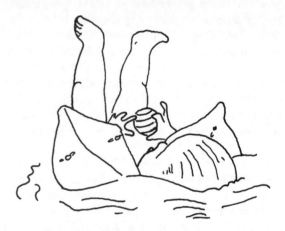

Figure 24.1   Independence!

Riding

Although many children I have treated have derived great benefit and enjoyment from riding, and I have attended many of their riding sessions, I have not been involved personally in a riding programme. I therefore asked a colleague of mine, Pippa Hodge, who has her own equestrian centre which I have visited, in British Columbia, Canada, if she would define the term 'riding' for me, in the context of the cerebral palsied child. The information is summarized in the following paragraphs.

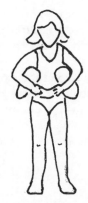

Figure 24.2 Simdyna swimming float

Hippotherapy

The purpose of hippotherapy is **not** to teach riding, but to **use the horse** and its movements to **meet therapy objectives** and goals. It is used to facilitate the development of symmetry, head and trunk control and sitting balance through the various movement progressions of the horse, and to promote mobility, muscle coordination, i.e. eye–hand control, improve muscle tone, and maintain joint range and gait pattern.

Horses and equipment are specially selected according to the child's needs. It is important to note that **the use of an unsuitable horse or improper equipment can cause problems such as overstretching or increasing muscle tone**. The session is taken by a **certified riding instructor**, each child works individually with a physical or occupational therapist and many positions on the horse are used, for example:

● lying over the horse to develop head and trunk control and relax extremities
● sitting backwards on the horse with hands flat on the rump, to develop weight-bearing
● lying supine over the rump, to mobilize the spine and shoulder girdle.

Therapeutic riding

In therapeutic riding the child is a member of a **small group**, usually no more than four children at a time.

Working as a member of a group is obviously more relaxing and challenging for the older child who neither wants nor needs a one-to-one situation. Their programmes at this stage will include more advanced sensorimotor skills including educational objectives, for example:

● identifying objects in the surrounding environment, other animals, flowers, etc.
● encouraging verbalization by voice-aids to the horse, communication with volunteers, instructor and other riders
● following tasks and directions
● recognizing their own body parts and those of the horse
● gaining sensory input, e.g. feeling the horse, saddle, and different textures
● learning the difference between left and right.

A therapeutic group is taken by a **specially trained** certified riding instructor. A physical therapist or occupational therapist may also be part of this team and he or she will be consulted as to the most suitable 'warm-up' and 'cool-down' exercises, as well as any specific group activities that will enable all the children in the group to participate.

Recreational riding (for the child who can ride independently)

Here, the **objective** for the child is to be **safe and have fun**. The horse chosen will be quiet but **not** specially trained, and equipment will vary. There are no specific therapeutic aims.

In time, the child will develop a rapport with his horse, not only by riding but through caring for the animal as he learns stable management, e.g. to groom, feed, water and rug-up. All these skills will promote his self-confidence and self-esteem.

As we mentioned when discussing swimming, when the child manages to reach a certain stage of proficiency, in this case in riding, he will have the opportunity to join a pony club and take part in competitions, and perhaps even go pony trekking with his friends and in some cases other members of the family.

Other recreational activities

Although not in the age range of his book, whenever practicable, skiing and camping are two outside activities that are highly recommended, either with the family or as a member of a special club.

If you should be fortunate enough to live near a river or a lake, fishing and sailing are two sports within the capabilities of many older children, **with the proviso that he can swim and that the correct flotation garment is worn**, especially if there is an enthusiastic member of the family who enjoys these sports. Clearly, extreme care must be taken to ensure that the child is secure and that all **safety precautions** have been taken.

Most of us enjoy having some outside hobby or sport, and if your child expresses a desire to try, he should be given **every encouragement and opportunity** to do so.

Appendix I

Illustrations of some of the terms used

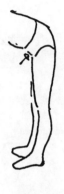 Hip flexion

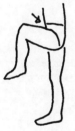 Hip flexion

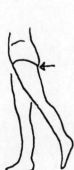 Hip extension

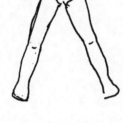 Abduction

Adduction

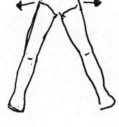 Inward rotation at the hips

Figure I.1

Figure I.2

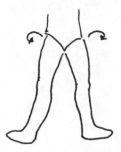

Outward rotation of the hips – legs extended and abducted

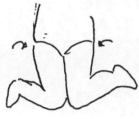

Inward rotation at the hips – legs flexed and adducted

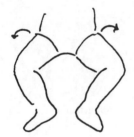

Outward rotation at the hips – legs flexed and abducted

Figure I.3

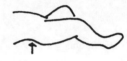

Flat back – hips and legs flexed

Pelvis tilted (posteriorly), legs flexed and together

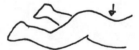

Pelvis tilted (anteriorly), legs extended

Pelvis tilted (anteriorly), legs flexed and abducted

Pelvis tilted (anteriorly), hips and legs slightly apart and flexed

Figure I.4

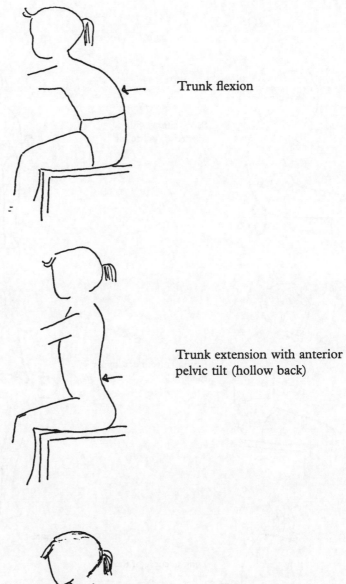

Trunk flexion

Trunk extension with anterior
pelvic tilt (hollow back)

Trunk extension with
a flat back

Figure I.5

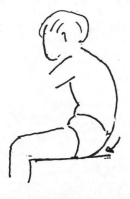

Sacral sitting with
(posterior) pelvic tilt

Pelvis elevated on the right

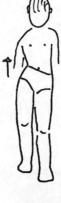

Kyphosis (rounded upper
spine)

Pelvis rotated to the right
(retracted hip) (head and feet
pointing forwards)

Figure I.7

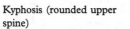

Long C curve of the spine

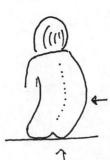

Weight

Figure I.6

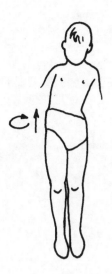

Pelvis elevated and rotated to the right (head and feet pointing forwards)

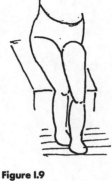

Windswept posture in sitting (this illustrates how one leg appears shorter than the other)

Figure I.9

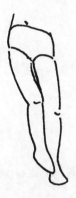

Windswept hip
Pelvis elevated on right, and rotated (retracted)
Hip – adducted
    – inwardly rotated

Figure I.8

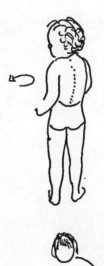

Trunk rotation to the left

Trunk side flexion to the right

Figure I.10

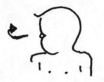
Head rotation to the right

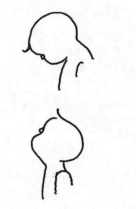
Head flexion

Head extension

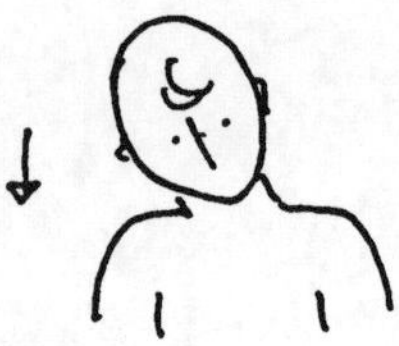

Head side flexion to the right

Figure I.11

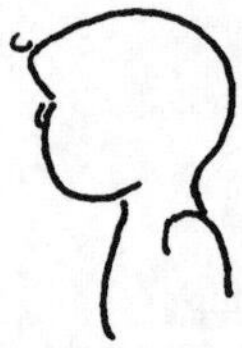

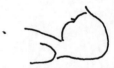
'Long' neck, chin tucked in

'Long' neck, chin tucked in (lying)

Figure I.12

Chin 'jutting' forwards, neck hyperextended (sitting)

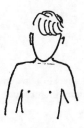

Shoulders level

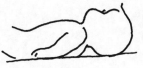

Chin 'jutting' forwards, neck hyperextended (lying)

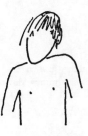

<u>Left</u> shoulder elevated (up)
<u>Right</u> shoulder depressed (down)

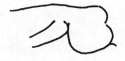

Head extended as part of a total pattern of extension

Figure I.13

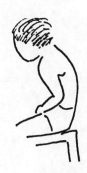

Protracted shoulders (forward)

Retracted shoulders (back)

Figure I.14

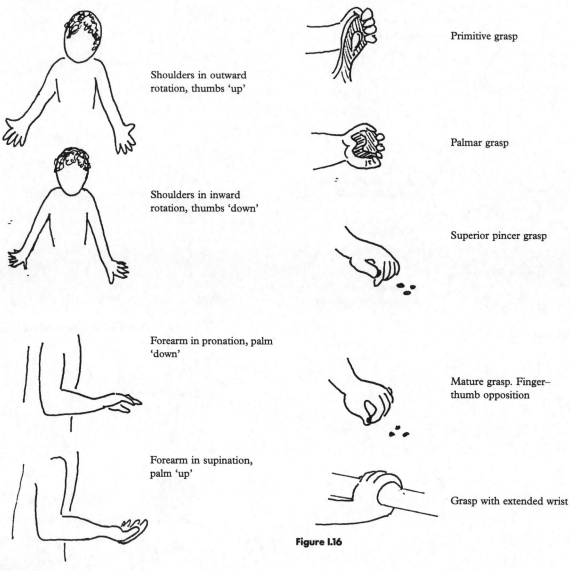

Shoulders in outward rotation, thumbs 'up'

Shoulders in inward rotation, thumbs 'down'

Forearm in pronation, palm 'down'

Forearm in supination, palm 'up'

Figure I.15

Primitive grasp

Palmar grasp

Superior pincer grasp

Mature grasp. Finger–thumb opposition

Grasp with extended wrist

Figure I.16

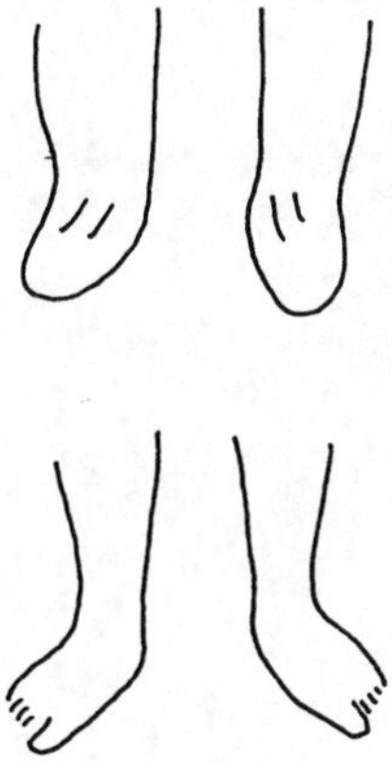

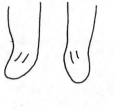

Feet in a varus position (pronated)
Weight taken on the inner border of the foot (seen from the back)

Left foot in the valgus position (supinated)
Weight taken on the outer side of the foot (seen from the back)

Feet in varus position (supinated) (seen from the front)

Left foot in a valgus position (supinated) (seen from the front)

Figure I.17

Figure I.18

Appendix II

An overview of the early stages of sensorimotor development

The purpose of this overview is to illustrate and emphasize that when helping a child with cerebral palsy towards independence in any functional skill, it is essential that we understand something of the sensorimotor patterns that underlie these skills

Given this understanding of the development of a baby as a basis, it will be easier to understand the differences between his development and that of the child with cerebral palsy, enabling us to appreciate how abnormal movement patterns interfere with future achievement. While obviously there are other stages in the sensorimotor development of a baby during the period we have covered, such as getting up to sitting, sitting to standing, standing and walking. I have only mentioned the most important early stages of development to provide examples of how the gross motor patterns of movement in supine, prone and sitting underlie the fine motor skills of the hands, and overlap with the development of vision, hearing and speech.

The posture of a baby during the first few months is predominantly one of flexion. At this early stage his head is rarely in the mid-line, he has no active head control other than the ability, when placed on his tummy, to turn his head sideways to breathe. His arms are usually bent with loosely closed hands, his legs bent and apart. His 'mass' movements are abrupt and follow no set pattern. He reacts to light and to loud sounds by blinking or by a Moro reaction, neither stimulus having any meaning for him.

Stage one

The first significant stage in motor development is that of mid-line orientation and the start of head control. Both of these activities make it possible for the baby to begin to make contact with his environment, first with his eyes and much later as he explores with his hands.

Rolling

For the first time the baby starts to move from one position to another, he does this by rolling to either side from his back. To begin with he will often hold his hands together while he rolls. The movement of rolling starts with the turning of the head which causes the body to follow (neck-righting reaction); later the baby initiates the movement himself.

Vision and the beginning of eye–hand regard

Gradually the baby starts to select what he sees. He can follow his mother as she moves around the cot, and follow a simple dangling toy 150–300 mm (6–12 in) above his face through a half-circle from side to side.

He begins to turn to the sound of a voice, smiling when his mother speaks to him. He is already learning to smile when he wants to be picked up, and to know that if he cries he will get attention.

Stage two

The next important pattern of motor development is the beginning of extension – abduction of the limbs (overlapping with flexion abduction) in conjunction with the extension of the whole body. He practises this extension in all positions, but at the same time is able to do activities in flexion.

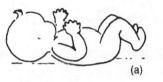

Figure II.1
(a) Supine
At this stage the baby prefers to lie on his back. His head is now usually in the mid-line. He brings his hands together over his chest, and looks at them. This combination of touch and vision is the first important step in self-exploration. He takes his hands to his mouth, at first accidentally and then purposefully to suck, later touching and exploring his lips, cheek and tongue with his fingers. His eyes start to coordinate and he becomes preoccupied with his mother's face, but to begin with only at a mother-to-child distance of 150 mm (6 in)

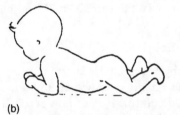

(b) Prone
Head control starts to develop first when the baby lies on his tummy. It should be noted that the top of the spine extends sufficiently to enable the baby to get his shoulders and arms forward. Weight is taken on the forearms which help him raise the upper part of his body. His hands remain loosely closed; one often sees the baby scratching the surface with his fingers. The pelvis which was previously up in the air when lying on his tummy is now flat on the support, his hips and legs are bent and apart, feet dorsiflexed

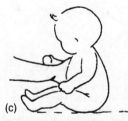

(c) Sitting
At this stage the baby must be supported when sitting. He holds his head erect but only for a few seconds. Even though his back is straight, *except for the lumbar region*, his body has to be supported in sitting long after he has complete head control in this position. His arms and legs are bent and abducted, feet dorsiflexed

Vision and the beginning of eye–hand coordination

The baby can, as it were, now 'grasp' an object with his eyes but is still *unable* to reach out and grasp it with his hands. He shows excitement and the fact that he wants something by kicking with both legs and waving both arms, *opening and closing* his fingers as he does so. At first he does this with his arms bent and near his body, but gradu-

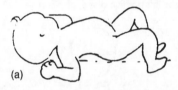

Figure II.2
(a) Supine
This is one of many ways by which the baby practises extension when lying on his back. Here, his shoulders are retracted, arms bent, hands loosely closed. His feet are flat on the floor and he lifts his bottom off the support. In no time he will learn to push himself back in this way. He also has the ability to *lift* his head *forward* despite the fact that his shoulders are retracted

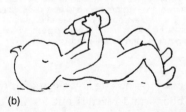

(b) We have included this sketch to illustrate that although so much time is spent practising extension, the baby is *also* able to bring his arms *forward* to place his hands on his bottle. Hand regard – playing with his hands and fingers and taking them continuously to his mouth – is a very important part of learning at this stage

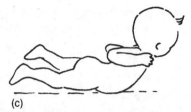

(c) Prone
We can see in this sketch how the 'high lifting' of his head facilitates the total extension of his body, including for the *first time the lumbar spine*. He lifts his arms, either bent and off the support as shown, or off the support with his arms extended sideways. The term 'swimming on his tummy' is often used to describe this activity.
It is important to note that although his legs are lifted and extended they are apart and the feet remain dorsiflexed

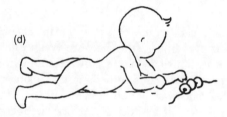

(d) We include this sketch to illustrate that the baby can *also* at this stage take weight on his forearms and reach out to touch a toy. His feet are dorsiflexed and toes bent pressing against the floor; later he will use this position of the feet when he starts to creep

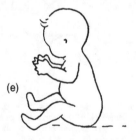

(e) Sitting
The baby's head is now steady, his body straighter including, for the first time, the beginning of *extension in the lumbar spine*. His arms are bent, abducted and retracted at the shoulders, or forward as shown. His legs are bent and apart, feet dorsiflexed. It is at this stage in his development that we often find it difficult to bend the baby's hips to sit him. He enjoys pushing himself back when in this position, and he still needs support

ally progresses to opening and closing his hands as he both follows and reaches out for the object – but he is still unable to grasp or to manipulate at this stage. It is worth noting that this is the first time that we see the baby making a deliberate attempt to move his arms *towards* an object with the intention of trying to get it.

He can follow an object if it is moved slowly from left to right in front of his face. If we place a rattle in his hand he grasps it strongly with the inner side of his hands and fingers. He can look at it for a *second* and then starts to wave his arms about in an uncoordinated way, often hitting himself and complaining loudly – *he cannot at this stage let go* (rattles are so varied in shape and sound these days that they are an excellent way of trapping the ears and eyes at this stage of development).

Hearing and speech

He responds momentarily to loud sounds, vocalizing as he moves and answering back in his way to sounds made by adults. In conjunction with the variation of pitch his repertoire enlarges, for example sounds of anger appear. He blows 'raspberries', syllables come into his babbling and he starts to make the sounds 'm' 'mm' and 'ddd'.

Stage three

The baby has progressed from being a flexed to being an extended individual and now he has perfect head control. He has now reached the *important stage in his development when he starts to break up these total patterns and a greater variety of motor patterns appear. This is the stage of strong extension* –

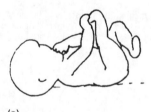

(a)

Figure II.3
(a) Supine
At this stage the baby starts making movements for a desired result, for example he reaches out with his arms when his mother approaches to pick him up. As the baby reaches out with his hands he has his hips bent and often his legs straight, a pattern he will use when getting up from sitting, and when he sits with his legs straight out in front. This pattern of reaching out is a very important one, coinciding as it does with his ability to grasp. He now finds his feet for the first time, and is able to integrate his ability to see, feel and grasp by holding onto his feet, becoming aware of how they look, both when still and when moving; he furthers his knowledge of himself by taking his feet to his mouth

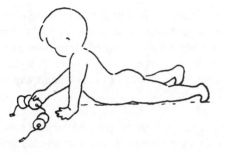

(b)

(b) Prone
When on his tummy the baby not only raises his head high with a completely straight back, but whereas a few weeks earlier he was taking weight on a closed hand, the hand is now open. Because of the mobility of the arms, when using them for support, he is very soon able to take his weight on one arm and reach out for his toys with the other – forward and later behind him

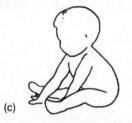

(c)

(c) Sitting
He sits now with his legs apart and straight out in front of him, his feet are dorsiflexed. He has no sitting balance, still tending to throw himself backwards when sitting. Because of lack of sitting balance and the lack of support sideways, he is often apt to fall over sideways. He begins to use his hands for support at this stage, but *only* in front of him

abduction of the limbs. Where before, movements of the limbs were taking place predominantly at the shoulders and hips, we now see active movements appearing at the elbows and knees. It should be noted that the development of the arms is still in advance of that of the legs.

Rolling

He can now roll over from his tummy onto his back, a movement that includes *rotation* and active extension of the whole body, so essential when he finally stands and walks.

Vision and manipulation

As head control is now complete the baby can follow objects with his eyes in all directions, he is also able to fix his gaze on small objects. Where before, when seeing his image in a mirror, he was puzzled, he is now aware of himself and will reach forward and pat his image. Self-exploration is now complete as the baby goes a step further and becomes aware of his feet.

Object exploration begins as he now has developed the ability to look, reach, touch and clutch an object with his whole hand. Manipulation is still very crude and for this reason everything is immediately taken to his mouth, the mouth playing an important part in providing information such as taste, shape and consistency.

He still has no fine movements of his fingers; flapping and scooping with his hands, having to open the whole hand widely before grasping, he succeeds in this way in picking up, for example, a 25 mm (1 in) wooden cube. His grasp is a 'palmar' one, i.e. with the whole hand. Movements at the wrist are becoming noticeably more refined. He can hold and transfer two cubes of 25 mm, but if he drops one he *takes no notice*. He will accept large objects with both hands, looking at them and immediately taking them to his mouth. Wooden spoons, bricks and cups are much preferred at this stage to soft toys.

Hearing and speech

He now turns immediately to sounds *except for* those that come from directly above his head, which tend to confuse him. He responds when spoken to by laughing, chuckling and squealing, vocalizing with variations in a tuneful way. The continuous sounds he makes are forerunners of future speech; his babbling is repetitive, using syllables such as 'ppp' and 'sss'.

Stage four

The baby now reaches the stage in his development when *his ability to rotate becomes well coordinated*. While rotation was present before when he rolled, reached across for an object when lying on his back, or when lying on his tummy supporting himself on one arm as he reached back with the other, now with arm support sideways developing

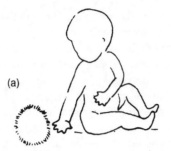

(a)

Figure II.4
(a) Sitting to prone
He now uses his ability to support himself on one hand, pushing himself up to sitting at the same time as he rotates his body and vice versa. He pivots on his tummy, also pushing himself backwards, the legs remaining rather inactive at this time, another example of how the development of the arms is still in advance of the legs. Later he will creep forward, his legs participating strongly in the movement, especially the feet

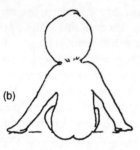

(b)

(b) Sitting
At first unsupported sitting is of short duration, probably no longer than a minute, the baby will then lean forward to support himself. With the gradual development of trunk control and sitting balance he learns to support himself sideways. Arm support is first done with a loosely closed hand and later the hand opens in preparation for bearing weight

as well as forwards, *spontaneous rotation, trunk control and sitting balance appear.*

Rolling

He now rolls from his back to his tummy in a well-coordinated manner where previously he was rather disorganized.

Vision and manipulation

As we have already pointed out, a baby's ability to reach and grasp objects is dependent on his balance and his ability to look at what he is doing. It is therefore not surprising, at this stage, to find him making exaggerated movements of his whole body and often overbalancing in his attempts to reach out for a toy. During the following months these exaggerated movements gradually diminish.

His ability to manipulate improves rapidly at this time; his grasp becoming more refined, he can now hold one object in each hand and transfer from hand to hand and bang two cubes together. He starts to take objects *out* of a container and tries unsuccessfully to pick up small objects. He starts to 'drop' large objects onto the floor, a basic pattern for future release, but once they have been dropped he has no further interest in them.

Speech

He uses sounds to express his anger and hunger and 'n-n-n' sounds to express dislikes, and imi-

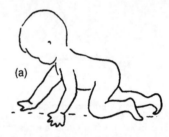

(a)

Figure II.5
(a) Crawling position
As we stated at the beginning of this section, moving is of prime importance at this time. The baby now only plays for short periods on his tummy, preferring to get on all fours where he rocks in preparation for crawling, a movement that requires both balance and reciprocal movements of the legs

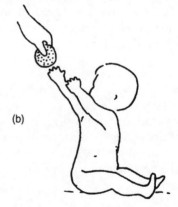

(b)

(b) Sitting
Backward protective extension of the arms is now starting. He has good balance in sitting and no longer relies on his hands for support. As illustrated, he can turn to look and grasp a toy with good rotation of the trunk, or alternatively pivot in the sitting position

tates dialogue using chains of sounds with intonation.

Stage five

The final developmental stage we shall deal with is the *acquisition of balance and the beginning of progression*. Most activities at this time start from the sitting position; moving around is the most important function for the baby at this stage – an opportunity to start exploring his environment and himself in relation to his environment.

Supine

On the rare occasions when he does lie on his back he does so now with his legs straight and slightly apart.

Eye–hand development

At this time *isolated movements* of the fingers are possible, enabling him to explore objects with his finger tips and poking them with his index finger. The *thumb and index finger* now play an important part in manipulation, small objects being picked up and inspected. It is important to note, at this stage, that although manipulation has now reached a more advanced stage, release of an object is still impossible, the baby attempts to release by pressing an object against a surface. Play now is more purposeful and the baby becomes engrossed for longer periods at a time; he is becoming aware of the permanence of objects and when he drops a toy on the floor will *look to see* where it is gone.

Speech

He vocalizes deliberately as a means of communication and understands the words 'no' and 'bye-bye' and enjoys copying adults, for example, when they cough.

Note

While obviously there are other stages in the motor development of a *normal* child during the period we have covered, such as getting up to sitting, sitting to standing, standing and walking, I have only mentioned the most important stages of early motor development to provide examples of how the gross motor patterns of movement in supine, prone and sitting underlie the fine motor skills of the hands, and overlap with the development of vision, hearing and speech.

The purpose of this Appendix is to illustrate and emphasize that when helping a child with cerebral palsy towards independence in any functional skill, it is essential that we understand something of the sensorimotor patterns that underlie these skills.

Given this understanding of the development of a *normal* child as a basis, it will be easier to understand the differences between his development and that of the child with cerebral palsy, enabling us to appreciate how abnormal movement patterns interfere with future achievements.

Appendix III

Glossary for parents – the terms we use

Abduction Movement of the limbs away from the mid-line of the body.

Active movements Purposeful spontaneous movements in accordance with a predetermined goal.

Adduction Movements of the limbs towards the mid-line of the body.

Agnosia Inability to recognize the relevance of sensory stimuli, i.e. the significance of objects seen, sounds heard, textures felt. A perceptual deficit.

Aphasia Impairment or loss of language.

Associated reactions Effort to achieve a task which increases tone. Sometimes actual movements of other parts of the body occur which are exaggerated in the presence of hypertonicity (increased tone).

Astereognosis Inability to appreciate size, shape, form or texture.

Asymmetrical When one side of the body differs from the other.

Asymmetrical tonic neck reflex Limbs on the face side extend and on the other side flex.

Ataxia Unsteadiness. This may apply to the limbs or trunk–movements are poorly-timed, graded and directed.

Athetosis Characterized by unpredictable fluctuating muscle tone, impairment of postural control causing involuntary movements. Static postural control absent, automatic reactions exaggerated.

Atrophy Wasting of muscles or nerve cells.

Audiotory Relates to the ability to hear.

Audiometry Process of measuring the activity of hearing.

Automatic reactions See Equilibrium; Protective reactions; Righting reactions.

Balance Maintaining equilibrium.

Bilateral Relating to both sides; having the ability to cross the mid-line.

Bite reflex A reflex that causes the baby to close his mouth tightly when touched on the lips, tongue or gums.

Body awareness Knowledge of one's body – in terms of both the idea of its different parts and their relation to one another.

Body image Appreciation of one's body parts. Plays a significant role in the development of motor and perceptual skills.

Cerebral palsy Movement and posture disorder resulting from a non-progressive defect of the brain.

Clonus Shaking movements of spastic muscles after the muscles have been suddenly stretched.

Cognitive Involving a learning rather than a physical process.

Colour perception Recognition and differentiation of hues and intensity of colour.

Concentration Interest in and understanding of a task.

Concept of space The body acts as a point of reference in relation to objects in the environment: up/down, under/over, in front/behind.

Conductive loss Hearing loss due to blockage or infection.

Contracture Permanently tight muscles and joints.

Contralateral Refers to the opposite side, usually refers to extremities.

Coordination Patterning of the action of the muscles of the body, i.e. right arm, left leg.

Cyanosis Blue discoloration due to circulation of imperfectly oxygenated blood.

Deformities Body or limbs fixed in abnormal positions.

Developmental scales Indicate mean ages at which various *skills* in all areas of development are achieved, but there is a *wide variation*.

Diplegia Descriptive term used to describe the motor involvement when the lower limbs are affected with milder upper limb involvement.

Dorseflexion Lifting of the foot up towards the body.

Dysarthria Difficulty in articulation due to an impairment of nerve muscular control. Speech is slow, sluggish and monotonous.

Dyslexia Difficulty in reading due to an inherent inability to understand or reproduce written symbols.

Dyspraxia Difficulty in planning movements and putting them in sequence.

Equilibrium State of balance.

Equinus Walking on the toes due to shortening of calf muscles.

Eversion Turning out of the foot – a valgus position.

Extension Straightening of any body parts.

Eye-motor coordination Ability to coordinate vision with motor activities.

Facilitation Term used to define specialized techniques used to obtain automatic movement patterns in response to handling, in contrast to movements performed at request.

Fine motor skills Grasp-release, finger movements, eye–hand coordination, and pincer grasp.

Finger grasp Grasping between thumb and one or more fingers.

Flexion Bending of any body parts.

Fluctuating tone Combination of high and low tone.

Form perception Ability to see a pattern of parts making a whole.

Function Ability to deal with tasks of daily living and future learning.

Gestures Movements used to communicate.

Gravity The pull of gravity cannot be seen but affects all our movements from birth onwards.

Gross motor skills Spontaneous physical activities that involve the whole body.

Handling Holding and moving with or without the help of the child.

Head control Ability to control the movements of the head.

Hemiplegia Descriptive term which is used to describe the motor involvement when one side of the body is affected.

Hypotonia Decreased tension in a muscle (low tone).

Hypertonus Increased tension in a muscle (spasticity).

Inhibition An attempt is made to shunt impulses from abnormal to normal patterns of activity as the child is handled. *See* Key points.

Intelligence Ability to understand the world, including information about the environment.

Inversion Turning in of the foot – a varus position.

Involuntary movements Uncontrolled movements.

Key points Proximal points from which one can influence postural tone and patterns of movement throughout the body, leaving the more distal parts free to move more actively.

Kinaesthetic Ability to perceive movement.

Language Inner language is used for thinking and talking to oneself; receptive language, an understanding of what is said to us; expressive language, the ability to communicate our ideas to others using words, gestures and written symbols appropriately.

Laterally Awareness of both sides of the body.

Locomotion Means of propulsion, to move freely through space.

Muscle tone State of tension in muscles at rest and when we move – regulated under normal circumstances subconsciously in such a way that the tension is sufficiently high to withstand the pull of gravity, i.e. to keep us upright, but it is never too strong to interfere with our movements.

Nystagmus   Continual oscillation of the eyeballs.

Otitis media   Glue ear.

Palmar grasp   When an object is grasped between the palm and two or more fingers.

Passive   That which is done to the child without his help or cooperation.

Pathological   Abnormal.

Patterns of movement   In every movement, or change of posture produced by it, the brain throws muscles into action, always in well-coordinated groups, i.e. in patterns.

Pelvic tilt   Anterior extension of the lumbar spine, the hips flex. Posterior tilt-flexion of the lumbar spine, the hips extend.

Perceptual behaviours   Process of organizing and interpreting the sensations an individual receives from internal and external stimuli; auditory, tactile, vestibular and kinaestheic.

Perseveration   Unnecessary repetition of movement and/or speech.

Phonation   Ability to utter vocal sounds.

Physiotherapy   Treatment of disorders of movement.

Pincer grasp   Use of thumb and index finger to grasp small objects.

Plantar flexion   Pointing of the foot downwards.

Plantar surface   Sole of foot.

Postural stability   An anti-gravity mechanism, essential if we are to move and balance in a smooth, controlled, coordinated manner from one position to another.

Postural tone   Potential a muscle has for action. The degree of muscle tension at a particular point in time constantly alters in response to a movement and changes in posture.

Posture   Position from which a child starts a movement and the positioning and alignment of the body.

Primitive movements   Baby movements.

Pronation   Turning in of the arm with palm of hand down.

Prone   Lying on tummy.

Proprioception   Information from the muscles, joints and vestibular systems (organs) providing us with information about body position and movement.

Protective reactions   Saving automatic reactions which protect the head and body following loss of balance.

Quadriplegia   Descriptive term which is used to describe the motor involvement when all four limbs are affected.

Reciprocal movements   Alternate movements of arms and legs.

Reflex inhibiting patterns   *See* Key points

Reflexes   Postures and movements beyond a child's control.

Retardation   Slowing down of physical and mental development.

Retraction   Drawing back of part of the body.

Righting reactions   Enable us to maintain the normal position of our head in space and in relation to our trunk, e.g. when the body moves, our face remains vertical, the mouth horizontal. Righting reactions underlie all our activities.

Rigidity   Very stiff posture.

Rotation   Movement taking place between the shoulder and pelvic girdles.

Scoliosis   Curvature of the spine.

Sensorimotor integration   Movements of the limbs send stimuli (message) to the brain to modify the strength, speed and frequency of limb movements.

Skilled activity   Programme of action directed towards the attainment of a specific goal.

Spasticity (Hypertonus)   The muscles in a varying state of cocontraction (stiffness), in a pattern of flexion of the upper limbs, extension of the lower limbs.

Speech   Process of producing sounds and combining these with words.

Stereognosis   Ability to recognize shape, size and/or weight of objects.

Stereotype   Unchanging.

Stimulation   Provides the desire to move, speak, etc.

Subluxation   Partial dislocation of the hip.

Supination   Turning of the arm up, with palm of hand up.

Supine   Lying on back.

Symmetry   Balance between body parts.

Trunk   The body as distinct from the limbs.

Unilateral   Relating to one side.

Valgus   Flat feet: a pronated position of the feet.

Varus   Supinated position of the feet.

Vestibular apparatus   Found in the inner ear, influencing posture, equilibrium postural tone and special orientation.

Visual memory   Ability to retain and reproduce shapes seen briefly.

Visual organization   Ability to scan and sequence.

Voluntary movements   Movements done with intention and with concentration.

Weight shift   Ability to shift one's weight against gravity, allowing adjustment in the trunk so that movements of the head and limbs can take place.

Appendix IV

Suppliers of equipment

Active Design Ltd, (Chailey standing support; Ramp cushion) Unit 68D, Wyrley Road, Witton, Birmingham B6 7BN (Tel. 0121 326 7506)

Anything Left Handed, 57 Brewer Street, London W1R 3FB (Tel. 0171 4373910)

AWP Woodworks, (Simple side-lyer) Unit G16, Belgravia Workshops, 157–161 Marlborough Road, London N19 4NA (Tel. 0171 281 7170)

Booster Electric Vehicles Ltd, Holly Bank Mills (Jan Pushchairs in UK), Lidget Street, Lindley, Huddersfield, West Yorkshire HD3 3JB (Tel. 01484 643444)

Britax-Excelsior Ltd, (car seats) 1 Churchill Way West, Andover, Hampshire SP10 3UW (Tel. 01264 333343)

Camp Ltd, (Jettmobile; Flexistand; Tumble Forms in UK), Northgate House, Staple Gardens, Winchester, Hampshire SO23 8ST (Tel. 01942 855248)

Cannon Babysafe Ltd, (Cannon Babysafe Trainer Cup), Lower Road, Glemsford, Suffolk CO10 7QS (Tel. 01787 280191)

Cris Lamb, (Truckle Truck) 18 Spoondell, Dunstable, Bedfordshire W6 3JE (Tel. 01582 601159)

Days Medical Aids Ltd, (DMA children's folding adjustable walker 246) Litchard Industrial Estate, Bridgend, Mid Glamorgan CF31 2AL (Tel. 01656 657495)

Everest & Jennings, (Munster Horse) Princewood Road, Corby, Northampton NN17 2DX (Tel. 01336 67667)

Glennoit UK Ltd, (spoons for bite reflex) Aberford Road, Woodlesford, Leeds LS26 8PX (Tel. 01532 826111)

Hamberman Feeders Ltd, 44 Watford Road, Radletts, Hertfordshire WD7 8LR (Tel. 01923 853544)

Hampshire Medical Developments Ltd, (snug seat) Appollo House, Lulworth Business Centre, Nutwood Way, Totton, Hampshire SO4 3WW (Tel. 01703 667700)

James Leckey Design, (Bambi standing frame; corner chairs/seats; Prone stander; side-lying boards) Design House, Kilwee Industri Estate, Dunmurry, Northern Ireland BT OHD (Tel. 01232 602277)

Jenx Ltd, (Roller seat; Side-lying Board; W Nutwood, 28 Limestone Cottage Lane field S6 1NJ (Tel. 01742 853376)

Maclaren Ltd, (Buggy Major) Stati Long Buckby, Northampton NN 01327 842662)

Mary Marlborough Disability tioning roll) Nuffield Ortho Headington, Oxford OX7 227600)

Mobility Aids Centre, 88D ground, Peterborough PE2

Mothercare UK Ltd (Boost seat) Cherrytree Road, Watt WD2 5SH (Tel. 01923 233577)

Newton Products, (Peto two-hand Bath seat), Meadway Works, Garrett Birmingham B33 0SQ (Tel. 01602 452345)

Nottingham Rehab, (Canvas corner seat; Columbia Bathing Aid with Hi-back; Columbia toilet support; Columbia Wrap Around bath support; Sunflower shallow bath; Thalia prone board Z1708/2; Tripp Trapp chair) Ludlow Hill

Road, West Bridgford, Nottingham NG2 6HD (Tel. 0115 9452345)

Possum Controls – Joncare Division Ltd, (Adaptor toilet seat; Munster horse; Tripp Trapp chair) Unit 8, Farnborough Close, Aylesbury Vale Industrial Park, Stockdale, Aylesbury, Buckinghamshire HP20 1DO (Munster Horse) (Tel. 01296 81591)

Quest 88 Ltd, (Kaye Products in UK, including posture control walker) Unit 1, Old Smithfield Industrial Estate, Aston St. Shifnal, Shropshire TF11 8DT (Tel. 01952 463050)

Rainbow Rehab., (Alvema 110) Unit 15, 7 Airfield Road, Christchurch, Bournemouth, Dorset BH23 3TG (Tel. 01202 481818)

Rehabilitation Engineering Unit, Chailey Heritage, North Chailey, Near Lewis, East Sussex BN8 42F (Tel. 01825 722112 ext 210)

Rifton, Robertsbridge, East Sussex TN32 5DR (Tel. 01580 880626)

S.K. Engineering, (Cheyne spoons and cup) Blaem Plwyf, Llanfair Road, Lampeter, Dyfed SA48 8JY (Tel. 0570 422183)

G. & S. Smirthwaite, (corner chairs/seats; Ladder back chair; Roller seat) 16 Daneheath Business Park, Heathfield, Newton Abbot, South Devon TQ12 6TL (Tel. 01626 835552)

Spencer (Banbury) Ltd, (Folding rotator) Spencer Division, Spencer House, Britannia Road, Banbury, Oxfordshire OX16 8DP (Tel. 01295 257301)

Swedish Rolo Plastics, Mig Grios Jo-plast, AB, Sweden (also available from Ikea Ltd, 2 Dury Way, London NW10 4QH (Tel. 0181 208 5600))

Taylor Therapy, (Pommel seat; head support) Woodlands Road, Pleck, Walsall WS2 9RN (Tel. 01922 27601)

Wilkinet Baby Carrier, P.O. Box 20, Cardigan, Dyfed SA43 1JB (Tel. 01239 831246)

Appendix V

Useful addresses

GENERAL

ACE Advisory Centre for Education, Aberdeen Studio, 22 Highbury Grane M5 2EA (Tel. 0171 3548318)

Advice on Government Benefits (Tel. Freephone 0800 666555)

Association for All Speech Impaired Children (AFASIC), 347 Central Markets, London EC1A 9NH (Tel. 0171 2363632 /6487)

Association of Professional Music Therapists, Diana Ashbridge, APMT Administrator, 38 Pierce Lane, Fulbourn, Cambridge CB1 5DL

Association of Swimming Therapy, 4 Oak Street, Shrewsbury SY3 7RH (Tel. 01748 344393)

Cerebral Palsy Helpline (SCOPE): 01800 626216 (call free – on all aspects of rights and benefits)

College of Speech and Language Therapists, 7 Bath Place, Rivington Street, London EC2A 3DR (Tel. 0171 6133855)

Crechendo, Freepost SW5373, London SW10 9YZ (Tel. 0171 2592727) (activity classes for children aged 4 months to 5 years)

Disabled Living Foundation 308–384 Harrow Road, London W9 2HY (Tel. 0171 2896111)

Handicapped Adventure Playground Association, Fulham Palace Road, Bishops Avenue, London SW6 6EA (Tel. 0171 7311435)

HEMI Help, 166 Boundaries Road, London SW12 8HG (excellent publications for parents)

(Tel. 0181 6723179, or 0171 3833555 (contact line for advice, support and access to their information database)

Mobility Aids Centre, 88D South Street, Stanground, Peterborough PE2 8EZ (Tel. 01733 344930)

National Association of Toy and Leisure Libraries (*Play Matters*), 68 Churchway, London NW1 1LT (Tel. 0171 3879592)

National Deaf/Blind and Rubella Association (*Sense*), 311 Gray's Inn Road, London W 8PT (Tel. 0171 2781005)

National Deaf Children's Society, 45 Road, London W2 5AH (Tel. 0171

National Library for the Handica Ash Court, Rose Street, Woking RG11 1XS (Tel. 01723 89110

Pre-school Playgroups Associ King's Cross Road, London 0171 8330991)

Riding for the Disabled A 'R', National Agricultural Warwicks CV8 2LY (Tel. 0

Royal National Institute (RNIB) Education Informatio Great Portland Street, London (including catalogue of toys for the blin partially sighted child) (Tel. 0171 3881266 ext. 2296)

Royal Society for Mentally Handicapped Children and Adults (MENCAP), 123 Golden Lane, London EC1Y 0RT (Tel. 0171 4540454)

Appendix V

Useful addresses

GENERAL

ACE Advisory Centre for Education, Aberdeen Studio, 22 Highbury Grane M5 2EA (Tel. 0171 3548318)

Advice on Government Benefits (Tel. Freephone 0800 666555)

Association for All Speech Impaired Children (AFASIC), 347 Central Markets, London EC1A 9NH (Tel. 0171 2363632 /6487)

Association of Professional Music Therapists, Diana Ashbridge, APMT Administrator, 38 Pierce Lane, Fulbourn, Cambridge CB1 5DL

Association of Swimming Therapy, 4 Oak Street, Shrewsbury SY3 7RH (Tel. 01748 344393)

Cerebral Palsy Helpline (SCOPE): 01800 626216 (call free – on all aspects of rights and benefits)

College of Speech and Language Therapists, 7 Bath Place, Rivington Street, London EC2A 3DR (Tel. 0171 6133855)

Crechendo, Freepost SW5373, London SW10 9YZ (Tel. 0171 2592727) (activity classes for children aged 4 months to 5 years)

Disabled Living Foundation 308–384 Harrow Road, London W9 2HY (Tel. 0171 2896111)

Handicapped Adventure Playground Association, Fulham Palace Road, Bishops Avenue, London SW6 6EA (Tel. 0171 7311435)

HEMI Help, 166 Boundaries Road, London SW12 8HG (excellent publications for parents)

(Tel. 0181 6723179, or 0171 3833555 (contact line for advice, support and access to their information database)

Mobility Aids Centre, 88D South Street, Stanground, Peterborough PE2 8EZ (Tel. 01733 344930)

National Association of Toy and Leisure Libraries (*Play Matters*), 68 Churchway, London NW1 1LT (Tel. 0171 3879592)

National Deaf/Blind and Rubella Association (*Sense*), 311 Gray's Inn Road, London WC1X 8PT (Tel. 0171 2781005)

National Deaf Children's Society, 45 Hereford Road, London W2 5AH (Tel. 0171 2299272)

National Library for the Handicapped Child, Ash Court, Rose Street, Wokingham, Berkshire RG11 1XS (Tel. 01723 891101)

Pre-school Playgroups Association (PPA), 61 King's Cross Road, London WC1X 9LL (Tel. 0171 8330991)

Riding for the Disabled Association, Avenue 'R', National Agricultural Centre, Kenilworth, Warwicks CV8 2LY (Tel. 0123 696510)

Royal National Institute for the Blind (RNIB) Education Information Service, 224 Great Portland Street, London W1N 6AA (including catalogue of toys for the blind and partially sighted child) (Tel. 0171 3881266 ext. 2296)

Royal Society for Mentally Handicapped Children and Adults (MENCAP), 123 Golden Lane, London EC1Y 0RT (Tel. 0171 4540454)

Road, West Bridgford, Nottingham NG2 6HD (Tel. 0115 9452345)

Possum Controls – Joncare Division Ltd, (Adaptor toilet seat; Munster horse; Tripp Trapp chair) Unit 8, Farnborough Close, Aylesbury Vale Industrial Park, Stockdale, Aylesbury, Buckinghamshire HP20 1DO (Munster Horse) (Tel. 01296 81591)

Quest 88 Ltd, (Kaye Products in UK, including posture control walker) Unit 1, Old Smithfield Industrial Estate, Aston St. Shifnal, Shropshire TF11 8DT (Tel. 01952 463050)

Rainbow Rehab., (Alvema 110) Unit 15, 7 Airfield Road, Christchurch, Bournemouth, Dorset BH23 3TG (Tel. 01202 481818)

Rehabilitation Engineering Unit, Chailey Heritage, North Chailey, Near Lewis, East Sussex BN8 42F (Tel. 01825 722112 ext 210)

Rifton, Robertsbridge, East Sussex TN32 5DR (Tel. 01580 880626)

S.K. Engineering, (Cheyne spoons and cup) Blaem Plwyf, Llanfair Road, Lampeter, Dyfed SA48 8JY (Tel. 0570 422183)

G. & S. Smirthwaite, (corner chairs/seats; Ladder back chair; Roller seat) 16 Daneheath Business Park, Heathfield, Newton Abbot, South Devon TQ12 6TL (Tel. 01626 835552)

Spencer (Banbury) Ltd, (Folding rotator) Spencer Division, Spencer House, Britannia Road, Banbury, Oxfordshire OX16 8DP (Tel. 01295 257301)

Swedish Rolo Plastics, Mig Grios Jo-plast, AB, Sweden (also available from Ikea Ltd, 2 Dury Way, London NW10 4QH (Tel. 0181 208 5600))

Taylor Therapy, (Pommel seat; head support) Woodlands Road, Pleck, Walsall WS2 9RN (Tel. 01922 27601)

Wilkinet Baby Carrier, P.O. Box 20, Cardigan, Dyfed SA43 1JB (Tel. 01239 831246)

Scope (formerly the Spastic Society), 12 Park Crescent, London W1K 4DA (Tel. 0171 6365020)

The ACE Centre, Ormerod School, Waynflete Road, Headington, Oxford OX3 8DD (Tel. 01865 63508)

Centre for Micro-Assisted Communications (CENMAC), Charlton Park School, Charlton Park Road, London SE7 8HY (Tel. 0181 3167589)

TECHNOLOGY EQUIPMENT SUPPLIERS

Liberator, Whitegates, Swinstead, Lincolnshire NG33 4PA (Tel. 01476 550391) (supply switches and communication aids)

Q.E.D. (Quest Enabling Designs), Ability House, 242 Gosport Road, Fareham, Hants PO16 0SS (Tel. 01329 828555) (supply switches, toy adapters and communication aids)

Toys for the Handicapped, 76 Barracks Road, Sandy Lane Industrial Estate, Stourport-on-Severn, Worcestershire DY13 0QB (Tel. 1299 827820) (supply switches, toy adapters d switch-controlled toys)

ity Playthings, Darvell, Roberts-ast Sussex TN32 5DR (Tel. 01580

g Centre, South Marston, Swin-(Tel. 01793 831300)
Grovenley Road, Christchurch, RQ (Tel. 01202 485834)

James Galt & Co. Ltd, Brookfield Road, Cheadle, Cheshire SK8 2PN (Tel. 0161 4288511)

Mike Ayres & Co., Unit 14, Vanguard Trading Estate, Britannia Road, Chesterfield, Derbyshire S40 2TZ (Tel. 01246 551546)

Nes-Arnold Ltd, Ludlow Hill Road, West Bridgeford, Nottingham NG2 6HD (Tel. 01602 452020)

Rompa, Goytside Road, Chesterfield, Derbyshire S40 2BR (Tel. 01246 211777) (therapy, leisure, play and sport customer service)

Toys for the Handicapped (TFH), 76 Barracks Road, Sandy Lane Industrial Estate, Stourport-on-Severn, Worcestershire DY13 9QB (Tel. 01299 827820)

SOCIAL SERVICES

In addition to the various medical services there are many organizations in Britain and in other countries which have been set up, either locally or at government level, to assist handicapped children and their families with literature, practical aid and financial assistance. The degree of assistance available obviously varies in different parts of the world and even in different areas of the UK. It is clearly impracticable in this book, which has been translated into many foreign languages, to provide details. **The purpose, however, is served by reminding you that if you need help it is available and that you are entitled to it. For information on all rights and benefits see under 'Advice on Government Benefits' and 'Cerebral Palsy Helpline', given in the above list.**

Further reading for parents

Carr, J. (1995) Helping Your Handicapped Child. Penguin: London.

Clarke, P. (1989) To a Different Drum Beat. Hawthorne Press: Stroud. A special guide to parenting children with special needs.

Douglas, J. and Richman, N. (1991) My Child Won't Sleep. Penguin: London.

*Featherstone, H. (1981) A Difference in the Family: Life with a Disabled Child. Penguin: London.

Green, E. M. Mulcahy, C. M. Pountney, T. E. Ablett, R. E. (1993) The Chailey Standing Support for Children and Young Adults with Motor Impairment: Developmental Approach. *British Journal of Occupational Therapy*, 56 (1).

Griffiths, M. and Clegg, M. (1996) Cerebral Palsy Problems and Practice. Souvenir Press: London.

Haskell, S. (1993) Education of Children with Motor and Neurological Disabilities. Chapman and Hall: London.

Lear, R. (1993) Play Helps. Toys and Activities for Children with Special Needs. Butterworth Heinemann: Oxford

*Mare, G. (1985) Working Together with Handicapped Children. Souvenir Press: London

*Newson, E. J. (1979) Toys and Playthings in Development and Remediation. Penguin: London.

SCOPE (1991) Your Child has Cerebral Palsy. SCOPE: London. A guide for parents livi and learning with young children.

Scrutton, D. (1984) Management of Motor order. Cambridge University Press: Caml ISBN 0521412102.

Sinason, V. (1993) Understanding yo capped Child. Rosendale Press: Lo

Stanton, M. (1992) Cerebral Palsy. and Co: London.

Winstock, A. (1994) The Practi of Eating and Drinking Diff Press Ltd: Oxford.

*Book out of print but may be found in libraries.

Scope (formerly the Spastic Society), 12 Park Crescent, London W1K 4DA (Tel. 0171 6365020)

COMMUNICATION AID CENTRES

The ACE Centre, Ormerod School, Waynflete Road, Headington, Oxford OX3 8DD (Tel. 01865 63508)

Centre for Micro-Assisted Communications (CENMAC), Charlton Park School, Charlton Park Road, London SE7 8HY (Tel. 0181 3167589)

TECHNOLOGY EQUIPMENT SUPPLIERS

Liberator, Whitegates, Swinstead, Lincolnshire NG33 4PA (Tel. 01476 550391) (supply switches and communication aids)

Q.E.D. (Quest Enabling Designs), Ability House, 242 Gosport Road, Fareham, Hants PO16 0SS (Tel. 01329 828555) (supply switches, toy adapters and communication aids)

Toys for the Handicapped, 76 Barracks Road, Sandy Lane Industrial Estate, Stourport-on-Severn, Worcestershire DY13 0QB (Tel. 01299 827820) (supply switches, toy adapters and switch-controlled toys)

TOYS

Community Playthings, Darvell, Robertsbridge, East Sussex TN32 5DR (Tel. 01580 880626)

Early Learning Centre, South Marston, Swindon SN3 4TJ (Tel. 01793 831300)

Escort Toys Ltd, Grovenley Road, Christchurch, Dorset BH23 3RQ (Tel. 01202 485834)

James Galt & Co. Ltd, Brookfield Road, Cheadle, Cheshire SK8 2PN (Tel. 0161 4288511)

Mike Ayres & Co., Unit 14, Vanguard Trading Estate, Britannia Road, Chesterfield, Derbyshire S40 2TZ (Tel. 01246 551546)

Nes-Arnold Ltd, Ludlow Hill Road, West Bridgeford, Nottingham NG2 6HD (Tel. 01602 452020)

Rompa, Goytside Road, Chesterfield, Derbyshire S40 2BR (Tel. 01246 211777) (therapy, leisure, play and sport customer service)

Toys for the Handicapped (TFH), 76 Barracks Road, Sandy Lane Industrial Estate, Stourport-on-Severn, Worcestershire DY13 9QB (Tel. 01299 827820)

SOCIAL SERVICES

In addition to the various medical services there are many organizations in Britain and in other countries which have been set up, either locally or at government level, to assist handicapped children and their families with literature, practical aid and financial assistance. The degree of assistance available obviously varies in different parts of the world and even in different areas of the UK. It is clearly impracticable in this book, which has been translated into many foreign languages, to provide details. **The purpose, however, is served by reminding you that if you need help it is available and that you are entitled to it. For information on all rights and benefits see under 'Advice on Government Benefits' and 'Cerebral Palsy Helpline', given in the above list.**

Further reading for parents

Carr, J. (1995) Helping Your Handicapped Child. Penguin: London.

Clarke, P. (1989) To a Different Drum Beat. Hawthorne Press: Stroud. A special guide to parenting children with special needs.

Douglas, J. and Richman, N. (1991) My Child Won't Sleep. Penguin: London.

*Featherstone, H. (1981) A Difference in the Family: Life with a Disabled Child. Penguin: London.

Green, E. M. Mulcahy, C. M. Pountney, T. E. Ablett, R. E. (1993) The Chailey Standing Support for Children and Young Adults with Motor Impairment: Developmental Approach. *British Journal of Occupational Therapy*, **56** (1).

Griffiths, M. and Clegg, M. (1996) Cerebral Palsy Problems and Practice. Souvenir Press: London.

Haskell, S. (1993) Education of Children with Motor and Neurological Disabilities. Chapman and Hall: London.

Lear, R. (1993) Play Helps. Toys and Activities for Children with Special Needs. Butterworth Heinemann: Oxford

*Mare, G. (1985) Working Together with Handicapped Children. Souvenir Press: London

*Newson, E. J. (1979) Toys and Playthings in Development and Remediation. Penguin: London.

SCOPE (1991) Your Child has Cerebral Palsy. SCOPE: London. A guide for parents living and learning with young children.

Scrutton, D. (1984) Management of Motor Disorder. Cambridge University Press: Cambridge. ISBN 0521412102.

Sinason, V. (1993) Understanding your Handicapped Child. Rosendale Press: London.

Stanton, M. (1992) Cerebral Palsy. Optima Little and Co: London.

Winstock, A. (1994) The Practical Management of Eating and Drinking Difficulties. Winslow Press Ltd: Oxford.

*Book out of print but may be found in libraries.

Index

Acceptance, 18–19
  of help, 20–1
  social, 21–2
Activity centre, 133
Ankle-knee-foot orthosis, 16, 259–60
Aspiration, 13
Ataxic cerebral palsy, type of, 8–9
Athetoid type of cerebral palsy, 8–9
  bouncing, 76–7
  carrying, 228
  chairs for, 234, 243
  dressing, 191–2
  feeding, 217
  handling recommendations, 69–77
  movement, 54, 55, 56–7
  play (the older child), 148
  standing, 60
  walking, 60–1
Attention problems, 41
Auditory awareness, *See* Hearing
Augmentative communication systems, 118–19
Automatic reactions, 50–1

Babies (early stages of hand function), 80–2
Baby baths, 181–3
Baby bouncers, 76–7
Baby seats, 239–40
Back care, parents, 186
Balance, 51
  equipment, 101–2
    inflatable therapy balls, 102, 103
    rolls, 101
Balls, 131–2
  inflatable therapy balls, 102, 103
Bambi Standing Frame, 100
Bathing, 180–9
  as learning situation, 186–7

baby, 180–1
baby baths, 181–3
bath seats, 183–5, 235
handling, 182–3
importance of balance, 180
independence, 187–9
interactive play, 182
older child, 184–6
problems, 180–1, 182–3
young child, 183–4
Beds, *See* Sleeping
Behaviour, 16–17
  behavioural problems, 29–30
    food fads, 28
    negativism, 28–9
    obstinacy, 27–8
    tantrums, 27–8
    toilet training, 28
  importance of play, 23
  social behaviour, 32
  See also Learning
Bladder control, 14–15
  See also Toilet training
Blankets, 165
  See also Sleeping
Body suits, 204
Books, 116–17, 130
Booster seat, 239
Boots, *See* Footwear
Bouncing, 76–7
Bowel problems, 14
Box chair, 240
Brothers and sisters, 31–2
Bunny-hopping, 57

Capes, 205
Car seats, 246

Carrying, 222–30
  athetoid child, 228
  normal child, 222
  spastic child, 223–8
  upright carriers, 228–30
  See also Handling the child
Cerebellar stimulation, 16
Cerebral palsy, 8, 49
  causes of, 9–10
  diagnosis, 10–11
  incidence, 10
  types of, 8–9
Chairs, *See* Seating
Chewing, 215
Clothing, 201–8
  fastenings, 203–4
  materials, 203
  safety regulations, 203
  suitable types of, 204–7
  See also Dressing
Colour awareness, 138–9
Columbia bathing aid, 185
Communication, 118–24
  alternative forms of, 41–2
  augmentative systems, 118–19
  between parents and professionals, 3–7
    exchange of information, 3–4
    setting goals, 6
    video tape recording use, 6–7
  development of, 118–19
  hearing problems and, 39–40
  non-verbal aspects, 118–19
  role in early learning, 110–11
  technology contribution, 118, 120–2
    choosing an aid, 120–2
    electronic communication aids, 120
    introducing pictures, 122
    motivation, 122
    using switches, 122–3
    writing and talking, 120
  See also Speech
Computerized tomography (CT), 11
Computers, 120–2
  early learning and, 121
  touch screen, 121–2
Concentration, 128
  attention problems, 41
Confidence, role in learning, 35–6

Constipation, 14
Continence, 14–15
  clothing, 173–4
  See also Toilet training
Contractures:
  basis of, 257–9
  sites of, 258
  See also Deformities
Convulsions, 12–13
Cots, *See* Sleeping
Creeping, 55–7
Cylinder chair, 241, 242

Daily routine, 5–6
Deafness, *See* Hearing impairment
Deformities:
  basis of, 257–9
  bony deformity at the hip, 258
  surgical correction, 260–1
    hand and wrist deformities, 260–1
    hip deformities, 260
Dental care, 220–1
  cleaning teeth, 220–1
  electric toothbrush, 221
Development:
  communication, 118–19
  feeding, 209–10
  hearing, 280, 281
  importance of play, 23
  motor development, 278–83
  normal development, 17, 278–83
  visual awareness, 278–80, 281, 282
  walking, 15
  See also Hand movements; Sensorimotor
    development; Speech
Diapers, 173–4
  changing of, 174
Diplegic (moderate/severe spasticity), 9
  abnormal posture, 59
  bathing, 183
  dressing, 200–1
  feeding, 217
  movements, 54, 55
  sitting up, 53
  surgical procedure, 260, 261 *See also* Handling
  walking, 259
Discipline, 25–9
  food fads, 28

negativism, 28–9
  obstinacy and tantrums, 27–8
  toilet training, 28
Dorsal rhizotomy, 16, 261–2
Dressing, 190–208
  athetoid child, 191–2
  handling, 191–5
  hemiplegic child, 197
  independence, 196–7
  position, 198–201
  problems, 195–201
    early cooperation, 195
    motor problems, 197
    self-help encouragement, 195–6
    skills needed, 196–7
  spastic child, 192–3
  See also Clothing
Dribbling, 14, 213–14
Drinking, 109–10, 215–17
  bottle-drinking, 214
  with polyester tube, 216–17
Drooling, 14, 213
Drug treatment, 16
Duvets, 165

Early infantile reactions, See Primitive reactions
Education:
  formal provision, 42–3
  playgroups, 39, 42
  schools, 39, 42–3
  See also Learning
Eezi Bath, 181, 182
Electric toothbrush, 221
Electroencephalogram (EEG), 11
Engine Seat, 236
Epilepsy, 12–13
Equilibrium reactions, 51
Equipment, See Therapeutic equipment
Eye-hand coordination development, 278, 279,
    282, 283

Feeding, 13–14, 209–21
  athetoid child, 217
  bottle-drinking, 214
  chewing, 215
  controlling mouth functioning, 212–13
  drinking, 209–10, 215–17
  food fads, 28

gadgets, 218
  hemiplegic child, 217–18
  hypersensitivity, 213
  independence, 217–20
  normal development, 209–10
  open mouth, 213–14
  positions, 210–12
  spastic diplegic child, 217
  spastic quadriplegic child, 217
  spoon-feeding, 214
Fits, 12–13
Flexistand, 100–1
Fluctuating tone:
  handling recommendations, 76
    carrying, 228
  sequences of movement:
  bridging and pushing backwards along floor,
    55
    creeping, 56–7
    rolling from supine to prone, 54
    walking, 60–1
Food fads, 28
Footwear, 193–4, 206–7
Fundoplication, 14

Gait, See Walking
Games, See Play; Toys
Gastro-oesophageal reflux, 13, 14
Gastrostomy, 14
Gestures, 116
Grasp, See Hand movements

Hammocks, 102–4
  description, 102–3
  suggested uses, 103–4
Hand movements, 80–95
  early development, 15, 62–3, 83–5
    early tactile experiences, 84–5
  eye-hand coordination development, 278, 279,
    282, 283
  further development, 281–83, 89–94
  grasp development, 86–8, 89
    getting an open hand, 84
    visually directed grasp, 62–3, 64, 86–8
  reaching and swiping, 89
  See also Touching
Handling the child, 65–79
  bath time, 182–3

bouncing on floor, 76–7
diaper changing, 174
dressing, 191–5
during routine activities, 77–8
handling methods not recommended, 75
helping to adjust to sleeping positions, 169
hypersensitivity to touch, 84–5
kicking encouragement, 77
pulling up to sitting from prone, 75–6
using hands, 65–6
vigorous play, 77
See also Carrying
Hearing:
development, 63–4, 280
role in early learning, 110–11
Hearing impairment, 12
learning and, 39–40
Hemiplegic, 9, 52–9
asymmetry, 52, 55, 56
chairs for, 235
dressing, 197
feeding, 217–18
handling recommendations, 69–73
movements, 55, 56
play, 155–9
sitting up, 52
surgical procedure, 259
Hip, 16
bony deformity, 258
surgical correction, 260
Hippotherapy, 267
Hospital visits, 263–4
Hypersensitivity:
during feeding, 213
to touch, 84–5

Imitative learning, 35
Imitative play, 136–7
Incontinence, 14–15
See also Toilet training
Independence, 23–4
bathing, 188–9
dressing, 196–7
feeding, 217–18
sleeping, 171–2
toileting, 177–89
washing, 187–8
Intelligence quotient (IQ), 11, 36–7

Involuntary movements, 8–9
See also Athetoid type of cerebral palsy

Jackets, 205
James-Leckey multi-adjustable bath chair, 185
Jog suits, 205
Joncare paediatric bath, 185

Kicking movements, 77

Ladderback chair, 243
Language difficulties, 12
See also Communication; Speech
Learning:
at bath time, 186–7
computer use, 121
concentration importance, 128
confidence importance, 35–6
difficulties, 11
attention problems, 41
subtle learning difficulties, 40
encouragement of, 37–8
handicapped child, 35–6
in child with additional impairments, 38–41
hearing problems, 39–40
visual problems, 38–9, 40–1
learning ability assessment, 36–7
mechanisms, 34–6
communicating, 110–11
listening, 110–11
looking, 109–10
touching, 108–9
normal child, 34–5
parents' contribution, 22–5, 107–11
parents' expectations, 36
play importance, 23
sensorimotor learning, 128–31, 187
See also Behaviour; Discipline; Education; Play
Lip reading, 39

Magnetic resonance imaging (MRI), 11
Makaton sign language, 39, 42
Materials, 203
Mattresses, 163–5
See also Sleeping
MENCAP, 19
Mobiles, visual awareness and, 82–3
Mobility aids, 247–8

Mother:
  as teacher, 22–4
  See also parents
Motor development, *See* Sensorimotor
  development
Motor disorder:
  assessment in babies, 4
  dressing problems and, 197
  treatment of, 15–16
    drugs, 16
    orthopaedic operations, 16
    orthoses, 16, 259–60
  See also Movement
Movement, 15–16, 47–9
  abnormal sequences of, 51–60
    athetoid child, 54, 55, 56–7
    spastic child, 51–4
  baby bouncers, 76–7
  bouncing, 76–7
  bridging and pushing backwards along floor, 55
  bunny-hopping, 57
  creeping, 55–7
  cruising, 58
  kicking movements, 77
  mobility aids, 247–53
  rolling from supine to prone, 53–4
  sitting up:
    from prone position, 53
    from supine position, 51–2
  standing, 57–8, 59–60
  walking, 15, 58–61
  See also Hand movements; Primitive reactions
Muscle activity, 48–9
Music, 125–6
  making music, 134
  music therapy, 126

Neck cushions, 165–6
Negativism, 28–9

Obstinacy, 27–8
Orthopaedic operations, *See* surgical procedures
Orthoses, 16, 259–60
Over-attachment, 30–1
Overalls, 205

Paget-Gorman signing system, 42
Parents:

acceptance of handicap, 18–19
accepting help, 20–1
adjustment, 19–20
communication with professionals, 3–7
  exchange of information, 3–4
  setting goals, 6
  video tape recording use, 6–7
educational role, 22–5, 107–11
  communicating, 110–11
  listening, 110–11
  looking, 109–10
  play, 23
  self-help skills, 23–4
  touching, 108–9
embarrassment, 20
expectations of, 36
helping now, 25
over-attachment, 30–1
preventative back care, 186
shame, 20
sharing the care, 44
social acceptance, 21–2
social isolation, 20
See also Discipline
Pillows, 165–6
See also Sleeping
Play, 23, 127–60
  bath time, 183
  books, 116–17, 130
  colour awareness, 138–9
  dos and dont's, 136
  equipment, 101–2
    inflatable therapy balls, 102, 103
    rolls, 101
  helping to adjust to sleeping positions, 169–70
    playing alone, 170–1
  imitative play, 136–7
  keeping a scrapbook, 134
  making music, 134
  movement and, 91–4
  sand play, 129–30
  sensorimotor learning, 128–9, 130–1, 187
  shape recognition, 133–4, 137–8
  siblings, 152–5
  simple games, 135–6
    for matching, 135
    manipulation, 135–6
  throughout the day, 130

transition to function, 131
vigorous play, 77
water play, 129
See also Toys
Playgroups, 39, 42
Pointing, 84
Position emission tomography (PET), 11
Postural reactions, 50–1
Postural tone, 50, 65
Posture, 8
    abnormal, 59–60, 65
    handling recommendations, 66–79
Potties, 175–6
Preventative back care, parents, 186
Primitive reactions, 49–51
Prone standers, 99, 100
Pushchairs, 243–6
    accessories, 245
    designs of, 245–6
Puzzles, 138
Pyjamas, 204

Quadriplegic (severe spasticity), 49, 52
    bathing, 185
    carrying, 225, 227
    dressing, 191, 194
    equipment, 98
    feeding, 205
    handling recommendations, 70, 71, 74, 75, 76, 77
    movement, 53, 55
    play, 129, 139
    sleeping, 166, 168, 171

Reflex-inhibiting casts, 261
Regurgitation, 13
Residential care, 31
Rhizotomy, 16, 261–2
Riding, 265, 266–7
    hippotherapy, 267
    recreational riding, 267
    therapeutic riding, 267
Rifton bath chair, 184
Righting reactions, 50
Rolls, 101

Sand play, 129–30
Saving reactions, 51

Schools, 39, 42–3
SCOPE, 19
Scrapbooks, 134
Seating, 231–43
    needs assessment, 232–3
    and tables, 247
    bath seats, choice of, 183–6
    car seats, 246
    chair inserts, 241–2
    home-made chairs, 240–1
        box chair, 240
        cardboard boxes, 241
        cylinder chair, 241, 242
        simple wooden chair, 240
    manufactured chairs, 233–40
        baby seats, 239–40
        bean bag chair, 237
        Booster seat, 239
        complete seating systems, 237–8
        corner chairs/sets, 234–5
        Engine Seat, 236
        folding canvas corner seat, 235
        inflatable chairs, 238
        ladderback chair, 243
        Roller chair, 236
        Safa bath seat, 184, 235
        S.A.M. seating system, 237–8
        Snug Seat, 233
        Tripp Trapp chair, 243
        Tumble Forms Deluxe Floor Sitter, 233–4
Selective posterior rhizotomy, 261–2
Self-help skills, *See* Independence
Sensorimotor development, 61–4
    See also Appendix II
Shapes:
    discovery of, 133–4
    recognition of, 137–8
Shoes, 193–4, 206–7
Siblings, 31–2
Side-lying boards, 197–9
    description, 197–8
    suggested uses, 98–9
Sign language, 39, 42, 118–19
'Sit-at-a-table' seat, 239
Sitting, 51–3, 231–2, 279, 281
    spastic child, 52–3
    See also Seating
Sleeping, 163–72

cot or bed, 163–6
   bedding, 165
   mattress, 163–5
   pillows, 165–6
   independence, 171–2
   problems, 166–8
   sleeping positions, 166
      adjusting to, 168–70
      playing alone, 170–1
Sleeping bags, 165
Snug Seat, 233
Social acceptance, 21–2
Social behaviour, 32
Social contact, 29–30
Socks, 193–4, 204
Sound, role in early learning, 110–11
Speech, 112–13, 118
   development, 23, 119, 280, 281, 282–3
      attempting speech, 116
      common problems, 114–15
      gestures, 116
      importance of personal interaction, 116–17
      major stages, 112–13
      preparation for speech, 113–14
      sensory input, 115–16
   difficulties, 12
   role in early learning, 110–11
   supplementation of, 119
   See also Communication
Spoon-feeding, 214
Standing, 57–8, 59–60
Standing frames, 99–101
Statement of Special Educational Need, 43
Sunflower shallow bath, 185–6
Surgery, *See* Treatment techniques
Swallowing, 13
Swimming, 265–6
Switches, use of, 222–3
Symbols, 118–19

Tables, 243
Tactile stimulation, *See* Hand movements;
   Touching
Tantrums, 27–8
Teaching, *See* Learning
Technology, *See* Communication; Computers
Teeth, 14
   See also Dental care

Tendo Achilles, 15–16, 259
Therapeutic equipment:
   inflatable therapy balls, 102, 103
   rolls, 101
   side-lying boards, 197–9
   standing frames, 99–101
   suppliers, 282–3
   wedges, 196–7
Thumb strap, 84, 85
Toilet training, 28, 173–9
   independence, 178–9
      toilet support systems, 177–8
   potties, 175–6
   volitional control, 176–7
Touch screen, 121–2
Touching:
   hypersensitivity to touch, 84–5
   role in early learning, 108–9
      See also Hand movements; Handling the child
Toys, 127
   books, 116–17, 130
   choice of, 131–4
   hand function development, 86, 89
   toy libraries, 135
   visual awareness and, 83
   See also Play
Treatment techniques:
   drugs, 16
   orthoses, 16, 259–60
   reflex-inhibiting casts, 261
   rhizotomy, 261–2
   surgical correction, 16, 260–1
      hand and wrist deformities, 260–1
      hip deformities, 260
Triangle inflatable chair, 238
Tripp Trapp chair, 243
Tumble Forms Deluxe Floor Sitter, 233–4

Upright standing frames, 99–101

Video tape recording use in communication, 6–7
Visual awareness, 80–3
   development, 278–82
   familiar objects, 81–2
   mobiles, 82–3
   outside, 82
   role in early learning, 109–10
   toys, 83

visual fixation, 80–1
visual following, 81
visually directed grasp, 86–8, 278–9, 281, 282
Visual impairment, 12
  learning and, 38–9
  visual perception difficulties, 40–1

Walking, 58–61, 259
  development of, 15

Washing, 187–8
  See also Bathing
Water play, 129
Waterproof pants, 173–4
Wedges, 196–7, 98
  cut-out foam wedges, 102–4
  description, 196–7
  suggested uses, 97
Wrap Around bath support, 185